# A
# Gui
# to
# Common
# Illnesses

Dr Ruth Lever qualified from St Mary's Hospital, London, with the degrees of MB, BS. Her career in orthodox medicine has included work in paediatrics, psychiatry and public health and she has an MSc in social medicine from London University.

For four and a half years she was Medical Officer in Charge of Troops at a large Army depot and it was during this period that she started to study and practise various complementary therapies including acupuncture, hypnosis, healing and nutrition counselling. Since leaving Army practice, she has written numerous articles on orthodox and complementary medicine, including an 'Ask the Doctor' column in a weekly woman's magazine. She appeared regularly on the TVS programme 'Problem Page' and is the author of *Acupuncture for Everyone* (Penguin, 1987) and *Hypnotherapy for Everyone* (Penguin, 1988).

She is married to a homoeopath and lives in Sussex.

# A
# Guide
# to
# Common
# Illnesses

Ruth Lever

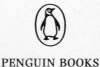

PENGUIN BOOKS

PENGUIN BOOKS

Published by the Penguin Group
27 Wrights Lane, London W8 5TZ, England
Viking Penguin, a division of Penguin Books USA Inc.,
375 Hudson Street, New York, New York 10014, USA
Penguin Books Australia Ltd, Ringwood, Victoria, Australia
Penguin Books Canada Ltd, 2801 John Street, Markham, Ontario, Canada L3R 1B4
Penguin Books (NZ) Ltd, 182–190 Wairau Road, Auckland 10, New Zealand

Penguin Books Ltd, Registered Offices: Harmondsworth, Middlesex, England

First published 1990

Filmset in Monophoto 10pt Photina

Printed in England by Clays Ltd, St Ives plc

*For my husband, John,*
*with my love*

# Contents

# Contents

## Hair Loss 197

The Mechanism of Hair Growth *197*
Male Pattern Baldness *198*
*Cause and symptoms 198*
*Orthodox treatment 198*

Female Baldness *199*
Telogen Effluvium *199*
Drug-induced Alopecia *200*
Alopecia Areata *200*
*Orthodox treatment 201*

Trichotillomania *201*
Secondary Hair Loss – Destructive or Scarring Alopecia *202*
Complementary Treatment *202*

## Herpes Simplex 203

Cold Sores *203*
Genital Herpes *204*
Complications of Herpes Infections *205*
Investigations *206*
Orthodox Treatment *206*
Recent Advances *206*
Complementary Treatment *207*
Self-help *207*
Organizations *208*

## High Blood Pressure (Hypertension) 209

Definition *209*
Essential and Secondary Hypertension *210*
Investigations *212*
Symptoms of Hypertension *214*
Dangers of Hypertension *215*
Orthodox Treatment *216*
*Secondary hypertension 216*
*Essential hypertension 216*

Complementary Treatment *221*

# List
### *of*
# Diagrams

# The
# Purpose
# *and*
# Structure
# of This
# Book

As the 'resident doctor' on the TVS programme 'Problem Page' and, now as the writer of an 'Ask the Doctor' column in a weekly magazine, I have become aware that, in the letters I receive asking for advice, certain questions come up again and again. They include:

*My doctor thinks I may have A and is sending me for tests. What will they entail?*

*My doctor tells me I have B. How will it affect my life?*

*I have just been told that I have C. What treatment will I have to undergo?*

*My doctor has prescribed D. What is it for and what are the side effects?*

*I have been treated by my doctor for E but nothing seems to help. Is there a complementary therapy I could try?*

> *I have F and feel it would help to talk to other*
> *sufferers. Is there an organization I can join?*

There are, of course, reasons why these questions keep cropping up. When a diagnosis is first made, it is not always easy for a patient to take in everything that is being said. Sometimes, the doctor uses language the patient doesn't understand. Sometimes he doesn't have time to explain everything thoroughly. Sometimes the patient's anxiety gets in the way of understanding. And, very often, so much is said that the patient can only remember a fraction of it. Unfortunately, there is also a limit to how much one can say in a few minutes on a television programme or in a couple of columns in a magazine. I began to feel more and more that what was needed was a full description of a number of common illnesses which would answer all these questions in depth and which the patient could keep for reference, to go back to and read again whenever necessary. And it was from that idea that this book stemmed.

Each chapter covers a common illness or group of illnesses although, in some cases, for the sake of completeness, I have mentioned one or two rarer conditions that fall within a common group. I have not included infectious illnesses that are self-limiting (such as the common cold and the childhood infections) as these do not generally cause problems. Nor have I included AIDS which, although it is of great importance, is, thankfully, not yet commonplace. I have tried to be guided in my choice of diseases by what the average GP would see in his surgery several times a year – at least.

The purpose of this book is not self-help but explanation. However, I have included a short 'self-help' section in some chapters where this is appropriate.

# Investigations

Having to go to hospital for investigations is always a little alarming and I hope that, by explaining what is likely to happen, this book will relieve some of the anxiety that patients naturally feel. Recently, however, I read an item in a magazine in which the writer commented that a friend of hers, having had some tests for cancer of the cervix, was unwilling to return to hospital, having been unprepared 'for the indignity of the procedure or the stinging pain'. I was horrified by this and wrote a letter to the magazine in which I said.

It is unfortunate, of course, that she found the colposcopy uncomfortable, but the stinging pain to which you refer is only momentary (and is not experienced by all patients) . . . As to indignity . . . doctors are not there to humiliate their patients but to help them and, wherever possible, to prevent them from becoming ill or to restore them to health. There is no indignity in this. It would be a tragedy if this woman failed to return for further investigations . . . To die from cancer which could have been cured is senseless.

It is inevitable that some investigations will be uncomfortable or unpleasant. It is therefore vital to remember that they are being done for the patient's benefit in order to restore him (or her) to health. The diseases which can, as a result, be diagnosed, treated and, in many cases, cured, are likely to be far more uncomfortable, unpleasant – and long term – than any investigations.

Someone who is anxious about an investigation (or any procedure) should ask the doctor to explain it as he goes along. This is usually very reassuring – and may even be interesting!

## Recent Advances

Most chapters have a paragraph or two on recent advances in diagnosis and treatment for that particular illness. I soon realized that writing this book could become like painting the Forth Bridge (finish one draft and then go back to put in the latest batch of recent advances)! I therefore called a halt at January 1989 and new discoveries which were published after that date have not been included.

## Diagrams

Some diagrams may be appropriate to more than one chapter

but, for reasons of space, can only be printed in one place. A list is therefore given at the beginning of the book for ease of reference.

## Organizations

Many of the organizations listed in this book are charities, working on a very limited budget. When writing to any of them for information, please enclose a stamped addressed envelope for the reply.

## The Appendices

Although I have tried to avoid jargon, there are some one-word medical terms that need eight or ten words to explain them. In such cases, I have used the medical term but an explanation appears in the glossary at the back of the book and, at least once, in the text. I have also tended to use medical terms where they are words that are finding their way into common usage (such as 'uterus' rather than 'womb') but, here again, an explanation is included in the glossary.

Nowadays most drugs are prescribed under their chemical names and it is these that I have used in the text. However, one drug may be made by a number of different companies and so have several different brand names, which are also sometimes used in prescriptions. I have listed all the drugs mentioned in the text, together with their various proprietary names, at the back of the book. If any do not appear here, it is because they are manufactured only under their chemical names. Some drugs are mentioned in several sections of the book but are detailed only once in the appendix; however, they are also listed in the index, which will direct the reader to the appropriate section of the appendix.

New drugs are being introduced all the time, while others are discontinued. It is possible, therefore, that by the time this book is published, one or two of the individual drugs I mention may no longer be in use and others will have taken their place.

Finally, I have also included a pronunciation guide, since

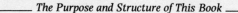

some of the medical terms I have included are very long and awkward to get one's tongue around and others, although shorter, may offer the possibility of being pronounced two or more ways.

## Terminology

I have generally used 'he' and 'she' in alternate chapters.

# How to
# Use
# This Book

The first few paragraphs in each section tend to relate to the whole section and should be read before going on to any individual part of it.

Some illnesses, diagnostic techniques and forms of treatment that are mentioned in passing in some sections may be dealt with in greater depth elsewhere. So please use the index to make sure you have found all the information relevant to any particular subject.

Before consulting the sections on complementary treatment, please read the introductory section on complementary therapies.

# Complementary Therapies

I have not attempted to list all the therapies that may be helpful in the treatment of an individual illness. Complementary therapies tend to treat the whole patient, not just the part that is diseased and therefore it is more a question of whether the individual patient will respond to a particular therapy rather than whether a certain illness will. Some therapies, like healing and radionics, can be helpful in an enormous range of problems but the treatment does not vary enormously from case to case so, on the whole, these are not listed as I have only mentioned an individual therapy for a particular illness where it has been possible to suggest what might be prescribed in such a case. This does not imply that therapies that are not listed would not be helpful.

Although I have mentioned specific complementary treatments (for example, herbs and homoeopathic remedies) this is not a recommendation for self-treatment, except as a first-aid measure. One will inevitably get the best results by going to see a therapist who has trained, usually for several years, in his speciality, rather than by trying something out from the health food shop. The exception to this is the Bach remedies, of which there are only thirty-eight and whose use is easily mastered.

# Acupuncture

Acupuncture has been used in China for thousands of years. It is based on the theory that the body's energy or vital force (called Chi) circulates through a series of channels or meridians. Each of these channels has the name of an organ of the body (such as the Heart channel and the Liver channel) and is specifically linked with that organ. Each organ has a special function, over and above the function that is recognized in Western medicine. Thus, for example, the energy of the kidney is said to control the reproductive system and hearing.

The channels can be invaded by 'harmful Chi', which takes the form of heat, damp, wind, cold and dryness. It is this invasion that causes illness, by disrupting the normal flow of Chi. Along the meridians are points which, when a needle is inserted into them, can be used to control the body's energy flow and to expel harmful Chi.

The acupuncturist will base his choice of which points to use on the patient's symptoms, on the appearance of his tongue and on his pulse.

# Alexander Technique

This is a system of posture training which can be invaluable when problems stem from or are made worse by a faulty posture.

# Aromatherapy

The life force of a plant is said, by aromatherapists, to be captured in its essential oil. Each of these has specific properties that make it valuable in the treatment of certain diseases. The oils may be taken by mouth, inhaled, used in the bath or massaged into the skin, depending upon the individual case.

# Bach Flower Remedies

These flower remedies were discovered by Dr Edward Bach, who was an eminent physician. He felt that some of his patients did not get well as fast as they should do and that this was due to their state of mind. He was convinced that flowers had properties that could affect the mind and he started to investigate these. The resulting thirty-eight remedies (and the combination 'Rescue Remedy' which is useful for all forms of shock and fright) are exceptionally gentle and very effective. Each is appropriate for a different negative state of mind, such as anxiety, melancholy, fear or exhaustion. They have no side effects of any kind, can be taken quite safely with any other type of medication and, what is more, can be taken as often as they are needed – every ten minutes if necessary. Four drops are put on the tongue and left for a few seconds before swallowing. They are best not taken within ten minutes of eating, drinking or smoking. Bach remedies are available from many health food shops or, by post, from the Bach Centre, Mount Vernon, Sotwell, Wallingford, Oxon, OX10 OPZ.

# Chiropractic

This is a system of manipulation which focuses primarily on the spine.

# Healing

There are many types of healers. Some believe their healing ability comes from God and that it is therefore a semi-religious experience. Others believe that they are merely acting as a channel for a natural energy. Some move their hands above the patient, others touch the patient. Some use visualization as part of their therapy, so that the patient is taking part in his own treatment. Healing can be remarkably effective in the treatment of many kinds of disease and, even in cases where a cure is not possible, can help to improve the patient's quality of life.

# Herbalism

Although herbalists use many herbs that are also used, in a refined form, by orthodox practitioners, the theory on which their use is based is somewhat different. For a start, herbalists believe that the whole plant is more effective in treatment than any one of its component parts. And they use herbs not to treat an individual symptom as such but rather to raise the level of health of the patient, clean toxins out of the body, restore normal function to the diseased part – and leave the body to heal itself, which it is then in a position to do.

## Homoeopathy

Homoeopathy is based on the premise of 'like cures like'. A substance which will produce a certain set of symptoms in a healthy person will, if given to someone who has developed those symptoms as the result of a disease, cure them. Homoeopathic remedies are used in enormous dilution and, because of this, produce few side effects, while at the same time being extremely powerful. There are over two thousand remedies, each of which has its own 'symptom picture'. The task of the homoeopath is to match, as closely as possible, the patient's personality and habits, as well as his symptoms, to a particular remedy.

## Hypnotherapy

Hypnotherapy is a form of deep relaxation which can be used in the treatment of any illness that has a psychosomatic component (that is, anything that can be brought on or made worse by mental factors such as stress or anxiety).

## Naturopathy

This is mainly based on a healthy way of life and much of the advice given by a naturopath concerns diet. I have therefore tended to include such ideas in the 'self-help' sections, as most of them are quite safe to follow on one's own. However, naturopaths sometimes recommend fasts and these should never be undertaken without the advice and guidance of a qualified therapist.

## Nutrition Therapy

Much of what we eat today is deficient in vitamins and minerals. Not only has a lot of the vegetable matter been grown in mineral-deficient soil, but the food itself has been harvested long before it reaches the supermarket shelves, so its vitamins have started to break down. Cooking and processing destroy vitamins still further but 'junk' foods increase our needs for these vital nutrients. It is scarcely surprising, therefore, that many nutrition therapists maintain that everyone nowadays needs to take vitamin and mineral supplements. A number of symptoms can be laid very firmly at the door of nutrient deficiencies and can be treated very successfully with nutritional supplements. I have tended to avoid giving dosages for supplements in the text, since these can vary enormously depending on the individual patient. However, the following is a suitable daily intake for the average adult: 7500 i.u. of vitamin A; 400 i.u. of vitamin D; 100 i.u. of vitamin E; 1000 mg of vitamin C; 25 mg each of vitamins $B_1$ (thiamine) and $B_2$ (riboflavin), and 50 mg each of vitamins $B_3$ (nicotinic acid), $B_5$ (pantothenic acid) and $B_6$ (pyridoxine); 5 mcg of vitamin $B_{12}$ and 50 mcg each of folic acid and biotin; 25 mg each of choline, inositol and PABA; 150 mg of calcium; 75 mg of magnesium; 10 mg each of iron and zinc; 2.5 mg of manganese; 25 mcg of selenium and 20 mcg of chromium. Several multivitamin/multimineral preparations contain quantities similar to these. Those that do not contain copper are preferable, since most people get adequate amounts of copper from their drinking water.

## Osteopathy

This is a form of manipulation which seeks to restore normal function to the joints and muscles of the body.

## Radionics

A form of absent healing, radionics uses a piece of the patient's hair as a 'witness' to link patient and practitioner. A well-known doctor once remarked that the most extraordinary thing about radionics is that it works. How it works no one knows – even the practitioners have no one theory. However, it can be extremely useful in a wide range of illnesses and, like healing, can help to improve the patient's quality of life even when a cure is not possible.

# Reflexology

Reflexology is a system of foot massage based on the theory that the entire body is reflected in the sole of the foot. Thus massage of a particular point will affect the organ with which it is linked. Not only is the treatment very soothing and relaxing but it can be remarkably effective for a wide range of ailments.

# Further Reading

A number of books have been published on complementary therapies in the 'Penguin Health' series. Among them are my own *Acupuncture for Everyone* and *Hypnotherapy for Everyone*.

Other books that I would recommend are:

*The Handbook of Complementary Medicine* by Stephen Fulder (Coronet) – a useful reference book

*Homoeopathy – Medicine of the New Man* by George Vithoulkas (Arco Publishing Inc., distributed in the UK by Thorsons)

*Homoeopathy: An Introductory Guide* by A. C. Gordon Ross (Thorsons)

*Practical Aromatherapy* by Shirley Price (Thorsons)

*Amino Acids in Therapy* by Leon Chaitow (Thorsons)

*Healing with Radionics* by E. Baerlein and A. L. G. Dower (Thorsons)

*Report on Radionics* by Edward W. Russell (Neville Spearman)

*Reflexology* by Anna Kaye and Don C. Matcham (Thorsons)

*Handbook of the Bach Flower Remedies* by Philip M. Chancellor (C. W. Daniel)

*The Family Nutrition Workbook* and *The Whole Health Manual* both by Patrick Holford, both published by Thorsons

A list of addresses of organizations holding lists of qualified complementary practitioners will be found at the back of the book.

# Acne

## Incidence, Cause and Description

Acne is a skin condition which probably affects 80 per cent of all adolescents to a greater or lesser degree. It usually begins around the time of puberty, affecting both boys and girls, and, in most cases, has cleared up by the early twenties. Boys are more likely to be severely affected, about 5 per cent continuing to have problems into their thirties, compared with 1 per cent of girls. Similarly, only one girl in 200 is likely to suffer from severe acne whereas, with boys, the proportion is about one in twenty-five.

Various factors are known to cause acne, such as contact with mineral or vegetable oils or crude petroleum (occupational acne), and, sometimes, the contraceptive Pill or the use of steroids. However, in the vast majority of cases it seems to be caused by androgens, sex hormones that are secreted for the first time at puberty.

Although androgens are the male sex hormones, they are also produced in small amounts by girls. Among other effects, they stimulate the production of facial and body hair which is kept soft by an oily substance called sebum. This is secreted by tiny sebaceous glands in the skin, which enlarge and become more active in response to these hormones. Acne occurs when the sebaceous glands become over-active and the exit from the gland is blocked by a deposition of keratin – the hard substance that forms an important part of the hair and nails and which helps to toughen skin. Sebum is therefore produced at a faster rate than it can leave the gland which, as a result, swells up. Normally harmless bacteria called *Propionibacterium acnes* tend to colonize in the swollen gland, where they feed on the sebum. Inflammation occurs and pimples and pus-filled spots (pustules) may develop. In severe cases, the glands may burst into the skin, producing cysts.

The first signs of acne are often whiteheads and blackheads. They are both caused by blocked sebaceous glands, the difference being that blackheads (whose colour comes from melanin, the pigment present in the skin and the hair) can be squeezed out or can work their way out of the duct, whereas whiteheads can't. In many cases, the condition doesn't progress any further and, after a few months or years, the skin becomes clear again. In more serious cases, in which pustules or cysts develop, scarring may occur as these heal.

The commonest site for acne is the face. Sometimes it may be months or even years before the condition spreads to the chest, back, shoulders or neck, but occasionally the chest may be the only area involved. Repeated pressure or friction on the skin may make the condition worse – for example, violin players may find that the area under the chin is most severely affected.

# Orthodox Treatment

Over 90 per cent of patients with acne respond to treatment. However, this often needs to be prolonged over months or even years. Two main forms are available – topical (applied directly to the skin) or systemic (taken internally).

*Topical Treatment*
Benzoyl peroxide is an exfoliating agent – that is, it helps the top layer of the skin to peel off – and it also prevents bacteria from multiplying. It is available as a gel, cream or lotion, sometimes in combination with sulphur, which is also an exfoliating agent. It needs to be used for a considerable time and may, at first,

produce redness and dryness of the skin, which will diminish after a while.

Tretinoin (or retinoic acid) is sometimes used alternately with benzoyl peroxide (one at night and the other in the morning) or it may be used alone. It is a derivative of vitamin A, which plays an important role in the maintenance of healthy skin, and it reduces the abnormal production of keratin at the mouth of the sebaceous glands. It is therefore very useful for the treatment of whiteheads and blackheads but is less effective in more advanced forms of acne. It can cause irritation and redness, especially if the skin is exposed to strong sunlight. Both benzoyl peroxide and tretinoin need to be used for a minimum of six months and it may take several weeks before any improvement is noticed.

Topical antibiotics are sometimes used in the treatment of acne, although some doctors avoid them because patients may become allergic to them.

In severe cases when cysts form, steroids injected into them may help them to resolve.

*Systemic Treatment*
The most popular treatment for acne is the antibiotic tetracycline. Used together with topical benzoyl peroxide, it is very effective. However, it is not well absorbed if taken with food, so the patient has to remember to take it between meals. Antacids, iron supplements and milk can also interfere with its absorption. It must be taken for a minimum of three months and often much longer, although some improvement is usually obvious after about two months. Other antibiotics are sometimes used and may be helpful when tetracycline has failed. These include co-trimoxazole, minocycline, doxycycline and erythromycin.

Although the initial changes of acne are brought about by androgens, nothing can be done about this in boys, since these are the hormones that transform them into men. However, in girls, whose development depends on the female hormones oestrogen and progesterone, anti-androgen treatment can be used. An anti-androgen, cyproterone acetate, is combined with the oestrogen ethinyloestradiol in a preparation called Diane. Although this needs to be taken for at least a year, it is very useful for patients who have responded to other forms of treatment but have not recovered fully. In addition, it is extremely useful for those young women who want to take the Pill, since it is also an effective oral contraceptive. Side effects are uncommon; they include nausea, weight gain and loss of sex drive.

The most recent innovation in the treatment of acne is isotretinoin (13-cis-retinoic acid) which, like the topical tretinoin, is a derivative of vitamin A. Its main effect is to reduce the production of sebum while at the same time stimulating the shedding of old skin cells. Because it can have serious side effects it is available only to those patients with severe acne who are referred to hospital skin departments. It commonly causes dryness of the lips and soreness at the corners of the mouth, a dry rash on the face, nosebleeds and conjunctivitis. Older patients may develop arthritis. It can also affect the liver and the levels of fat in the blood, so blood tests are taken every six weeks during treatment in order to monitor this. Any abnormalities would mean that the patient would be taken off the medication straight away. Normally, however, treatment is continued for about four months. Facial acne improves in between 80 and 90 per cent of patients, while acne on the back and chest improves in about 60 per cent. The effect of one course may last up to six years. Because isotretinoin can cause malformations in an unborn child, sexually active women must use adequate contraception throughout the course of treatment and for two months afterwards.

## Recent Advances

An Italian chemist has developed a method of getting rid of acne scars that is said to be effective in 80 per cent of cases. It is available from qualified beauty therapists under the trade name AS-43 Suntronic treatment. A pad soaked in a liquid that contains protein is put over the affected area and a very small electric current is passed through it, stimulating the skin to repair itself. The treatment is marketed by the Mediform Clinic, 22 Harcourt House, 19 Cavendish Square, London, w1. It is also widely available in Europe and the United States.

It may, one day, be possible to vaccinate youngsters against acne. Scientists at the Medical Academy in Krakow, Poland, prepared a vaccine from the bacteria proprionibacterium, which is known to colonize the sebaceous glands of patients with acne. This vaccine was then used in a double-blind trial involving 320 adolescents. In the group given the vaccine, definite improvements were noticed in the skin.

## Complementary Treatment

*Acupuncture*
Points are used to relieve the stagnation of Chi in the channels of the face, said to be the cause of acne.

*Aromatherapy*
Chamomile, lavender, juniper and bergamot are among the oils that may be helpful.

*Herbalism*
Herbs are used to reduce toxicity, which is believed to be associated with any chronic skin condition, and to restore the function of the skin to normal. Among those that may be prescribed are dandelion root and burdock root. Echinacea and poke root are used for their anti-inflammatory properties; red clover, which is also used, may have oestrogenic action.

*Homoeopathy*
Kali brom. may help patients who have pustules and blind boils, especially on the face, neck and upper part of the back. For those with oily skin, blackheads and pimples, selenium may be prescribed, while for patients whose pustules are painful and discharge yellow pus hepar sulph. may be appropriate.

*Nutrition*
Supplements of B complex (particularly $B_6$), C and E, and of the mineral zinc may be recommended since these are very important for the health of the skin, as is vitamin A, which may be added to the list for patients who are not already taking isotretinoin.

Eating foods that are rich in sulphur such as eggs, onions and garlic may be helpful. Patients are likely to be advised to avoid sugar, cigarettes and fried and fatty foods.

## Self-help

Ultraviolet light or sunlight may sometimes improve acne but its effect is only temporary.

Excessive washing is not helpful.

# Anorexia
## *and*
# Bulimia

These are two potentially life-threatening disorders of eating, which mainly affect young women. They are thought to be caused by psychological factors but, as yet, comparatively little is known about them. Indeed, it is only in the past few years that bulimia has been recognized as a separate disease entity, although both conditions can occur together.

## Anorexia Nervosa

DEFINITION, INCIDENCE, CAUSES AND SYMPTOMS

The word anorexia is used by doctors, without the 'nervosa' suffix, to describe loss of appetite due to any cause. However, anorexia nervosa is defined as a disease in which the patient, who has an intense wish to be thin and an overwhelming fear of fatness, starves herself so that she weighs less than 75 per cent of the standard weight for her height and build.

Surveys have shown that anorexia nervosa affects between 1 and 2 per cent of schoolgirls and female university students. However, it is thought that many more have less severe degrees of the disease. Ninety-five per cent of cases begin in late adolescence, usually between the ages of sixteen and seventeen. The condition is rare over the age of thirty and affects twenty females for every male.

Various theories have been put forward as to its cause. Some specialists see it as an attempt by young women to escape back into childhood, away from the problems of adolescence. Others suggest that it occurs mainly in girls who do not feel in control of their lives and that starvation is their way of trying to gain control over themselves and the people around them. One symptom of the disease is an absence of periods (amenorrhoea) but, in about 20 per cent of cases, this occurs before there is any dramatic weight loss. This has led some authorities to suggest that, in such cases, the condition may be caused by a hormonal imbalance.

Anorexia nervosa is more common among the daughters of professional people and seems to affect girls in certain occupations, such as nursing or ballet, more frequently than others. It is also far more common in those cultures where thinness is equated with beauty than in those where there is less stress on weight-watching. Often the patients have been slightly overweight in the past. Having decided to lose weight, their dietary controls become more and more strict until they eat hardly anything. Carbohydrate, in particular, is avoided. In addition, the patient does exercises, takes purgatives and may make herself vomit after eating. Her fear of being fat does not diminish as she continues to lose weight and she is unable to see how thin she has become or to recognize the fact that she has problems. She has no sex drive, her skin may become mottled and her body covered by a fine soft hair (lanugo) and she is likely to have a low body temperature, a low heart rate and a low blood pressure.

The disease may take the form of one prolonged episode or may fluctuate, with the patient seeming to get better for a while and then relapsing again.

ORTHODOX TREATMENT
Some patients may be treated at home but, in most cases, especially if the patient is severely malnourished, she will need admission to hospital. If she refuses to go in and it seems that

her life is in danger, she can be made to enter hospital under a psychiatric court order.

Treatment consists mainly of a high calorie diet together with psychotherapy. Usually the patient is told on admission to hospital that she will be allowed no privileges but can earn them by putting on weight. She will be watched carefully to ensure that she does not take purgatives and does not make herself vomit. Support and counselling are offered and, in some cases, antidepressants may be helpful.

PROGNOSIS

The outlook for patients with anorexia nervosa is variable. The longer they have been ill and the more severe their weight loss, the poorer are their chances for a complete recovery. Patients who purge themselves or make themselves vomit, who suffer from bulimia, who have problems in their relationships with others or whose illness began at a relatively late age are also less likely to do well. Follow-up studies of patients, done between four and ten years after the onset of the disease, have shown that about 2 per cent had died from starvation, 16 per cent were still seriously underweight and 19 per cent were moderately underweight; 29 per cent still had no periods and in 17 per cent the periods were irregular; 36 per cent were still using purgatives. Recently an American study has suggested that anorexic women are more likely than others to develop osteoporosis at an early age. In the long term, between 2 and 5 per cent of patients with chronic anorexia nervosa may commit suicide.

COMPLEMENTARY TREATMENT
*Aromatherapy*
Bergamot, clary sage or rose may be helpful.

*Herbalism*
Several herbs are appetite stimulants and condurango may be especially helpful in the treatment of anorexia nervosa.

*Homoeopathy*
Remedies that may be helpful include natrum mur., silica

(especially for pale, cold patients with sweaty hands and feet) and arg. nit. (particularly when anorexia is associated with phobias).

_Hypnotherapy_
Hypnosis may be of limited use in anorexia. It can be used to discover the cause of the patient's anxieties and to help her to overcome them by expressing them in another, less harmful, way. However, it is only possible to hypnotize a willing patient, so the many anorexic women who refuse to believe that there is anything wrong with them would not be suited to this therapy.

_Nutrition_
Anorexia may be associated with a raised level of zinc in the body. If tests show that this is the case, it can be corrected by taking supplements of other minerals such as copper, iron, calcium and manganese. However, these supplements should be prescribed by a qualified nutrition therapist as it is essential to get the balance correct.

# Bulimia Nervosa
SYMPTOMS, INCIDENCE AND COMPLICATIONS
This condition may occur together with anorexia nervosa or as a separate entity. The patient is preoccupied with food and indulges in episodes of bingeing after which she makes herself vomit. She has a fear of not being able to stop eating and uses drugs such as laxatives, diuretics, appetite suppressants or thyroid extracts to control her weight.

Bulimia affects a slightly higher age group than anorexia, the average age of onset being eighteen. In the USA, between 5 and 30 per cent of girls in high schools, colleges and universities are said to be suffering from it to a greater or lesser degree. Like anorexia, it is far more common in females than in males.

Patients are often depressed and may at times become suicidal. They may indulge in anti-social behaviour, such as stealing, and may become addicted to alcohol or to drugs.

There are many physical problems that may result from persist-

ent bingeing and vomiting, including inflammation of the oesophagus (gullet), distension of the stomach, pancreatitis, poor
kidney function, swelling of the salivary glands and rotting of
the teeth (due to repeated contact with acid from the stomach).
The loss of acid from the stomach causes an imbalance in the
body chemistry and this, in turn, may result in abnormal heart
rhythms and muscle spasm or paralysis. Complete loss of periods
is rare but they are usually irregular.

ORTHODOX TREATMENT
Because bulimia has only recently been recognized as a disease
in itself, doctors are, as yet, unsure about the best treatment and
the likely outcome. However, a form of psychotherapy in which
the patient keeps a diary of what she eats and tries to identify
and avoid anything in her life that seems to act as a stimulus to
bingeing seems to be having good results.

RECENT ADVANCES
Research in the United States has suggested that, in some cases,
bulimia may be associated with a hormonal problem. It seems
that cholecystokinin, the enzyme which produces a feeling of
satisfaction after a meal, is secreted in abnormally small amounts
in patients with bulimia, which may account for their bingeing
in an attempt to feel satisfied. It is not clear, however, whether
the low cholecystokinin level is the cause of bulimia or results
from it but, either way, it seems likely that it perpetuates the
disorder. Tricyclic antidepressants which boost the secretion of
cholecystokinin can be a very effective treatment.

# Organizations

The Eating Disorders Association at The Priory Centre, 11 Priory
Rd, High Wycombe, Bucks., HP13 6SL (tel. 0494 21431), and at
Sackville Place, 44–8 Magdalen St, Norwich, NR3 1JP (tel. 0603
621414) offers support, information and advice to sufferers from
anorexia and bulimia, their families and friends.

# Anxiety
# *and*
# Phobias

## Anxiety

DEFINITION AND INCIDENCE

Everyone feels anxious from time to time but the medical condition known as anxiety is one in which the patient constantly feels anxious, has physical symptoms related to the anxiety and may, from time to time, have sudden panic attacks during which the symptoms worsen considerably. Often a patient feels anxious and apprehensive without having any clear idea what is causing these symptoms – this is known as free-floating anxiety.

Anxiety affects some 5 per cent of the adult population, women twice as often as men. It usually begins between the ages of fifteen and forty and, in most cases, is mild. Hospital admission is rarely necessary. However, the condition may be a long-term one and there is a danger that patients may become dependent on tranquillizers or on alcohol.

SYMPTOMS

Physical symptoms of anxiety may be due to muscle tension, to overbreathing or to excessive activity of the sympathetic nervous system. This part of the nervous system, which is not under voluntary control, governs the way in which the body reacts to a threatening situation. The bodily changes that are temporarily brought on by fear (such as diarrhoea, pain in the chest, dry mouth, dizziness and a wish to pass water) may continue to trouble the patient suffering from anxiety over a long period of time. Other symptoms include excessive sweating, sleeplessness, unpleasant dreams, palpitations, breathlessness, indigestion, impotence or loss of the sex drive, ringing in the ears, blurred vision, restlessness and inability to concentrate. Panic attacks in which there is a sudden feeling of terror and impending doom may be associated with overbreathing, or hyperventilation. Rapid breathing in and out expels more carbon dioxide from the lungs than is normal and this upsets the balance of oxygen to carbon dioxide in the bloodstream, which has the result of making the blood more alkaline – a condition known as respiratory alkalosis. This, in turn, produces other chemical changes in the blood which cause various symptoms such as dizziness, tingling (especially in the arms and legs) and spasm of the muscles in the hands and feet. A patient who develops these symptoms, particularly if associated with palpitations or chest pain, may think that she is having a heart attack, which will increase her anxiety still further.

INVESTIGATIONS
Occasionally, a patient may develop the physical symptoms of anxiety without the mental symptoms and may have to go through numerous investigations of her digestive system, heart, lungs and so on before the diagnosis of anxiety is made. However, in most cases, the diagnosis is clear. For a patient who hyperventilates, there is a simple test that is most useful in demonstrating to both patient and doctor that it is this that is causing the unpleasant symptoms. The patient is asked to overbreathe deliberately for two to three minutes. As she does so, she will develop the tingling, chest pain, dizziness and so on of which she has been complaining. She is then given a paper bag and asked to breathe in and out of that. By doing this, she rebreathes the carbon dioxide that she has just breathed out. This brings the level of the blood gases back to normal and the symptoms subside. Not only does this reassure the patient but it also offers her a way in which she can control her attacks in future.

## ORTHODOX TREATMENT

As well as the 'paper-bag' technique, patients who suffer from hyperventilation can be offered training in how to breathe slowly and in relaxation techniques.

Psychotherapy takes several forms. The simplest form – supportive psychotherapy – may help to minimize the symptoms of an anxious patient until the condition clears up of its own accord (which, in many cases, it does). Recurring attacks, however, may warrant behaviour therapy (in which the patient's behaviour patterns are changed in order to help her cope with her condition) or even psychoanalysis (in which the root cause of the problem is investigated). However, psychoanalysis is very lengthy and expensive, and not all patients are suited to this form of treatment.

Tranquillizers such as diazepam, chlordiazepoxide, nitrazepam, oxazepam, temazepam and lorazepam may greatly reduce symptoms of anxiety and, taken at night, may give the patient a good night's sleep. However, they cannot be taken for more than three or fours weeks without the risk that the patient will become tolerant of them (needing a higher dose for the same effect) and addicted to them. Side effects include drowsiness, confusion and unsteadiness. Patients who have been on such tranquillizers for a long time and suddenly stop taking them are likely to develop withdrawal symptoms such as insomnia, anxiety, trembling and muscle twitching. Patients who suddenly stop taking a high dose may even have convulsions. It is important, therefore, when stopping tranquillizers after a prolonged period to come off them gradually over the course of several weeks.

Because of the problems associated with tranquillizers, some doctors prefer to treat patients suffering from anxiety with beta blockers (described in the section on high blood pressure). The effect of these is to reduce overaction of the sympathetic nervous system and thus to relieve the symptoms that this produces.

Very rarely, when anxiety is chronic and severe, brain surgery may be the only answer. This consists of destroying a tiny area of brain tissue at a specific site, which is located with great accuracy using special instruments. The patient's symptoms may not disappear entirely after the operation but she is usually better able to cope with them.

# Phobias

DEFINITION AND SYMPTOMS

A phobia is an irrational intense fear of a specific object, activity or situation. The patient is aware that the fear is irrational and tries to fight against it, but this only brings on extreme anxiety and, in the end, the attempt is given up.

The condition usually appears before the age of forty and affects two or three times as many women as men. Probably some 20 per cent of the population are affected by what are known as simple phobias – fear of dogs, cats, spiders and so on – but few of these are disabling. These types of phobia often begin in childhood. Agoraphobia – a fear of leaving one's home (literally a fear of the market-place) – affects between 3 and 7 per cent of the population and usually begins in early adult life. It may be very disabling and result in the patient becoming housebound.

Closely related to the phobias are the obsessions. These are irrational actions which the patient feels compelled to carry through. Failure to do so brings on anxiety. For example, a woman living alone may feel herself compelled to lock up all her kitchen knives every night in case someone should break in and stab her. Or a patient may be unable to leave her house without checking five or six times that she has turned the stove off or locked the front door. A hand-washing obsession is not uncommon, with the patient constantly feeling that her hands are dirty and, as a result, washing them twenty or thirty times a day. Obsessional phobias, in which the patient is constantly afraid that she may do something terrible against her will, may also occur.

ORTHODOX TREATMENT

Desensitization therapy consists of asking the patient to imagine the thing of which she is afraid and, as the fear develops, teaching her how to relax and reduce her anxiety. Very gradually, over a period of weeks or months, she imagines more and more intense situations until finally she can cope with the object of her phobia.

Flooding treatment is based on the fact that if an animal cannot escape from the thing of which it is frightened, it loses its fear. The patient is asked to imagine situations which produce a considerable amount of fear until, ultimately, the fear is exhausted. Implosion is a variation on this, in which the situation imagined is exaggerated so as to be the worst possible. Although successful, there is little evidence that these forms of treatment are any better than desensitization.

The best treatment for agoraphobia is programmed practice, in which the patient is taken outside her house and exposed to situations which produce a limited amount of anxiety. She is taught how to cope with this and, practising for at least an hour each day, gradually becomes able to deal with situations that, previously, she could not face.

Obsessional phobias are sometimes helped by drug treatment. The drugs used include chlorpromazine, trifluoperazine and clomipramine. Chlorpromazine and trifluoperazine, although useful, have a wide range of side effects, not least of which are trembling, restlessness and abnormal body movements. However, not all patients are affected and, for those who are, adjusting the dose can usually minimize the problem. Clomipramine may cause dry mouth, drowsiness, blurred vision, constipation and excessive sweating, all of which usually decrease as treatment continues.

# Complementary Treatment

*Acupuncture*

In the Chinese theory of energy flow around the body, the heart is said to be the seat of the mind and the spirit. Thus disturbances of the mind such as anxiety are seen as being due to a dysfunction of the heart. This may be due to a deficiency of Chi or to the presence of phlegm and heat. In the first case, points will be chosen to stimulate the Chi of the heart and, in the second, to eliminate phlegm and heat. In both cases, points will also be used to strengthen and pacify the spirit.

*Aromatherapy*
Lavender, geranium and marjoram are among the oils that may be recommended for patients with anxiety.

*Bach Flower Remedies*
Agrimony is for the person who is calm and cheerful on the outside but anxious on the inside and who tries to keep active as a way of coping with the anxiety.

Aspen will help someone who is anxious for no apparent reason and whose fears may be associated with death or with sleep; she may also suffer from faintness, headaches and trembling. Red chestnut is useful for the sort of person who can always find something to worry about and who tends to worry about other people's problems and the problems of the world.

Cherry plum is for the treatment of severe anxiety where the patient is suicidal or worries that she is going insane. It may also be helpful in the treatment of obsessions.

Mimulus is used to treat specific fear such as fear of animals, the dark or being alone. Rock rose is for sudden fear and is useful in the treatment of panic attacks and as a sedative after nightmares.

White chestnut treats what the medical profession calls 'rumination' – the constant thinking over minor worries and building them up into major anxieties. Patients may also complain of insomnia, depression and feeling of guilt.

Rescue remedy is a combination of cherry plum, clematis (which revives faintness), impatiens (for stress and nervous tension), rock rose and star of Bethlehem (for shock, grief and distress) and is a wonderful emergency treatment for all manner of experiences, ranging from anxiety before going to the dentist to shock following a car accident.

*Herbalism*
A number of herbs act as relaxants and tranquillizers and may be useful in the treatment of anxiety. These include scullcap, valerian, vervain and lemon balm.

*Homoeopathy*

Calc. carb. may be prescribed for someone who readily becomes anxious and discouraged, who is apprehensive, forgetful or confused, and who may have palpitations. Phosphorus may be appropriate for the oversensitive patient who constantly needs reassurance and ignatia for the person who over-reacts to situations and tends to exaggerate her problems. For the patient who is greatly lacking in confidence and covers up by being irritable and touchy, lycopodium may be helpful. Severe anxiety associated with restlessness may be treated with arsenicum alb. Phobias may respond to arg. nit. or gelsemium.

*Hypnotherapy*

This can be extremely helpful in the treatment of patients with anxiety and phobias. Hypnosis itself is a form of deep relaxation which can have a considerable calming effect. When in a hypnotic trance, the patient is given suggestions that she will feel more relaxed and is taught how to hypnotize herself to reinforce this training. In the treatment of phobias, hypnosis may be combined with the desensitization techniques described above and, in addition, with analytical techniques which may enable the patient to discover the cause of her phobia and thereby to overcome it.

*Nutrition*

Magnesium is a natural tranquillizer and may be recommended.

# Organizations

Phobic Action, Greater London House, 547–51 High Rd, Leytonstone, London, E11 4PR (tel. 081-558 6012), offers support and advice for patients suffering from anxiety and phobias by means of local self-help groups.

The Phobics Society, 4 Cheltenham Rd, Chorlton-cum-Hardy, Manchester, M21 1QN (tel. 061-881 1937), has a number of branches throughout the United Kingdom, publishes a newsletter six times a year and offers help and advice to phobic patients.

MIND (the National Association for Mental Health) has its headquarters at 22 Harley St, London, W1N 2ED (tel. 071-637 0741).

# Arthritis

## Definition

Literally, arthritis means inflammation (-itis) of a joint (arthr-), but in some arthritic conditions inflammation does not play a large part. The term is used to include any condition in which one or more joints become painful, stiff or limited in function for a prolonged period of time, and encompasses gout and joint infections as well as rheumatoid arthritis and osteoarthritis (the two commonest forms). Some patients suffering from psoriasis develop arthritis and the condition may also occur as part of a generalized reaction to an infection, as in the case of Reiter's syndrome, which predominantly affects men and in which other symptoms may include a discharge from the urethra and conjunctivitis.

Because there are so many facets to arthritis and because some of its forms are quite uncommon, this section will be restricted to osteoarthritis, rheumatoid arthritis and gout. Over eight million people in the UK suffer from arthritis and, of these, some five million have osteoarthritis. Psoriatic arthritis is mentioned in the section on psoriasis.

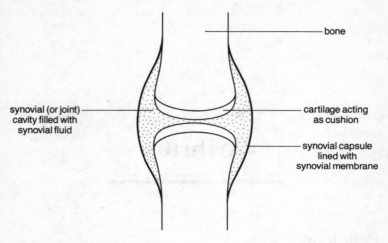

*The structure of a joint*

# Rheumatoid Arthritis

Although rheumatoid arthritis (RA) primarily attacks the joints, it also affects other parts of the body. It is thought to be an auto-immune disease – that is, one in which the body is attacked by its own immune system. Why this should happen is not known although there are theories that it may be precipitated by a viral infection. Whatever the cause, it is of comparatively recent origin since archaeologists have found that, although a number of ancient skeletons show evidence of having suffered from gout and septic arthritis (infection of a joint by bacteria), there is no convincing evidence of rheumatoid arthritis occurring before about 1800.

Nowadays, RA is a common disease, affecting between 2 and 4 per cent of the population and usually starting between the ages of thirty and fifty. Among young adults, it is six times more common in women than in men, but in older patients the sexes are more equally represented.

Affected joints become inflamed and swollen, causing pain and, sometimes, deformity, and the lining of the joint cavity

(synovium) becomes thickened. The disease may also affect the
heart, lungs, eyes and nervous system.

## SYMPTOMS AND COURSE

The main symptom of rheumatoid arthritis is usually increasing
stiffness and pain in the small joints, of which those of the hands
are often the most severely affected. In about 10 per cent of cases
the patient has a single attack and then recovers completely, and
in about 25 per cent the disease remains relatively mild with
long symptom-free periods elapsing between attacks, but in 65
per cent the symptoms are moderate to severe, with a flare-up
every few months.

RA may start in a number of different ways. The patient may,
for a time, simply be aware that her joints are stiff when she
wakes in the morning. Gradually the stiffness worsens and more
joints become involved. However, in some cases, the onset can
be much more acute and a previously healthy patient may,
literally overnight, develop severe arthritis affecting a number of
joints. Another mode of onset, commoner in younger people, is
that in which the joint symptoms are comparatively minor but
the patient is quite ill with more general symptoms such as
fever, weight loss and anaemia. In one quarter of patients, the
disease begins in a single joint, often the knee, and later spreads.
In the early stages of RA many patients complain of tiredness,
loss of appetite and weight loss, which are sometimes
accompanied by fever and sweating.

Rheumatoid arthritis usually affects the hands, wrists and
knees but can involve almost any joints, including those of the
spine. The hands may become deformed as the muscles waste,
the joints swell and the muscle tendons contract and pull the
bones out of their normal position. Typically, the fingers are
pulled sideways, away from the thumb (this is known as ulnar
deviation). The fibrous sheaths in which the tendons are encased
may also swell, causing pain when the fingers are moved;
sometimes the tendons themselves rupture, so that the patient
can no longer move her fingers. The skin of the hands may
become very thin and fragile, and prone to infection or ulceration.

The bones in the feet may become displaced, giving the patient the sensation of walking on pebbles. Deformity of the toes may occur and this may result in ulceration, because the tips of the toes, which are not normally weight-bearing, now have pressure put on them during walking.

About 30 per cent of patients, usually those whose arthritis is more severe, develop small nodules under the skin. These tend to occur near joints and over areas that are subject to pressure, being commonest just below the elbow. They are not tender but may persist for months or years. Two thirds of all patients have a moderate degree of anaemia, which may be made worse if aspirin is used to treat their arthritis.

About 10 per cent of patients recover completely from RA. In 40 per cent the condition persists but causes no disability. Another 40 per cent suffer from a moderate degree of disability while 10 per cent become severely disabled. When the disease starts slowly at an advanced age it usually remains relatively mild.

Younger women who suffer from rheumatoid arthritis often find that the condition improves when they become pregnant and recent research undertaken at the London Hospital has shown that the contraceptive Pill seems to have a protective effect against the disease. According to this study, women who have taken the Pill are only half as likely to develop RA as women who have never taken it. Those who had been on the Pill for four years or more seemed to have slightly less risk than those who had taken it for less than two years.

DIAGNOSIS
The diagnosis of rheumatoid arthritis is often made from the symptoms and an examination. However, it is sometimes necessary to differentiate it from other forms of arthritis. Eighty per cent of patients have what is known as rheumatoid factor (RF) in their blood, but this test is not specific, RF being found in other diseases as well. Anaemia is often present and needs to be diagnosed so that it can be treated. X-rays are very helpful in establishing the diagnosis of RA.

## ORTHODOX TREATMENT

In recent years, many new drugs have been developed for the treatment of arthritis, most of them falling into the NSAID (non-steroidal anti-inflammatory drug) category.

### NSAIDs

These include drugs such as ibuprofen, indomethacin and naproxen. They are very effective in many cases but can cause unpleasant side effects, usually affecting the stomach and intestines. Occasionally a patient has to stop taking the medication because of symptoms such as indigestion, nausea and abdominal pain. A recent study looked at a group of patients who had been taking NSAIDs long term and discovered that over 70 per cent of them had inflammation of the small intestine. Specialists are unsure whether the use of NSAIDs can actually cause an ulcer to form in the stomach or duodenum but have no doubt that they can delay healing once an ulcer has occurred. Some doctors, therefore, are very cautious about giving these drugs to patients who have a history of ulceration. Elderly people, in particular, need to be watched closely since, if they develop ulcers, they are more likely to suffer from complications than those in a younger age group. In some cases, where the patient seems at risk of developing an ulcer but where an NSAID is essential, additional anti-ulcer medication may be prescribed as a preventive measure.

Patients who take anticoagulants may have to reduce their dosage if they start to take NSAIDs as well, since the latter can interfere with blood clotting. They can also induce water retention which may make them unsuitable for patients with certain heart conditions. And some preparations may need to be avoided by asthmatic patients as they tend to increase the irritability of the lungs.

### Aspirin

This is an effective painkiller and anti-inflammatory drug but, like NSAIDs, it may upset the stomach and may cause bleeding from the stomach or intestines.

*Gold*

Gold is given by injection as the compound sodium aurothiomal-
ate or by mouth as auranofin, and tends to be used only if
aspirin and NSAIDs have been unsuccessful. It takes between
six and twelve weeks to work and provides relief in 40–60 per
cent of cases. Sometimes this relief is only partial, but in other
cases a total remission occurs. However, the results after a single
course may be only temporary and up to 50 per cent of patients
develop side effects. The commonest of these is a rash which,
although usually mild, may occasionally cause severe peeling of
the skin. Mouth ulcers can also occur. Much less common is
suppression of the bone marrow, with a consequent reduction in
the number of blood cells and platelets (vital for the process of
clotting) in the blood. Monthly blood tests are essential and,
since gold may also damage the kidneys, the urine is regularly
checked for the presence of protein.

*Other 'Second-line' Drugs*

One of these is penicillamine which, like gold, may take twelve
weeks or more to work. Its success rate and side effects are also
similar to those of gold and monthly blood tests and urine tests
must be done.

Drugs that suppress the immune system, such as azathioprine,
may be used (usually together with steroids) if gold and penicillamine have failed.

Methotrexate is a drug that prevents the rapid turnover of
cells and, as such, is used successfully in the treatment of both
cancer and psoriasis. However, in the past ten years it has also
been used to good effect by rheumatologists. Short-term side
effects include gastro-intestinal upsets, hair loss and soreness of
the mouth.

*Steroids*

These are normally kept for cases in which the patient is suffering
from a more generalized illness and in which other parts of the
body, such as the heart, blood vessels or spleen, have been
affected. In younger patients they are used only if all other forms
of treatment have failed. However, they are sometimes prescribed

36

in less severe cases when one or two joints are particularly troublesome; in such cases they are not taken by mouth but are injected directly into the joint. Usually this relieves pain and stiffness for a week or two only, but for some patients the effect is long-lasting. Unfortunately, steroids don't prevent the disease from continuing to destroy the joint.

*Surgery*
In some patients, the disease continues to progress despite treatment, and surgery may become necessary to restore function to the joints or to relieve pain. A commonly used operation, particularly for the fingers and knees, is synovectomy in which the lining of the joint capsule (the synovium) is removed. This regrows within three or four weeks but the operation seems to delay the rheumatoid process, sometimes for several years.

Other operations include repair of ruptured tendons which may restore movement to the fingers, and fusion of joints which, while preventing all movement, will relieve pain. Nowadays, operations to replace joints (arthroplasty) are quite common and may give good results.

RECENT DEVELOPMENTS
A cream has been developed, containing an NSAID, which can be applied topically to an inflamed joint. The NSAID penetrates the skin but remains localized and can therefore treat the affected area without causing any unpleasant side effects. At the time of writing, the cream (diclofenac gel) has not yet been given a licence in the UK but it is already available in West Germany and Switzerland.

Recently the interest of orthodox practitioners has been caught by the use of evening primrose oil (EPO) and fish oils in the treatment of arthritis. Both these oils contain essential fatty acids which are converted by the body into substances that are important for the control of inflammation. Research at the University of Glasgow has proved conclusively that both EPO and fish oils can make a dramatic difference to patients with RA. Fifty-two patients who were taking NSAIDs were divided into three groups and given EPO or EPO and fish oil or a placebo. All of those on

EPO and fish oil and 94 per cent of those taking EPO alone said they felt better and 94 per cent and 83 per cent respectively of these groups were able to stop or dramatically reduce their dosage of NSAIDs. Of the patients given placebo, only 34 per cent stopped or reduced their NSAIDs. When the patients who had been given the oils were changed on to a placebo, most of those who had improved began to deteriorate again. Although the results of this trial are very encouraging, the treatment itself is rather more expensive than standard drug therapy.

## COMPLEMENTARY TREATMENT
### Acupuncture
According to Chinese acupuncture theory, arthritis is caused by a blockage to the flow of energy, or Chi, around the body. If Chi cannot flow normally, the body cannot function properly. In chronic arthritis the blockage is said to be due to cold and damp. In acute forms, when the joints are red and swollen, it is said to be due to heat and wind. In either case, the aim of treatment is to rid the body of the causative factors and to restore the flow of Chi to normal.

### Aromatherapy
Pain and inflammation may be reduced by use of a number of essential oils. Commonly used are juniper, thyme, rosemary and chamomile.

### Herbalism
Like orthodox medicine, herbal medicine treats RA by reducing inflammation and pain but also aims to rid the body of those toxins which have accumulated and which are preventing recovery. Among the many herbs that may be prescribed, dandelion root and burdock root are used to cleanse toxic conditions, while white willow is a painkiller, containing salicylates – chemical relatives of the orthodox drug, aspirin.

### Homoeopathy
Because RA can present in a multitude of ways, there are many remedies that may be appropriate for its treatment. Bryonia, for

example, may be prescribed if the pain is worse on movement and at night but is better for rest and cold. Rhus tox. may be given if the pain is worse for rest, cold and damp but better for heat and continued movement. If the patient complains of pain moving from joint to joint and being easier when the joint is exposed to the air, pulsatilla may be needed.

*Nutrition*
In some cases, arthritis seems to be an allergic process which can either be brought on or made worse by certain foodstuffs or drinks, notably wheat, sugar, salt, coffee, tea, dairy products or citrus fruit. A nutritionist may recommend an exclusion diet to see whether avoiding any of these results in a lessening of symptoms.

Some patients with arthritis have low levels of copper in their blood, while others seem to have an excess. The former group may benefit from taking a multi-mineral tablet containing copper or from wearing a copper bracelet. (It seems that molecules of copper can actually be absorbed through the skin into the bloodstream.) However, an assessment of the patient's copper status will be made before such treatment is recommended, since additional copper may make the symptoms worse for someone whose levels are already high. For such a patient, supplements of vitamins A, C and E, together with the mineral zinc, will help to reduce their copper to within normal limits.

Supplements of vitamins A, C, D and $B_5$ may be helpful in some cases, as may dolomite, a tablet containing calcium and magnesium.

Some patients with RA will respond to the amino acid histidine, taken together with vitamin C.

## SELF-HELP AND PARA-MEDICAL ASSISTANCE
A vegetarian diet containing no refined carbohydrate may sometimes be recommended by a naturopath.

Some years ago it was found that an extract from the New Zealand green-lipped mussel could be very effective in the treatment of rheumatoid arthritis, although it must not be taken by anyone who is allergic to shellfish. This substance is available from health food shops under various trade names.

It is very important for a patient with rheumatoid arthritis to keep mobile and, to this end, special exercises may be taught by a physiotherapist. However, when joint pain is severe, bed rest, for a short period, may be helpful. It is also important to maintain a good posture – patients should sleep on a firm mattress with only a small pillow and should sit on chairs that have firm seats and straight backs.

Heat can reduce pain and spasm, and paraffin baths are especially good for relieving pain in the hands and wrists. Using a splint at night, especially for the wrists, helps to rest the joints and to prevent deformities from occurring.

Special adaptations to the home may be essential. These include tap handles that are easy to turn on and off, a raised toilet seat, and rails to assist walking and to enable the patient to get in and out of the bath or shower.

Patients whose hands are affected by arthritis may find it very difficult to open 'child-proof' medicine bottles. A special plastic exemption card is available free (with stamped addressed envelope) from the Arthritis and Rheumatism Council. This states the patient's need for 'old-fashioned' bottles, and can be handed in to the pharmacist with the prescription.

# Osteoarthritis

Osteoarthritis is usually said to be a disease of wear and tear. It affects less than 1 per cent of people aged twenty but over 80 per cent of those aged seventy. The cartilage which cushions the articulating surfaces of the bones becomes soft and splits and then gradually wears away. The bone underneath the cartilage gets thicker and new bone is formed around the edges of the joint. Gradually the joint becomes stiff and painful. Osteoarthritis usually develops in middle-aged women and may involve one joint or several. It tends to run in families and, in the majority of cases, is a mild disease.

SYMPTOMS AND COURSE
The joints most frequently affected by osteoarthritis are the knee, hip, spine (particularly in the neck and lower back), the fingers,

elbows, thumbs, ankles and big toes. The shoulders and wrists are seldom involved. Osteoarthritis of the knee is more likely to affect women than men but for the hip the position is reversed. Joints that have been damaged are particularly susceptible and may become osteoarthritic within ten years of the original injury.

Osteoarthritis affects only the joints and is not a systemic (generalized) disease. Another way in which it differs from rheumatoid arthritis is that hand function does not become impaired since it is the finger joints nearest the nails that are likely to be involved, whereas in RA it is the second finger joints and the knuckles. However, characteristic bony swellings, known as Heberden's nodes, may form on the affected finger joints and these may be painful.

The symptoms of osteoarthritis are pain, limitation of movement and stiffness. Most cases progress slowly and only a small proportion of patients develop any major disability. The pain is usually worse on exercise but is often mild and aching in character. The stiffness is worse after rest but wears off after a few minutes' movement; the severe morning stiffness associated with rheumatoid arthritis does not occur.

The joints may look quite normal but sometimes they are enlarged and, in such cases, may be tender. Often only one joint is affected.

When it affects the hip, osteoarthritis causes pain, generally in the groin or the buttock, but occasionally in the thigh. It is usually worse when the patient stands or walks and may keep him awake at night when the muscles relax. The hip may become distorted, partly due to muscle spasm around the joint and, as a result, the gait may be affected. The leg may become shortened and this, in turn, may put a strain on the spine.

Perhaps some 60 per cent of all people over sixty-five in Great Britain have osteoarthritis in the spine (spondylosis). Sometimes no symptoms occur but patients may complain of pain, which is due to a nerve being trapped between the affected bones. Occasionally, a nerve in the chest may become trapped, producing a pain which may be mistaken for angina.

Most people over the age of fifty have some degree of

osteoarthritis, which can be demonstrated on X-ray. But symptoms occur only in about 20 per cent, of whom two thirds are women, although the disease probably affects the two sexes equally. By the age of eighty, some 85 per cent of the population are affected but may often be symptom-free despite quite considerable joint deformities. However, injury may cause sudden severe pain in a joint which was previously symptomless. Symptoms are likely to be made worse by obesity and are also more likely to occur during the menopause or when the patient is suffering from another disease, such as chronic depression or thyroid deficiency.

DIAGNOSIS
This is made by X-ray, which shows the joint spaces to be smaller than normal, with extra lips of bone growing around the edges of the joint surfaces.

ORTHODOX TREATMENT
*NSAIDs*
Although these can be useful in an acute flare-up of osteoarthritis, some specialists think that they may, if used long term, make the condition worse. Many patients need only simple painkillers such as aspirin or paracetamol to control their pain.

*Steroids*
As with RA, an injection of steroid into an acutely painful joint may give temporary or long-lasting relief from pain.

*Surgery*
Sometimes if the joint becomes swollen, it is necessary to insert a needle and draw off the fluid.

Synovectomy can be combined with a clearing out of debris from the joint – fragments of cartilage or bone that have broken off. This is particularly useful for the treatment of the knee joint.

Another operation used is osteotomy in which the bone below the affected joint is divided and then allowed to heal again. How this works is unknown but it may dramatically relieve pain and the effect may last for several years. However, the result is unpredictable and not all patients respond well.

Fusion of a joint (arthrodesis) is the best way to relieve severe pain, especially in young people, but inevitably causes some disability.

About 30,000 total hip replacements are done each year in the UK, many of which are to relieve severe pain or disability in patients suffering from osteoarthritis. The results, on the whole, are extremely good. About 5000 knee replacements are also performed.

COMPLEMENTARY TREATMENT
Those therapies listed in the section on rheumatoid arthritis may also be beneficial to sufferers from osteoarthritis. Since most complementary prescriptions are based on the patient's symptoms and appearance rather than on the orthodox diagnosis, many of the same treatments may be appropriate for all forms of arthritis. In addition, osteopathy or chiropractic may be useful for patients with osteoarthritis, helping them to retain maximal possible movement in the joints and to maintain good posture. However, manipulative therapies are not usually suitable for those whose joints are inflamed as a result of rheumatoid arthritis.

SELF-HELP
It is important for patients to avoid long periods of immobility. Swimming is an ideal form of activity to keep the joints mobile.

Overweight patients may find it helpful to lose weight, thus relieving their joints of some extra stress.

# Gout
CAUSE
Gout is a condition in which an excessive amount of the waste product uric acid circulates in the blood. Because it is impossible for all this acid to be held in solution, it is deposited in the body tissues in the form of urate crystals. It is these urates which, when deposited in the joints, cause the symptoms of gout.

The cartoonist's picture of a person with gout is that of an elderly man who drinks excessively, but this is not necessarily the case. Five per cent of patients are women and the condition can occur in young people, although it is rare under the age of forty. Also, the patient does not have to be a heavy drinker. However, in those who are prone to gout anything that causes the body to manufacture uric acid – and this includes red meat and liver as well as alcohol – may precipitate an attack. The condition may run in families and, for some reason, is rare in Scots and in patients suffering from rheumatoid arthritis.

## COURSE OF THE DISEASE

Gout usually affects the hands and feet, especially the great toes, and sometimes the wrists, ankles, knees, elbows and shoulders. The first attack tends to involve only a single joint (the big toe in 50 per cent of cases) but, later, others may be affected. The joint suddenly becomes very painful and swollen and is usually red and impossible to move. Attacks seem to occur more often in the spring time and may be accompanied by a slight fever. The first episode subsides gradually over a period of a few days to a few weeks but there are likely to be recurrences. These may occur at intervals of a few months or of several years. Repeated attacks will damage the joints involved, so that full function will not be regained when the inflammation has died down. As well as dietary indiscretions, attacks may be brought on by stress or trauma, surgical operations and some antibiotics. The rapid turnover of skin cells that occurs in psoriasis also raises the level of uric acid in the blood, so patients suffering from both conditions may find that a flare-up of the rash brings on an attack of gout.

As well as being deposited in the joints, urate crystals are also laid down in the soft tissues (particularly those of the ear lobes, hands and feet) of some 25 per cent of patients. Here, after a number of years, they form hard little lumps, known as tophi, which are relatively painless but which may cause progressive stiffness and aching and, ultimately, deformities. If they become large, they may ulcerate through the skin. Sometimes urates are deposited in the kidneys where they may form stones or, if they are laid down within the body of the kidney, may interfere with its function and cause the blood pressure to rise.

## DIAGNOSIS
Blood tests usually show a raised level of uric acid although, occasionally, this may be normal. There may also be increased amounts of uric acid in the urine during an attack. X-rays may show rounded erosions, caused by the crystals, near the edges of affected joints.

## ORTHODOX TREATMENT
### Colchicine
This drug is so specific for gout that if the patient takes it and gets better this is considered to confirm the diagnosis. It usually relieves the pain within 24–48 hours but it is unpleasant to take and often causes diarrhoea, nausea, vomiting and cramps.

### NSAIDs
These may be useful in an acute attack. Azapropazone dihydrate may be particularly effective in both acute and chronic cases, since it increases the excretion of uric acid by the kidneys.

### Steroids
Injected into a joint, hydrocortisone usually relieves pain within 24–36 hours.

### Allopurinol
This is used in cases of chronic gout to lower the level of uric acid in the blood. Because there is a risk that, initially, it may increase the number of acute attacks, it is often given together with colchicine for the first six months. It works by preventing the formation of uric acid from its precursor, xanthine, which is a more soluble substance.

### Uricosuric Drugs
These work by increasing the concentration of uric acid that is excreted in the urine. The patient needs to take them regularly and to drink plenty so that the uric acid can be flushed out. They should not be taken by people with kidney stones since they may precipitate an attack of renal colic – allopurinol is usually used instead. Other side effects include stomach upsets and rashes.

Uricosuric drugs include probenecid and salicylates (the aspirin family of drugs). However, aspirin itself should not be taken by patients with chronic gout since it can cause retention of uric acid.

## COMPLEMENTARY TREATMENT

*Acupuncture*
Gout is treated in a similar way to an acute attack of rheumatoid arthritis.

*Aromatherapy*
Juniper, benzoin, chamomile, rosemary and basil are among the essences that may be used.

*Herbalism*
Celery seed and nettle are specific herbs that increase the body's excretion of uric acid. Other herbs are also used to reduce pain and inflammation. Colchicum autumnale is related to the refined product, colchicine, used by orthodox practitioners.

*Homoeopathy*
A wide range of remedies is available. These include calc. carb. for patients who develop gout whenever the weather changes, nux vomica for a first attack coming on after drinking a lot of wine, and ledum for pain situated in the ball of the big toe that is worse for warmth but is associated with little swelling. Homoeopaths, too, use colchicum when the big toe and heel are very painful, red and tender, the pain moves from one joint to another and the patient is irritable and feels weak.

# Organizations

The Arthritis Association, 1 Park View, 6 Park Avenue, Eastbourne, East Sussex, BN22 9QN (tel. 0323 500288), is a self-help association which aims to relieve arthritis using diet and herbal remedies.

Arthritis Care, 6 Grosvenor Crescent, London, SW1X 7ER (tel.

071-235 0902), provides information and practical aid for sufferers.

The Arthritis and Rheumatism Council, 41 Eagle St, London, WC1R 4AR (tel. 071-405 8572), publishes information on various aspects of arthritis and supplies the 'request for old-fashioned medicine bottles' card mentioned above.

# Asthma

## Incidence and Cause

Asthma affects between 10 and 12 per cent of all children in Britain and is a major cause of absence from school. Fortunately, many of them grow out of the condition, which affects only 3–5 per cent of adults; 50 per cent of all cases begin before the age of ten and only one sixth after the age of thirty. In young children asthma is twice as common in boys as in girls, whereas in adult life it affects as many women as men. Usually the attacks are intermittent, but some patients have persistent symptoms.

Inhaled air enters the windpipe (trachea) which divides to form the two main bronchi. These, in turn, divide many times, forming the bronchi leading to the even narrower bronchioles which finally end in little sacs, called alveoli. In the alveoli, the air is separated from the bloodstream by only a single layer of cells. Oxygen diffuses through this layer to enter the blood and is carried to the body tissues, while the waste product, carbon dioxide, diffuses out into the alveoli and is exhaled. All but the smallest bronchioles have in their walls a layer of muscle which constricts and relaxes in response to certain stimuli to regulate the breathing. However, in an asthma attack, this muscle contracts dramatically, narrowing the air passages. The patient finds breathing is difficult (typically, it is harder to breathe out

48

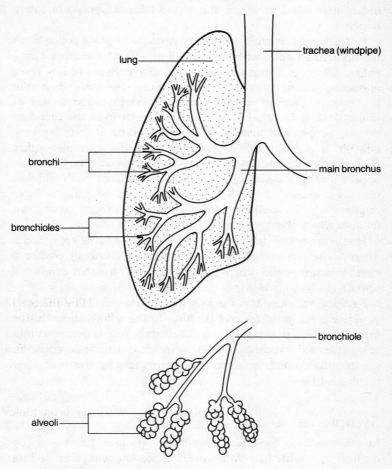

*The lungs: bronchi and bronchioles*
*A terminal bronchiole*

than to breathe in) and wheezing can be heard as the air is forced down the narrowed tubes. As the attack continues, the lining of the tubes may become inflamed and swollen and mucus is secreted, which narrows the passages still further. An asthmatic attack in a very young child may be more severe than in an older child in whom the bronchioles are proportionately larger.

In children, it is often an allergy (usually to grass pollen or to the house dust mite) which sparks off an attack of asthma. Grass pollen allergy is also responsible for the symptoms of hay fever and some patients may suffer from this too. The house dust mite is a minute creature which is found everywhere and thrives in house dust. It has no harmful features apart from the fact that certain people are allergic to it. Eradicating it can be very difficult, if not impossible. Asthmatic patients may also suffer from another disease associated with allergy – eczema. This may appear during the same period as the asthma or one condition may be superseded by the other. One third of patients have relatives who have suffered from asthma, and many come from families where there is a history of hay fever or eczema.

However, not all asthma attacks are due to an allergy. Some 40 per cent are precipitated by an infection – a heavy cold or a chest infection – and others may be brought on by an emotional upset.

Asthma accounts for two to three deaths per 100,000 total population per year in Great Britain. On the whole, these deaths are more likely to occur in older patients whose chronic asthma is complicated by chronic bronchitis. Most asthmatic children, on the other hand, are free from symptoms by the time they reach adulthood.

## Symptoms

In acute asthma the attack may come on quite suddenly, often during the night, in which case the patient wakes up feeling breathless. Or it may be preceded by a head cold or a dry, hacking cough. The main symptoms are a tight feeling in the chest and difficulty in breathing out. The breathing becomes wheezy and the patient may cough, without bringing anything very much up from the chest. As the attack progresses, the breathing becomes rapid and shallow, and the patient looks pale and anxious and avoids the effort of speaking. In a severe attack the breathing becomes irregular and the wheeze may be less noticeable as less air goes in and out of the lungs. The patient becomes increasingly restless and the relative lack of oxygen in the blood may turn his lips blue. His pulse may race, but only if the attack has been brought on by an infection will he have a fever. An attack may last for minutes or hours, or rarely, for days. Sometimes the patient will vomit and, following this, his breathing may become easier.

Effort of any kind makes the symptoms worse, as does anxiety, so that a vicious circle may arise as the patient becomes more and more anxious over his inability to breathe normally. He is usually most comfortable sitting, leaning forward, with his arms resting on something that is at the same level as his shoulders, since this is the position in which breathing is easiest. A number of extra muscles (the so-called accessory muscles of respiration) are brought into play at the top of the rib cage, around the base of the neck, in order to keep the chest moving and on breathing in the spaces between the ribs may appear to be sucked in. A patient suffering from chronic asthma often has a distended barrel-shaped chest with very little movement visible on respiration. After a prolonged attack the patient will be very tired, his chest and abdomen may be sore, due to the over-use of muscles, and he is likely to cough up a great deal of mucus including worm-like 'casts' – the plugs of mucus which have formed in the small bronchioles.

Normally there are no symptoms between attacks but adult patients who suffer from chronic asthma may become breathless on slight exertion, may wheeze frequently, may have a cough which is particularly troublesome during the night and may bring up quantities of sputum first thing in the morning. The cough may persist for months, especially during the winter. Superimposed on these symptoms, acute attacks of asthma can be brought on by a chest infection and these patients often suffer from chronic bronchitis in addition to asthma. Some children who have acute asthma may also have a recurrent dry cough which is usually worse in the evening or early morning. Sometimes this is their only symptom and they do not proceed to the full-blown asthma attack.

# Status Asthmaticus

This is a condition in which an attack continues for many hours or days and is not relieved by the patient's usual medications. It is a life-threatening condition and usually requires hospital treatment.

Because the attack progresses without any let-up, mucus accumulates in the smallest of the bronchioles and may block them completely, adding to the patient's breathing difficulties. If a whole section of the lung becomes plugged, it may collapse and pneumonia may develop. Finally, the amount of oxygen being taken in may become so small that the patient can die from suffocation.

# Investigations

Between attacks, the asthmatic patient may appear perfectly normal. However, tests of lung function may become abnormal after exercise. A child who is suspected of having asthma may be told to run around for a few minutes before being asked to blow into a machine, known as a spirometer, which will measure the capacity of his lungs. The two measurements that are generally used are the FEV1 and the FVC. The FEV1 is the forced expiratory volume in one second – the patient is asked to take a very deep breath, hold it and then breathe out forcibly as hard as he can into the spirometer tube. The amount of air that he forces out during the first second is measured by the machine. The FVC is the forced vital capacity – the total amount of air that the patient can force out of his lungs after taking the largest possible breath in. On the whole, spirometers are used by hospital doctors, whereas GPs have smaller, portable, machines called peak flow meters. Such a machine measures the peak expiratory flow or PEF – the maximum rate at which the air can flow from the lungs – a measurement comparable to the FEV1. Here again, the patient is asked to breathe forcibly into the machine, which he holds in his hand, after filling his lungs as deeply as he can.

People who are in the throes of an acute asthma attack, those who suffer from chronic asthma and most asthmatic patients who have just exercised will have levels of FEV1, FVC and PEF that are lower than normal. If, however, they are given a drug to relieve the constriction in the lungs (a bronchodilator), the FEV1 usually rises fairly quickly.

Other investigations that may be done are chest X-ray which will show up any areas of lung infection or collapse, skin tests to check for allergies which may be precipitating attacks and, in status asthmaticus, blood gases. This last test shows the levels of oxygen and carbon dioxide in the arterial blood, which reflects the balance of gases in the lungs. It serves as a guide to the severity of the attack and monitors the efficacy of the treatment being given. The blood is usually taken from the femoral artery (in the groin) or from the carotid artery (in the neck).

## Orthodox Treatment

Nowadays it is possible to give drugs that will prevent asthma attacks from happening as well as drugs to relieve and cut short attacks when they do occur.

Sodium cromoglycate is a commonly used drug with practically no side effects whose action is to inhibit the release from the tissues of histamine and other chemicals involved in the development of an allergic reaction. Its action is entirely preventive and it has no effect once these substances have begun to act and an asthma attack is under way. It has to be taken regularly up to four times a day and is usually prescribed only for patients who have frequent asthmatic attacks, but it may also be useful for those in whom asthma is brought on by exercise, in which case it should be taken ten to fifteen minutes before the activity begins. Another, similar, preventive drug is nedocromil sodium which, however, is only suitable for patients over the age of twelve, whereas sodium cromoglycate seems to be particularly effective for children. Nedocromil needs to be taken for at least a week before the full effect is seen.

Bronchodilators are given once an attack has started, to relieve the spasm in the lungs. They may be divided into two main groups, the xanthine drugs, such as theophylline and aminophylline, and the beta adrenergic drugs, such as isoetharine, salbutamol, fenoterol and terbutaline. The xanthine drugs, although effective, may have considerable side effects such as irritability, hyperactivity, abdominal pain, an increased heart rate and vomiting of blood. However, if a small dose is taken first and then, if necessary, followed by gradually increasing doses, the side effects are usually minimal. A long-acting form of theophylline is said to be particularly helpful in controlling attacks that occur during the night, but may cause nausea, headache and digestive problems. Among the beta adrenergic drugs, terbutaline and fenoterol seem to have a longer-lasting action, so these too may be useful for patients who have nocturnal asthma.

Steroids are also effective against asthma but, because of the dangers of long-term side effects, are usually prescribed for limited periods, except in the case of patients whose asthma is incompletely controlled by any other drugs. Used regularly to prevent attacks from occurring, they have few side effects and are usually tailed off slowly after about a year of treatment. As in the case of nedocromil, it may be at least a week before their full benefit is seen.

Many of the drugs mentioned here can be given either by mouth or through an inhaler, the latter method often being preferred since it is likely to have fewer side effects. There are various forms of inhaler and even quite young children (over the age of four) can usually manage to use one of them successfully.

If a patient fails to respond to basic treatment in an asthma attack, hospital admission may be necessary. The treatment of status asthmaticus includes the administration of oxygen, intravenous steroids and a bronchodilator, either inhaled or in the form of aminophylline given intravenously. The patient is likely to be considerably dehydrated (because rapid, shallow breathing results in the loss of a great deal of moisture from the lungs) so he will need plenty of fluids and, if he is unable to drink due to the severity of the attack, a drip will be put up. If the attack has been brought on by an infection, antibiotics will also be necessary. In a very severe case, the patient may need to have his breathing assisted by a mechanical respirator for a short period.

Most asthmatic patients are kept under review by a hospital specialist, although those whose attacks are mild and infrequent are usually looked after by their GPs. In either case, regular check-ups are important.

In some cases, where the attacks are shown to be brought on by an allergy to grass pollen or to the house dust mite, desensitizing injections may be effective.

# Recent Advances

Measuring the lung function of small babies has always been difficult but now an inflatable jacket has been developed in Australia which makes this possible.

For patients whose asthma attacks are related to allergies, a new antihistamine, cetirizine, offers hope. A French study found that it was particularly effective for those whose symptoms were worse during the grass pollen season.

Some asthmatic patients may be suffering from an allergic condition without realizing it. The Professor of Allergy at the University of Virginia in the USA has found that patients who have both asthma and athlete's foot are likely to be allergic to the ringworm fungus that is causing their foot condition. When the athlete's foot is treated, the patients' need for asthma medication is reduced.

An experiment carried out at St Thomas's Hospital in London showed that when men increased the amount of salt in their diet, their bronchi and bronchioles became more sensitive and more likely to go into spasm. However, the same effect was not demonstrated in women. These results suggest that men who suffer from asthma might be well advised to reduce their salt intake to a minimum.

At the University of Natal in Durban, South Africa, doctors have found that when asthmatic children lie down it is more difficult for them to breathe and that they are likely to cough and wheeze less during the night if they sleep propped up. This applies particularly to children in the two-to-three age range.

Methotrexate is a drug which has been used for some time in the treatment of cancer because of its ability to kill abnormal cells. It is also used successfully in severe cases of psoriasis and has been found useful in the treatment of arthritis. Now researchers in the United States have found that giving it once a week to fourteen patients with severe asthma allowed them to reduce their dose of steroids. The only side effects seemed to be transient nausea and, in one patient, a rash. Other studies will be needed to confirm these results.

# Complementary Treatment

_Acupuncture_

Asthma is divided into three types – the cold type (acute asthma), the hot type (acute asthma associated with an acute chest infection) and the deficiency type (chronic asthma).

For the cold type, points will be chosen which have the effect of warming and strengthening the lungs, expelling the cold and clearing phlegm. For the hot type, the aim of treatment is to cool the heat and clear phlegm. For chronic asthma, in which there is said to be a deficiency of energy or Chi in the lungs, points will be chosen which will strengthen the lungs and their Chi. In all three types, points are also used which produce relaxation of the bronchi.

_Alexander Technique_

Improving the patient's posture may have the added benefit of helping him to breathe more easily.

_Aromatherapy_

A large number of essential oils may be used including eucalyptus, hyssop, lavender, aniseed, cajuput, lemon and thyme.

_Herbalism_

Among the herbs used to treat asthma are ephedra (which relaxes the bronchi), coltsfoot (which soothes the irritated airways and which is an expectorant, helping the patient to cough up mucus), grindelia (an expectorant and antispasmodic), lobelia (which has expectorant and anti-inflammatory properties), and skunk cabbage, thyme, bloodroot and sundew (all of which are expectorants).

*Homoeopathy*

The patient may be given one of a large number of remedies that are appropriate for different types of asthma. Ipecac. may be helpful for patients whose attack is associated with a rattling in the throat, sweating, anxiety, nausea and a feeling of chill. Patients who require arsenicum are often elderly and are usually worse after midnight and worse for lying down or for movement. Kali carb. is useful if the patient is worse for movement, especially walking, and suffers from dizziness and diarrhoea. Lobelia may be prescribed if the attack is associated with nausea, vomiting, giddiness and a feeling of heaviness in the chest and abdomen. If the attack follows an upset stomach or a period of great mental exertion, nux vomica may be appropriate, but if it follows exposure to wind or to cold, the patient may require aconite. Sambucus is especially useful for children who develop an acute attack during the night.

*Hypnotherapy*

Very often a mild asthma attack may be made worse by the patient's anxiety, which causes additional spasm in the bronchi. Under hypnosis, a patient can be taught how to relax when the first symptoms of breathlessness arise. Once this has been learned and used on a few occasions, he will begin to feel confident in his ability to control an asthma attack and this will reinforce the power of the technique. For some patients, it may be possible, by using self-hypnosis, to prevent an attack from developing altogether. Often additional techniques are taught which are used in conjunction with self-hypnosis, such as one in which the patient visualizes his bronchi relaxing and performs some action (such as unclenching clenched fists) to mirror this and 'cause it to happen'.

*Manipulation*

Patients who have had asthma for many years may develop a curvature of the spine and a pigeon chest. Manipulation can improve the mobility of the spine and loosen the rib cage so that breathing becomes easier and deeper.

*Nutrition*

The lining (mucosa) of the bronchi and bronchioles needs vitamin A in order to stay healthy. A supplement of this may be recommended, together with vitamin C, which helps to inactivate any inhaled substances which may spark off an asthma attack.

# Self-help

Measures should be taken to reduce the house dust mite population – feather pillows and quilts should be replaced by others with synthetic filling and a plastic cover should be put over the mattress. Reducing humidity, in which the mites thrive, is also important. Wood-fuelled or calor-gas heating, condensation in the bathroom and drying clothes indoors, all of which raise humidity, should, wherever possible be avoided. A paint called Artilin 3A can be used on woodwork to kill the house dust mite. Details of this are given in the section on chronic rhinitis and hay fever.

Some children seem to be allergic to milk, so exclusion of milk from the diet may be helpful. However, a calcium supplement, in the form of dolomite, will need to be taken regularly. In some cases, goat's milk can be substituted. Fish, eggs, nuts and berry fruits may also bring on attacks, especially in the very young. Some children are allergic to animals and will have to be denied the pleasure of keeping a pet.

Garlic is effective in reducing mucus and may be taken in capsule form.

Because steroid inhalers may promote the growth of monilial infections (thrush – see separate section) in the mouth, patients should brush their teeth after using such preparations in order to minimize the risk of this occurring.

Patients, especially children, who wish to undertake some form of exercise should opt for something such as swimming or walking rather than a sport which necessitates sudden bursts of activity and which may more readily bring on an attack of asthma.

# Organizations

The Asthma Society and Friends of the Asthma Research Council has over 150 local branches that offer advice and information. The association, which has its headquarters at 300 Upper St, London, N1 2xx (tel. 071-226 2260), also publishes a magazine, *Asthma News*, three times a year.

# Back Pain

## Incidence

Every year about two million adults in Great Britain see their GPs because they are suffering from back pain and every day 50,000 people are off work for the same reason. This, however, is only the tip of the iceberg – it is estimated that for every one of these patients there are another eighteen who do not seek medical advice. Fortunately, nearly half of all those affected are better within a week and over 90 per cent have recovered within two months. The majority of sufferers are women but, in many cases, the problem is related to the patient's occupation: 64 per cent of all those who are involved in heavy work will suffer at some time from back pain, and, each year, one sixth of all nurses will be affected to some extent.

## Types of Pain

Back pain is not a single entity – it can have many different causes – and so the types of pain that patients may experience can differ quite considerably.

Pain can be sharp or aching, constant or intermittent, localized or diffuse, and may be relieved by a variety of postures. If a nerve is irritated, as well as a relatively sharp pain at the site of irritation, a dull ache may be felt further along the length of that nerve. So, for example, a prolapsed ('slipped') disc which is pressing on the nerve that runs down the leg and into the foot may cause an ache in the toes. This is known as referred pain.

## Causes of Back Pain

There are many causes of back pain. However, the commonest single cause is a prolapsed intervertebral disc (PID), which accounts for 20 per cent of cases. A further 15 per cent are caused by a number of uncommon conditions, while the remaining 65 per cent are labelled 'non-specific' – in other words, the patient's symptoms and the findings on examination do not point to any particular physical cause.

Specific causes of back pain, apart from a prolapsed disc, include fractures of the vertebrae, dysfunction of the joints, arthritis, inflammation, ligament problems and osteoporosis. Muscle spasm can cause considerable pain and often exacerbates that due to another cause. Occasionally, pain originating in the abdomen may be felt in the back – for example in patients suffering from pancreatitis (inflammation of the pancreas). Rarely, back pain may be caused by an infection or a growth in the bone itself.

Fractures of the vertebrae (the bones making up the spine) are usually the result of injury. However, a child or adolescent who takes part in a lot of sports may sustain a spontaneous stress fracture in one of the lower lumbar vertebrae, and elderly people may develop crush fractures as the result of osteoporosis (see section on osteoporosis).

## Prolapsed Intervertebral Disc (Slipped Disc)

The disc which cushions adjacent vertebrae is made up of two parts – the tough outer annulus fibrosus and the jelly-like inner nucleus pulposus. With age, the disc degenerates. It is possible that this occurs unevenly, setting up stresses in the annulus fibrosus, making it more likely to tear. If it does tear, the nucleus

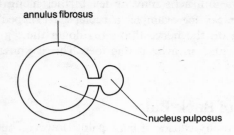

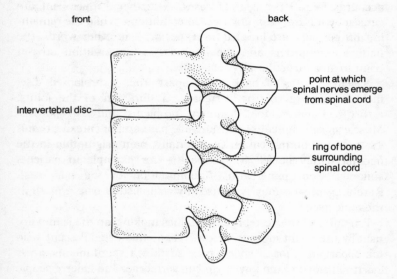

_A prolapsed disc_
_Vertebrae_

pulposus flows out, producing symptoms by stretching the annulus fibrosus and pressing on the adjacent nerves.

Usually the patient is young or middle-aged and the first attack strikes suddenly when, after twisting, bending or coughing, she suddenly finds herself in severe pain and unable to move. There is often a history of injury to the back at some time in the past. However, sometimes the pain comes on in a less spectacular manner, increasing gradually over the course of a day. The patient may also be aware of pain running down into her buttock, thigh or leg, and, occasionally, may just have pain in the leg with very little in the back. Normally only one side is affected and the patient may take up a lopsided posture in an attempt to relieve the pain.

Prolapsed discs seem to occur most frequently in those parts of the spine that are the most mobile. Thus they are commonest in the lumbar spine (lower back), fairly common in the cervical spine (neck) and quite rare in the thoracic spine (chest region). It is customary to refer to a disc by the numbers of the vertebrae between which it lies. Thus the disc lying between the fourth and fifth lumbar vertebrae is known as L4/L5, while that between the fifth lumbar and the first sacral vertebrae is L5/S1. It is L5/S1 that is found to have prolapsed in the majority of cases of PID.

DIAGNOSIS OF PID

The doctor will make his diagnosis of a prolapsed intervertebral disc primarily on the patient's history of sudden pain and locking, together with referred pain down the leg. The location of the pain will allow him to decide which disc is involved. He will diagnose a prolapse of L4/L5 if the patient is experiencing pain in the region of the hip and groin, running down to the back of the thigh, the outer surface of the lower leg, the back of the foot and the first or second and third toes. Tingling, soreness or numbness may be associated with the pain and the patient may find it difficult to point her toes due to weakness of the muscles involved. Occasionally the knee reflex or the ankle reflex is reduced in vigour.

A prolapse of L5/S1, on the other hand, is suggested if the patient has pain running from the buttock down the back of the leg to the underside of the foot and the fourth and fifth toes. This patient, too, may have tingling, soreness or numbness in the lower leg or the outer toes and a reduced ankle reflex, but the movement that is likely to be difficult is that of bending the foot upwards. Pain running down the leg from the back is often called sciatica.

On examination, the doctor will look for specific points of tenderness in the back and leg, and will probably try the 'straight leg raising test'. In this, the patient sits on the couch with her legs stretched out in front of her. The leg in which she feels the pain is slowly raised and, if she has a prolapsed disc, this will bring on the pain before the leg is raised to an angle of 45°. If the prolapse is severe, raising the symptomless leg may also aggravate the pain in the affected leg. In addition, the doctor will check the patient's flexibility – she is likely to have restricted movement in bending forwards although she may be able to bend fully to the sides.

An X-ray is seldom taken since there is usually nothing to be seen until the patient has had her problem for several years, at which point there may be evidence that the space occupied by the disc between the vertebrae is narrowed. However, if surgery is proposed, a myelogram, in which a radio-opaque dye is injected into the spinal canal, may be done to show up distortion of the affected disc.

## Spondylosis

This is the name given to a severe form of osteoarthritis affecting the spine, associated with degenerated intervertebral discs. Spondylosis affects older patients, who complain of pain, stiffness and limited movement which is relieved by rest. The pain occurs in either the neck or the lower back and may radiate to the arms or the legs. Often the patient will have periods when the pain suddenly gets worse and movement becomes more difficult.

An X-ray will show the characteristic appearance of an arthritic spine. However, many older people have these changes without suffering from any symptoms and it is not known why this condition should cause pain only in some and not in others.

## Spondylolisthesis

This is a condition in which one vertebra becomes displaced and slips forward, causing pain that is relieved by stooping. It is responsible for 15 per cent of cases of back pain that occur in people under the age of twenty and may, in some cases, be due to a slight deformity in the vertebra itself, although, in others, it is caused by injury. In the elderly, L4 may slip forward on L5 as a result of osteoarthritis. Diagnosis can be made on an X-ray.

# Rheumatoid Spondylitis (Rheumatoid Arthritis of the Spine)

This is comparatively rare. It often begins in the sacro-iliac joints situated between the lower part of the spine, or sacrum, and the pelvic bones. The patient complains of a continuous ache and stiffness in the back or the buttocks and thigh, often accompanied by other symptoms of rheumatoid arthritis (see section on rheumatoid arthritis). The pain is often worse after resting and eased by exercise, and it commonly occurs at night or in the early hours of the morning. It is frequently aggravated by changes in the weather.

# Ankylosing Spondylitis

This is a form of arthritis which is mainly a disease of young men, although it sometimes attacks women and may begin at any age before fifty. It affects 1–2 per cent of the population and is the commonest of the so-called seronegative arthritides (in other words, arthritis where the diagnostic rheumatoid factor, found in the blood of patients with rheumatoid arthritis, is absent). It is thought to be a reactive arthritis, triggered off in a genetically susceptible individual by a particular stress such as an infection.

It causes recurrent episodes of stiffness together with low back pain which may be aching in character and may radiate down the legs. Unlike the one-sided pain from a slipped disc, that of ankylosing spondylitis is usually symmetrical. One third of patients also develop arthritic changes in the shoulders, hips, knees and ankles, and one quarter suffer from recurrent inflammation of the eyes. Other symptoms may include fever, fatigue, weight loss, chest pain, pain in the sole of the foot and the Achilles tendon, and a skin rash.

It used to be thought that ankylosing spondylitis was always a progressive disease in which the bones of the spine gradually fused and the patient was left with a rigid 'poker back', often in a stooped and deformed position. However, in very few cases does the spine fuse completely and modern treatment can control the symptoms in the majority of patients.

In early cases, the diagnosis usually has to be made from the history, since it may be some time before the classical picture of blurring of the sacro-iliac joints and calcification of the ligaments of the spine are visible on X-ray. Morning stiffness which is relieved by exercise suggests this diagnosis, as does a finding of tenderness over the sacro-iliac joints.

# Spinal Stenosis

In this condition, the spinal canal and the canals through which the spinal nerves leave the vertebral column are narrowed as the result of osteoarthritis, a prolapsed disc, previous surgery, spondylolisthesis or a disease of the bone itself. Pain is felt in the back and the buttock, is eased by bending over and is made worse by standing up straight or walking downhill. It may be accompanied by referred pain, numbness, tingling or weakness in the affected part, all of which may be brought on by walking and relieved by sitting down.

# Non-specific Back Pain

In the majority of cases of back pain no particular cause can be found. One specialist believes that many of these patients are suffering from spinal stenosis, which may be hard to diagnose. In some cases, the pain may be due to ligament strain or muscle spasm caused by awkward movement or incorrect use of the back when lifting. The episodes may be recurrent but usually settle within two weeks. The pain may radiate to the buttocks and thighs, often gets worse with prolonged walking, sitting or standing, and is usually most severe in the evenings.

# Orthodox Treatment

This varies according to the diagnosis that has been made. In all cases painkillers are helpful. Anti-inflammatory drugs (NSAIDs) such as indomethacin and flurbiprofen are effective in rheumatoid spondylitis and in ankylosing spondylitis.

It is customary to recommend a period of bed rest on a firm mattress until the acute symptoms have disappeared but a study carried out in the United States in 1986 showed that two days in bed was as effective as seven and in some ways better, since prolonged bed rest allowed the back muscles to become weak, adding to the patient's problem. Spinal support, in the form of a corset, may be used following bed rest and may be particularly helpful as a long-term treatment in patients with spondylosis and spondylolisthesis.

Manipulation and stretching the spine with traction may be used, especially for patients with a diagnosis of a prolapsed disc. In some cases injections into the spinal joints or the spinal canal of steroid and local anaesthetic can be effective. Physiotherapy in which the patient is taught exercises to strengthen the back muscles will often help not only to relieve the pain but also to prevent further episodes.

Patients suffering from spinal stenosis can be helped by physiotherapy, exercises and posture training, and over half find relief from the use of transcutaneous electrode nerve stimulation (TENS). This is a gadget which is strapped to the skin in the affected area and delivers a tiny electrical stimulus to the nerve in such a way as to anaesthetize it.

In many cases of prolapsed disc, the basic treatment of bed rest and painkillers, possibly with some traction, will suffice. However, when attacks occur frequently and are both prolonged and severe, doctors may consider surgery to be appropriate. Because the results of surgery cannot be guaranteed, caution must be exercised when offering operative treatment and it is usually only suggested for certain categories of patient.

The most commonly performed operation is partial removal of the prolapsed disc, or laminectomy. This reduces pain in up to 96 per cent of patients but the relief is total in only 15 per cent.

Such an operation may have to be performed as an emergency if a disc has prolapsed in such a way that it is pressing on the nerves that run to the bladder, resulting in paralysis of the muscles of the bladder wall and consequent retention of urine. Extensive weakness of the leg muscles is also a clear indication for surgery.

A more recently introduced form of treatment is chemonucleolysis in which the disc is dissolved by injecting into it an enzyme called chymopapain. A general anaesthetic is not necessary, the procedure being performed under local anaesthetic and sedation. It is done in the operating theatre, and the surgeon checks the position of his needle by using X-rays, which means that this technique cannot be used for pregnant women. After the treatment, the patient is kept in bed for forty-eight hours, during which time her back pain may be severe and she may need powerful painkillers. She is then allowed up, wearing a corset, which she continues to wear for four weeks.

One per cent of patients have a severe allergic reaction to chymopapain and, although this is easily dealt with, the treatment involves the use of adrenaline. This makes chemonucleolysis inadvisable for people who have recently had a heart attack or who have liver or kidney disease, since adrenaline might be harmful to them should it need to be given, A second injection of chymopapain increases the risk of such a reaction to 12 per cent, so this form of treatment is very rarely offered a second time.

Since the discs dry up of their own accord with age, chemonucleolysis is inappropriate for older patients. It is also unsuitable for adolescents who may still be growing. The ideal patient is aged between twenty and forty, has three or more attacks of back pain a year, lasting over a month each time, with leg pain that is eased by bed rest. A myelogram or scan will be done before treatment and it is important that the location of the patient's symptoms correspond exactly to the disc that is seen to be prolapsed. In this way, the surgeon will have no doubt that he is treating the correct disc. Because it is vital that the enzyme is injected into the centre of the nucleus pulposus and because it is sometimes difficult to do this with an L5/S1 disc, patients with a prolapse at this level are more likely to be offered surgery.

If all these conditions are adhered to and if chemonucleolysis is offered only to patients who are perfectly suitable, it is said to have an 80 per cent success rate. However, 10 per cent of those treated may need surgery at a later date and 2 per cent may have severe backache for up to a year following the procedure. In the United States, some surgeons no longer offer this form of treatment since they consider the long-term results to be inferior to those of laminectomy.

# Recent Advances

A new method of treatment has been introduced for prolapsed discs that looks as though it will be very effective for selected patients. One English surgeon has reported that he has used it on fourteen patients; in thirteen cases it was highly successful and only one patient still needed a laminectomy. Known as nucleotomy, the technique consists of inserting a special needle into the centre of the prolapsed disc and using it to cut through the disc material and suck out the debris. As a result of this procedure, the pressure inside the disc is relieved and the prolapsed section can fall back into the space that has been cleared. Done under local anaesthetic, and aided by X-rays, nucleotomy takes only an hour and the patient can go home the same day. Relief of pain is almost immediate in successful cases. However, because not all patients are suitable for this operation, laminectomy is likely to remain the standard procedure for the treatment of a prolapsed disc.

# Complementary Treatment

*Acupuncture*
Back pain is associated with stagnation of the flow of energy or Chi in the affected area. This may be due to blockage of the channels by wind, cold and damp. Treatment consists of using points to warm the channels, to dispel the wind, cold and damp, and to restore the normal flow of Chi. Specific points can also be used to relieve pain.

## Alexander Technique

This is a system of posture training whose aim is to relieve the body of all unnatural tensions. Back pain is always associated with muscle spasm and abnormal posture, so Alexander training can be very effective, helping not only to relieve the pain but to prevent its recurrence.

## Aromatherapy

Ginger, juniper, marjoram, sage, geranium and lavender are among the essential oils that may be used in treating back pain.

## Chiropractic

A chiropractor offers manipulative treatment for musculo-skeletal disorders, especially where these are related to spinal problems. Some forms of back pain may respond very well because manipulation improves the flexibility of the spinal joints and muscles, even if it is incapable of curing the degenerative process which is causing the trouble. Treatment also aims to improve the strength of the muscles that support the spine.

A chiropractor will examine the patient's back in the same way as a doctor and will take X-rays. The manipulation used is localized on the exact area in which the problem lies and is accompanied by massage, exercises and advice on posture. Several sessions of treatment may be necessary, depending on the individual patient.

## Herbalism

Herbs may be used to reduce muscle spasm, such as yarrow, cramp bark or lobelia, or to reduce inflammation and relieve pain, such as white willow (which contains aspirin-like compounds) and vervain. Lady's slipper has all these actions.

## Homoeopathy

Of the many remedies that may be suitable for patients with back pain, rhus tox. is one of the most commonly used. It is often prescribed when the pain has resulted from straining and is associated with stiffness on first moving; the pain is usually better for heat, firm support and continued movement. Other remedies include bryonia, which may be indicated when the pain is severe, shooting in quality and travels from the lower back down to the ankles; the patient tends to feel cold and to walk stooped over. Arnica is useful when the pain is due to injury, especially if there is a lot of bruising. Sulphur may help patients with chronic sciatica which is worse for warmth, especially if it is on the left side. Patients whose low back pain is dull, severe and usually worse in bed and in the morning may be helped by nux vomica.

*Osteopathy*
Osteopathic manipulation is different from that used by chiropractors but equally effective, especially in the treatment of prolapsed discs. Chronic or recurrent back pain that is associated with a previous injury or that is worse for rest and better for exercise is also likely to respond well, as is pain due to strain or muscle tension. Several sessions of treatment may be necessary.

# Organizations

The Back Pain Association, 31–3, Park Rd, Teddington, Middlesex, TW I I OAB (tel. 081-977 5474), is involved in fund-raising for research into the causes and treatment of back pain and offers leaflets on ways of preventing back pain from occurring.

# Bed-wetting

## (Nocturnal Enuresis)

### Incidence and Causes

This is a very common problem among children but, in the great majority of cases, the cause is unknown. In about 5 per cent of cases, there is some underlying physical disorder such as a urinary tract infection, diabetes, chronic constipation or epilepsy, but these children almost always have other symptoms so that diagnosis is made easier.

The age at which children 'should' be dry is difficult to assess, but most doctors will not start treating for bed-wetting before the age of five or six. On average about one child in five wets the bed more than once a week at the age of three, one in ten at the age of five and one in thirty-five at the age of fourteen. Bed-wetting is commoner in boys than in girls and commoner in children who are emotionally deprived, such as those living in institutions. Some 10 per cent of bed-wetters will also have trouble controlling their bladders during the day.

In 70 per cent of cases, bed-wetting runs in the family, with the mother, father or a brother or sister having been affected. It is customary to divide patients into two groups – those who have never been dry (primary enuresis) and those who were dry but have started to wet again (secondary enuresis). Primary enuresis is commoner than secondary, but since both types

72

are treated in the same way, the distinction is purely academic.

Sometimes when a child who is dry starts to wet again, it is at a time when something important is happening in his life, such as starting school or the birth of a new brother or sister. However, this does not necessarily mean that the child is worried or upset by the event and some specialists deny that bed-wetting is associated with stress. Often when a child goes on holiday or stays with relatives he will suddenly become dry again but the reason for this is unclear.

## Investigations

Before any treatment is offered, the urine will be checked to rule out any infection and, if necessary, a few basic tests of balance, coordination and sensation will be done to see whether there might be anything wrong with the nervous system. If an underlying organic disease is suspected, this will be investigated and treated.

## Orthodox Treatment

There are many methods that have been used to treat bed-wetting, some more successful than others. In the first place, the child needs to understand that the mechanism that controls the bladder is very complex and that bladder control is something that has to be learned in the same way that he must learn to swim or ride a bicycle. Keeping a star chart (with a gold star for every night that he is dry) and praising or rewarding him as he gains better control can be very productive. Admonishing or punishing him when he is wet, on the other hand, can be very counter-productive and parents should try, as far as is possible, not to express their annoyance or anger to the child on the occasions when the bed is wet.

Lifting the child at night is sometimes helpful but the time at which he is roused should be varied or he will just tend to wet at that particular time. Fluids before bedtime should not be restricted because it is important that the bladder learns to cope with normal amounts of urine. If less is given, it just gets used to holding less.

Drug treatment is available in the form of the tricyclic anti-depressant imipramine or the antispasmodic propantheline, both of which seem to have the effect of relaxing the bladder muscle so that it does not contract abnormally. This has a 50 per cent success rate but, unfortunately, up to 70 per cent of those helped relapse again later. However, it is useful in the short term, for example if the child is going on holiday.

The most effective treatment the doctor can offer is the enuresis alarm. This consists of a urine-sensitive pad which is put (depending on the model) either on the bed or inside the pyjamas with, wired up to it, an alarm which is placed by the bedside or attached to the pyjama top. As soon as the pad becomes wet, the alarm goes off, causing the child to jump. This results in automatic contraction of the muscles at the base of the bladder and the flow of urine stops. While the alarm is still sounding, it is necessary for a parent to come into the room and wake the child so that he can turn the alarm off himself. Eventually, a reflex will develop in which the sensation of starting to wet will cause the child to jump and wake up. The alarm has an 80 per cent success rate after about three months' treatment, with only a 13 per cent relapse rate. Some children who do not respond straight away may do so with a different type of alarm – some respond better to bells, others to buzzers. If the parent wakes the child each morning by pressing the test button on the device, this will also help him to associate the sound of the alarm with waking up. The child should keep a record chart to show the nights on which he stays dry. But, in the early stages, encouraging signs are smaller wet patches in the bed and wetting later at night. Nylon sheets, pants and pyjamas should be avoided, as should duvets, since these tend to make the user sweat and sweating can dampen the pad and lead to false alarms. After two weeks of consecutive dry nights, in order to reduce the risk of relapse, the child should be given more to drink in the hour before bedtime and continue to use the alarm until he has had another two weeks of dry nights.

# Recent Advances

It is thought that some children who wet the bed do so because of a deficiency of antidiuretic hormone or ADH, which results in the production of abnormally large amounts of urine. ADH controls water secretion by the kidney and, if inadequate amounts of the hormone are produced, the bladder fills up faster than normal. Based on this theory, a synthetic form of ADH, desmopressin, has been produced as a nasal spray. One puff into each nostril at night should be enough to control bed-wetting in suitable children.

# Complementary Treatment

*Acupuncture*
As in the case of incontinence (see separate section), bed-wetting is said to be due to a lack of Chi in the kidney and treatment uses specific points which will strengthen the kidney and restore its energy flow to normal.

*Aromatherapy*
Cypress or pine may be recommended.

*Herbalism*
St John's wort, which is used to treat anxiety states, may also be very helpful in the treatment of bed-wetting where the problem seems to result from stress. Horsetail and cornsilk act by making the lining of the bladder less irritable. Other herbal remedies may also be prescribed.

*Homoeopathy*
For a child who wets the bed quite early in the night, bella-donna may be helpful, whereas one who passes large amounts later on and is anxious and irritable may benefit from lyco-podium. Gelsemium may be prescribed if the child is of a ner-vous disposition and wets himself during the day as well as at night.

*Hypnotherapy*

Children over the age of about six may often benefit from treatment by hypnosis. Some paediatricians treat them in groups, while others see them individually. The aim of treatment is to convince the child that his bladder can expand to hold more urine than it now manages to cope with at night and to enable him, if it really does become full, to wake and go to the toilet, rather than wetting the bed. It also reduces the anxieties that the child may have about his inability to stop wetting.

## Self-help

The National Enuresis Resources and Information Centre (ERIC), 65 St Michael's Hill, Bristol, BS2 8DZ, provides information about specialist clinics around the country which treat bed-wetting and offers a twelve-page guide for parents and a newsletter for children.

# Breast
# Lumps

There are a number of conditions that can produce lumps in the breast, but most of them are fairly rare. The only common causes are fibroadenosis, fibroadenomas and cancer. Any woman who finds a lump in her breast tends to think that it must be cancer but, in fact, in every ten cases of breast problems seen by GPs, only one turns out to be malignant.

## Fibroadenosis (Chronic Mastitis)

This condition, in which the breasts are lumpy and tender, is ten times commoner than cancer of the breast. The tenderness and lumps are most noticeable just before a period and are often confined to the upper outer quadrant of the breast and the segment that stretches up into the armpit. Also known as chronic mastitis, fibroadenosis occurs between the ages of fifteen and fifty and is thought by some specialists to affect most women to a certain extent.

The hormonal changes that occur at the time of ovulation each month act on the lining of the womb and on the breast to prepare them for pregnancy. The breast tissue enlarges but, if pregnancy does not occur, it subsides again until the next ovulation. Because this happens every month, the breast may

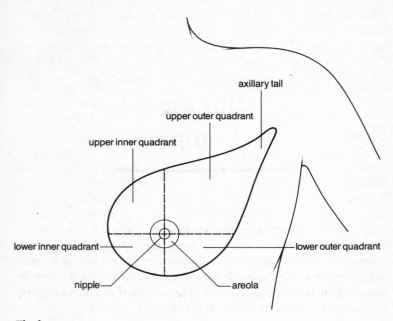

*The breast*

become increasingly lumpy and cysts may form. The condition is more common in women who have never had babies and in those who have not breast-fed, and it may become less of a nuisance after a woman has fed her first baby. Although symptoms may be particularly severe around the time of the menopause, the condition tends to disappear after this, since the monthly hormonal changes are no longer occurring.

It is usual for one breast to be more severely affected than the other and the pain may be made worse by moving the arm. The glands under the arm may be tender as well. Sometimes the lumpiness of the breast may be the first sign to appear or there may be a discharge from the nipple, which may be blood-stained, yellow, green or brown. Occasionally, the first sign is a smooth, spherical swelling which may be quite large.

# Fibroadenoma

This is a very mobile lump with well-defined margins which tends to slip away from the examining fingers. Also known as a 'breast mouse', it occurs primarily in women between the ages of fifteen and thirty-five and usually grows to a size of 1–3 cm in diameter. Rarely, there may be more than one in the same breast.

# Cancer

Breast cancer is common in most developed countries, affecting between one in twelve and one in fifteen women. In the United Kingdom it accounts for one quarter of all cases of cancer in women, with about 19,000 new cases each year. It tends to occur in older age groups, and 75 per cent of patients are over fifty. Rarely, breast cancer occurs in men.

There seems to be an environmental factor in the development of breast cancer, since Japanese women in the United States are affected much more frequently than those who live in Japan. Similarly, it is commoner in Danish women than in their near neighbours, the Finns. It is relatively uncommon in Africa and Asia.

The risk of breast cancer seems to be increased, to a greater or lesser extent, in women who are obese, who eat a diet high in saturated fat, who have never been pregnant, whose first pregnancy occurred at an advanced age, whose first period was at a comparatively early age, who have had benign breast disease previously or whose mother or sister has had breast cancer.

Usually the first sign of breast cancer is a painless lump, although occasionally there may be pain or discomfort which is pricking in character. Sometimes the first sign is an indrawing of the nipple or a blood-stained discharge. The lump is usually hard and may be fixed to the overlying skin or to the chest, so that it is immobile.

# Phylloides Tumour

This relatively rare variant of the fibroadenoma occurs mainly in women over the age of forty. It feels tender, warm and cystic, grows quite rapidly and can become very large. The skin over the tumour may become thin and the veins on the surface of the breast may dilate. Very rarely, it may break through the skin, forming an ulcerating mass. Unlike cancer, it rarely attaches itself to the skin or to deeper structures but remains mobile. Occasionally there may be a clear discharge from the nipple.

# Intraduct Papilloma

This is an uncommon little growth that occurs within the milk ducts of the breast, just under the nipple. It affects women in the 20–50 age range, being rare under the age of twenty-five and commonest in the over-thirty-fives. The first sign is usually a blood-stained discharge, sometimes with a lump detectable under the areola (the dark skin around the nipple). Occasionally there may be more than one papilloma present.

# Fat Necrosis

Necrosis means death of the tissue involved. Fat necrosis in the breast occurs after injury, and bruising may be visible although, occasionally, the woman may not remember having hurt herself. The patient is usually an overweight middle-aged woman. A painful lump is often the first sign, although pain may be absent. The lump may then become smaller and, being attached to the skin, may pull it inwards, producing a dimple.

# Breast Abscess

This is a fairly rare condition that most often occurs in women who are breast-feeding. The cause is commonly a cracked nipple, through which bacteria have entered the milk ducts. This is why breast care and hygiene are so important for nursing mothers. The breast becomes red, hot, swollen and very painful, and, if incorrectly treated, the abscess may become chronic.

## Mondor's Disease

In this uncommon condition, the veins that run across and under the breast become thrombosed (that is, the blood within them clots). The cause is unknown, although it may occur after injury. The affected veins may be felt as long cord-like strands, some 3 mm across, in the outer part of the breast, often extending up into the armpit or down towards the abdomen. They are usually tender at first and may remain noticeable for up to a year.

## Retention Cyst

This is similar to a sebaceous cyst anywhere else on the body and occurs in the areola around the nipple.

## Papilloma of the Nipple

This is a small benign growth that arises from the areola or the nipple. It may grow to the size of a cherry and is always attached to the breast by a thin stalk.

## Investigation of Breast Lumps

Some breast lumps – such as papilloma of the nipple and Mondor's disease – are easy to diagnose, but most of the others will need further investigation in order to differentiate the benign tumours from cancer. Very often a doctor can make a diagnosis of fibroadenosis just from examination of the breast but, sometimes, when there is an obvious lump, mammography and biopsy may be suggested.

A cyst is a fluid-filled swelling which may occur without there being any other indication of breast disease. However, it is most frequently associated with fibroadenosis. It is often easy to diagnose. If the doctor holds a torch pressed to one side of the breast lump and the light shines through it, this is a clear indication that there is fluid in the lump. This technique is called trans-illumination. A further test is to insert a needle into the lump and extract all the fluid possible; if the fluid is clear and if the lump has completely vanished by the end of the procedure, this will confirm the diagnosis of a simple cyst. However, if the fluid is blood-stained or if a lump can still be felt, further investigations are necessary, although in many cases the condition will be found to be benign.

Mammography is a fairly simple procedure in which the breast is squeezed between two X-ray plates and either one or two pictures are taken. Cancer may show up as a darker patch on the X-ray. However, benign tumours may also look dark and so, if any abnormality is seen, a biopsy is usually performed as well.

## Orthodox Treatment

Most benign tumours will not recur if removed, but it is not uncommon for cysts to recur in a breast with fibroadenosis. Forty per cent of all phylloides tumours grow again unless they are removed with a wide margin of normal breast tissue so that, if the tumour is very big, a mastectomy may have to be performed. In the case of multiple intraduct papillomas, it may be necessary to remove all the major milk ducts leading from the breast to the nipple, which means that breast-feeding will no longer be possible.

Mondor's disease needs no treatment and will subside of its own accord in time. Fibroadenosis usually needs no treatment, if there is no obvious lump, but if the patient complains of persistent pain, hormone treatment may be given for four to six months. Among the agents commonly used are danazol and bromocriptine.

A breast abscess that has only just started to form will often subside if the patient is treated with antibiotics. However, for those whose abscesses are beginning to 'ripen' and for those who do not show a fairly immediate response to antibiotics, drainage is necessary. This is done under general anaesthetic. The abscess is cut open and the pus cleaned out. The wound is packed with a dressing which will prevent the resulting hole from closing over. Healing thus occurs from the base of the wound, and this helps to guard against a recurrence of the infection. The dressings are changed daily, less and less being packed into the wound as it becomes smaller.

The treatment of cancer depends very much on how advanced the tumour is and on who is treating the patient, since different surgeons have their own preferences. However, nowadays, many specialists are happy just to remove the lump with a wide margin of normal tissue ('lumpectomy') rather than to remove the entire breast. In most cases lumpectomy is combined with radiotherapy. Recent studies suggest that life expectancy following this form of treatment is as good as it is after mastectomy. Usually, a radioactive implant is inserted into the breast during the operation and is removed forty-eight hours later. Then a course of radiotherapy is given in the out-patients' department. Because the first 'port of call' for a cancer that is spreading is the lymph glands in the armpit, it is usual to remove these, whatever type of operation is being performed.

Mastectomy may be of three kinds. In the simple mastectomy just the breast tissue (plus the lymph glands) are removed. In a radical mastectomy the muscle on which the breast lies is taken in addition. In an extended radical mastectomy, the lymph glands that run down the front of the chest are also removed. These more mutilating types of operation are less commonly performed nowadays than in the past.

Some forms of breast cancer are hormone dependent – in other words, they thrive on oestrogen. In such cases a drug that suppresses oestrogen may be given or, in a premenopausal patient, the ovaries may be surgically removed. In post-menopausal women, the anti-oestrogen drug tamoxifen, which has a minimum of side effects, is commonly used. It has been shown that treatment with tamoxifen is as effective as surgery for breast cancer occurring in women over the age of seventy – a fortunate finding, since many elderly patients tolerate operations badly. Hormone therapy may also be valuable when cancer which seemed to have been cleared recurs; radio-therapy, too, can be useful in such cases. Chemotherapy (the use of drugs which kill cancer cells) is also effective, particularly in non-hormone-dependent tumours or when the cancer has spread to other parts of the body.

In the few men who develop breast cancer, a radical mastec-tomy is performed and this usually necessitates a skin graft to cover the wound. If the tumour is hormone-dependent, removal of the testes (orchidectomy) may be required.

Two per cent of breast cancers occur in pregnant women. In the first half of pregnancy, the treatment is the same as for non-pregnant women and, if radiotherapy or chemotherapy is used, the pregnancy may have to be terminated, since both of these can cause severe deformities in the unborn child. If, however, the patient is nearing the end of her pregnancy, it may be feasible to induce labour and deliver the baby before beginning treatment. In some cases, it may be possible to wait a few weeks before starting treatment in order to allow the foetus to become a little more mature before it is delivered.

Patients are followed up at regular intervals following an operation for cancer of the breast so that any recurrence may be treated immediately.

Breast cancer is classified according to stages, stage one includ-ing all those cases in which the cancer appears to be confined solely to the breast itself, without any evidence of spread. **At least 80 per cent of patients who are treated at this stage are still alive five years later, but for more advanced growths, the outlook is less good. This is why it is so important for a woman to see her GP immediately she discovers a lump in her breast, just in case it turns out to be malignant.**

## Recent Advances

Trials of lumpectomy plus radiotherapy have shown how success-ful this treatment is. Doctors at the University of Kansas Medical Centre treated 110 cases of breast cancer in this way and found only two recurrences during the following four years, while doctors at the Albert Einstein College of Medicine in New York observed a recurrence rate of 14 per cent within five years, when they followed up 201 patients.

At the time of writing, plans are going ahead to introduce a nationwide screening programme in which all women over the age of fifty will be offered mammography. The age limit has been chosen for two reasons. One is that breast cancer is commoner in older women and the other is that, before the menopause, the density of the breast tissue reduces the reliability of the test. It has been estimated that some 10 per cent of women who have mammograms will have to be recalled for reassessment and further tests, although only a small proportion of these will be found to have cancer.

However, some younger women are at higher risk of developing breast cancer than others, because the disease seems to run in the family. A Family Cancer Clinic has been set up by the Royal Free and University College Hospitals in London to offer screening to any woman over the age of thirty whose mother or sister developed breast cancer before she was fifty.

There has been some debate in the medical press as to how effective mammography is as a screening process, but in a New York survey of 62,000 women over a period of eighteen years it was found that in those who were offered mammography the death rate from cancer of the breast fell by one third. Similarly, both Holland and Sweden reported a 30 per cent drop in mortality following the introduction of mammography.

A technique which has been developed at the Royal Marsden Hospital in London is able to show whether or not an abnormality that has shown up on a mammogram is malignant, without a biopsy being necessary. The new technique records blood flow within the breast and shows it on a screen. Normal breast tissue and benign tumours appear blueish, while cancers, which always have an increased blood flow, appear red. Cancers as small as half a centimetre across can be picked up and the intensity of the colour shown can guide specialists as to the kind of treatment required.

The need for biopsies may also be reduced by a technique which is now being used in a few centres across the world. This is needle aspiration. A tiny needle is inserted into the lump and a small section of the tissue is removed and examined under a microscope.

Other methods of screening which will pick out women who are particularly at risk of developing breast cancer are constantly being sought. At the Christie Hospital in Manchester, doctors took tiny pieces of skin from women whose mothers and grandmothers had had breast cancer. Then, in the laboratory, they grew some of the cells (the fibroblasts) contained in the skin samples and found that, in half of the cases, they took on the character of cancer cells and became invasive. The women are now being followed up to see whether those whose tests were abnormal are those who develop cancer.

In another study at the University of California school of medicine, breast fluid was drawn off through the nipple from 3194 women. The cells contained in the fluid were abnormal in 420 cases, and researchers were able to follow up 335 of these. Subsequently nineteen of these women developed breast cancer, compared with six in a similar-sized group who had had normal results.

At the Royal Liverpool Hospital, surgeons found virus-like particles in the white blood cells of thirty-one out of thirty-two patients with early breast cancer but only in three out of twenty-seven healthy women. The particles were also seen in the breast, in the macrophage cells which, like the white cells, are part of the body's defence against foreign tissues such as bacteria, viruses and cancer. Further research is going to be necessary to determine whether the virus itself is causing the cancer or whether it just reduces the effectiveness of the white cells and macrophages, making them less able to fight cancer when it arises. If it turns out that the virus is a causative factor, it may be possible, at some time in the future, to develop a vaccine against it.

At Rockefeller University in New York, it was found that patients with breast cancer had 50 per cent more 16-alpha hydroxy oestrone in their blood than healthy women. This oestrone is a breakdown product from oestrogen and it is thought that it becomes bound to the nuclei of the cells making up the breast tissue, stimulating them and increasing the risk of abnormal growth. It has been found that women who have a high dietary intake of saturated fat have higher blood levels of 16-alpha hydroxy oestrone, whereas those who have low intakes and who regularly eat fatty fish or take fish oil supplements tend to have low levels.

In Toronto, two groups of women considered to be at risk of developing breast cancer were observed over a period of five years. One group followed a low fat diet and only one member developed cancer, while the others ate a normal diet and produced six cases over the five years. Very recently results of another study have seemed to show that women who drink heavily have a greater risk of developing breast cancer than occasional drinkers.

It has also been suggested that taking the contraceptive Pill may have some effect on the breast and increase the risk of developing cancer. But although a recent study carried out at Oxford University confirmed the findings of the Imperial Cancer Research Fund epidemiology unit that women who took the Pill for four or more years before having their first full-term pregnancy had more than double the risk of those who had not, several other studies, including a much larger one in the United States, showed no such risk. And since new, low-dose Pills are being introduced constantly, none of these studies has really been able to determine the true effects of the modern Pill.

Tests which can assess the severity of a cancer are also important since they can ensure that appropriate treatment is given. Normally, the lymph glands under the arm are removed in all operations for breast cancer, since there is no way of knowing whether or not the tumour cells have spread there. However, doctors working for the Imperial Cancer Research Fund have discovered a method of detecting spread which may, eventually, mean that it will be possible to pick out those women in whom spread has not occurred and avoid having to do this extra piece of surgery. The test makes use of an antibody which sticks to tumour cells. This is attached to a mildly radioactive substance and injected into the patient. A special camera is then used to detect the antibodies – if they are clustered in the glands, this is a clear indication that the glands should be removed.

## Complementary Treatment

The use of complementary therapies in the treatment of cancer is described in the section on cancer of the cervix.

## Organizations

The Breast Care and Mastectomy Association offers help and advice to women undergoing treatment for cancer of the breast through its 16,000 volunteers, all of whom have had breast surgery. It has also published a leaflet entitled *Living with Breast Surgery*. The Association's headquarters are at 26a Harrison St, London, WC1H 8JG (tel. 071-837 0908).

Organizations associated with cancer care are listed in the section on cervical cancer.

# Bronchitis

The word bronchitis simply means inflammation of the air passages of the lungs – the bronchi and bronchioles. (See the diagram showing the structure of the lungs on p. 49.) Bronchitis can be acute or chronic.

## Acute Bronchitis

Acute bronchitis is caused by an infection, probably 90 per cent of cases being due to viruses and 10 per cent to bacteria. It usually begins with a hacking cough and after 24–48 hours the patient begins to bring up phlegm, which is white if the infection is viral or yellow or green if it is bacterial. Children tend to swallow phlegm rather than spit it out and the irritation this causes to the stomach lining may cause vomiting.

In many cases the patient is feverish and often a wheeze can be heard as he breathes in and out, forcing air through bronchial tubes that have become narrowed by inflammation and excessive mucus secretion. The cells that form the lining of the bronchi possess microscopic finger-like projections called cilia, whose function is to sweep mucus upwards out of the respiratory tract. These cilia are paralysed by cigarette smoke, so smokers may take much longer to recover from an attack of acute bronchitis than non-smokers. If infected mucus settles low down in the respiratory tract, it may cause pneumonia. Among non-smokers, this is more likely to occur in the very young and the very old.

It is not uncommon for children to develop acute bronchitis, those suffering from measles or whooping cough being particularly susceptible. Viral bronchitis, which often attacks children under the age of five, tends to occur in localized outbreaks. Although infants may appear to be seriously ill with bronchitis, the infection is very seldom fatal. However, after recovering from the condition many children will continue to have a dry cough for several weeks.

## Chronic Bronchitis

This is altogether a more serious illness than acute bronchitis. Traditionally, it is defined as a condition in which the patient coughs, bringing up phlegm, on most days during a period of three consecutive months for more than two successive years. In other words, the condition is long term and recurrent.

The most important causative factor is cigarette smoking. Whereas only five non-smokers in every 100,000 will die each year from chronic bronchitis, forty-nine who smoke under twenty-five a day and 106 who smoke more than this will die each year. Stopping smoking, even quite late in the disease, may make a difference to the patient's life expectancy, the average death rate from bronchitis of ex-smokers being thirty-eight per 100,000.

Chronic bronchitis is commoner in older people and in men. Exposure to air pollution is also a factor in its development. In Britain it affects one middle-aged man in ten and causes the loss of 30 million working days a year. It is often known as 'the British disease', since its severe forms are very much more common in Britain than elsewhere, possibly because it is exacerbated by the climate. Deaths from bronchitis are commoner in winter and in urban areas, and are more likely to occur among unskilled and semi-skilled workers than among the professional classes. This is probably because the former tend to smoke more heavily than the latter and are more likely to be exposed to atmospheric pollution in their place of work.

Chronic bronchitis usually begins between the ages of thirty and sixty. The symptoms may come on very gradually or may follow on from an attack of acute bronchitis or pneumonia. To begin with, persistent phlegm, requiring frequent clearing of the throat, may be the only symptom. This phlegm is produced by over-activity of the mucus-secreting glands that are found in the lining of the air passages. As more and more is produced, the patient starts to cough some up each morning when he wakes. Eventually the cough may continue throughout the day. At first the phlegm is clear, although it may contain black specks which are particles of carbon left in the lungs from smoking. The cough is likely to become worse towards the end of the day, particularly if the patient has been exposed to dust or cigarette smoke, or has been in crowds or has drunk alcohol. There may also be a feeling of discomfort in the sinuses, across the cheek bones and forehead, together with a dripping of mucus from the sinuses down the back of the throat, making it sore. Coughing may come in fits, particularly at night or on waking in the morning, and may be started off by taking a deep breath.

Acute chest infections in patients suffering from chronic bronchitis (acute on chronic bronchitis) are not uncommon, particularly in advanced cases. In healthy lungs there are no infective organisms present in the air passages but the excessive mucus produced in chronic bronchitis makes it easier for viruses and bacteria to live there. Viral infections increase the mucus secretion still further and encourage bacterial growth. If a bacterial infection takes hold, the mucus thickens and becomes yellow or green and the air passages become acutely inflamed. This may cause permanent damage to the lungs, especially if it is not possible to eradicate the bacteria from the phlegm completely, in which case repeated episodes of infection are likely to occur. The final picture of a patient with severe chronic bronchitis is one in which any form of exertion is impossible since it causes bouts of coughing, wheezing and breathlessness.

For those patients who give up smoking early in the course of the disease and who manage to avoid recurrent chest infections, the outlook is good. However, the poorer the lung function becomes, the more likely the patient is to die from respiratory failure or from heart failure.

91

# Emphysema

This condition often occurs in conjunction with chronic bronchitis and may be responsible for much of the breathlessness experienced by patients. In emphysema, damage to the air passages results in dilation or destruction of the alveoli – the tiny air sacs through which oxygen diffuses into the blood and carbon dioxide diffuses out into the lungs. The normal elasticity which aids breathing out is lost, the lungs become over-inflated, and the patient is constantly breathless.

# Pulmonary Heart Disease

The word pulmonary is used to describe anything related to the lungs, such as their blood supply (pulmonary circulation) or tests of how they are working (pulmonary function tests). Pulmonary heart disease may occur as a result of poor air flow from the lungs into the blood. If inadequate amounts of air get through to the alveoli because of narrowing of the air passages, insufficient oxygen enters the bloodstream, which remains overloaded with carbon dioxide. As a result, the blood vessels that carry the blood to and from the lungs constrict. This occurs as an automatic reaction which may be reversed in the early stages if the condition of the lungs improves. However, if there is no improvement, pulmonary hypertension may eventually occur, in which the blood pressure in these vessels is a great deal higher than it should be. This, in turn, puts strain on the right side of the heart whose function is to pump blood through the pulmonary circulation, and it may cease to function effectively.

# Investigations

Investigations are usually unnecessary in acute bronchitis since the diagnosis is easily made on examination. However, tests may be needed for patients with chronic bronchitis, not only to confirm the diagnosis but to ascertain the extent of the lung damage that has occurred.

A chest X-ray taken early in the course of the disease is likely to be normal, as are X-rays of the sinuses. A culture of the sputum may show bacteria growing there. Lung-function tests (described in the section on asthma) may also be normal at first.

Occasionally the doctor may suspect that there is a more sinister cause for the patient's chronic cough and, in such cases, may suggest bronchoscopy or bronchography. In the former, a small tube with a tiny inbuilt camera is passed into the patient's lungs under anaesthetic. Through this the specialist can see whether there are any localized problems such as a foreign body that has been inhaled, TB or a tumour. In bronchography, the air passages of each lung in turn are filled with a substance that will show up on X-ray. A film can then be taken which will demonstrate any abnormalities. In chronic bronchitis, it may show the wide mouths of the many over-active mucous glands together with narrowing of the smaller airways.

At a later stage in the disease, a chest X-ray may show enlargement of the right side of the heart, indicating a degree of pulmonary heart disease. This may also show up on an electrocardiogram. Results of the lung-function tests will begin to deteriorate and a blood count may show an excess of red cells. Production of these cells, whose function is to carry oxygen in the bloodstream, is stimulated by a continuing lack of oxygen in the blood. Increased numbers are also to be found in the blood of people who spend their lives at very high altitudes where the atmosphere is thin.

# Orthodox Treatment

## Acute Bronchitis

Although 90 per cent of cases are viral and therefore will not respond to antibiotics, it is customary to prescribe these in all cases. There are two reasons for this. Firstly, it is not always easy to determine which cases are viral and which are not, and, secondly, tissue that has already been damaged by a virus is susceptible to superimposed bacterial infection.

## Chronic Bronchitis

The most important form of treatment is to persuade the patient to stop smoking, since this, more than anything else, will help to prevent the rapid deterioration of his health. Other preventive measures include vaccination against influenza every winter and avoidance of dusty and smoky atmospheres and fog. Overweight patients should attempt to diet, since obesity puts further strain on the heart. Physiotherapy to help the patient to clear his lungs of mucus is also beneficial.

Antibiotics are given when acute bacterial infections occur and some patients may need regular small doses throughout the winter months in order to prevent acute attacks. Some patients find bronchodilators helpful; these reduce spasm in the bronchi and are usually prescribed in the form of inhalers. If right-sided heart failure occurs, this will need to be treated, usually with diuretics (as in hypertension). If the heart beat becomes erratic, the patient may need digoxin.

In severe cases, oxygen given over a period of at least fifteen hours in every twenty-four may help to relieve the patient's symptoms. Some patients with severe breathlessness may be helped by the use of steroids, usually in an inhalable form.

# Complementary Treatment

*Acupuncture*
Acute bronchitis is said to be due to invasion by wind and cold or by wind and heat which obstruct the flow of energy, or Chi, in the lungs. Specific points will be used to eliminate phlegm, wind and either cold or heat, and to restore the flow of Chi to normal. Because the lung is intimately related, in the Chinese system of energy flow, with the spleen and kidney, treatment for chronic bronchitis will include the use of points to strengthen these organs.

Acupuncture can also help patients to give up smoking.

*Alexander Technique*
Correct posture may help the patient with chronic bronchitis to breathe more easily.

*Aromatherapy*
Thyme may be useful in acute bronchitis, and niaouli, origanum,

rosemary, sandalwood and sage in chronic bronchitis. Other oils such as cajuput, eucalyptus, hyssop and pine may be effective in either type.

## Herbalism

This may be helpful in both acute and chronic bronchitis. A variety of herbs may be used. Coltsfoot relaxes the bronchial tubes, acts as an expectorant (helping the patient to cough up phlegm) and soothes the inflamed airways. Hyssop in acute bronchitis encourages sweating, so lowering the fever, reduces the inflammation and also acts as an expectorant. Other expectorants include aniseed and elecampane (both of which are particularly useful in chronic bronchitis), garlic and thyme.

## Homoeopathy

The remedy needed by an individual patient will depend on his symptoms. In the early stages of acute bronchitis, when he is restless and feverish and has a dry, painful cough, aconite may be appropriate, whereas a spasmodic cough with rattling of mucus in the chest and an inclination to vomit may indicate a need for ipecac. Phosphorus may improve the condition of a patient who has tightness across the chest, wheezing and hoarseness, and who is worse for talking and fresh air. Antimony tart. is particularly useful for children and old people who have a lot of loose phlegm in the chest and rattling wheezy breathing, but who cough up very little and are afraid of suffocating during a coughing fit.

## Hypnotherapy

By helping patients to give up smoking, hypnosis may be a valuable adjunct to the treatment of chronic bronchitis. However, since it works only by strengthening the patient's resolve and reducing or preventing withdrawal symptoms, it cannot make someone give up if he doesn't really want to.

## Manipulation

Both chiropractic and osteopathy may help the patient to increase the air space in his chest cavity and thus to use his lungs more effectively.

*Nutrition*
Vitamins A, B complex, C and E and the minerals selenium and
zinc strengthen the immune system and help the body to fight
against infections. Supplements may be recommended to prevent
recurrent attacks of acute or acute on chronic bronchitis. Vitamins A and C also help to maintain healthy lung tissue. A
nutrition therapist may suggest that a patient avoids dairy
produce, which encourages the formation of mucus.

# Cervical
# Cancer

## Incidence and Risk Factors

Cancer of the cervix, or neck of the womb, primarily affects women between the ages of thirty and fifty, although it can occur both earlier and later than this. It is commonest in married women and in the lower socio-economic classes, and seems to be more likely to occur in those who started having sexual intercourse at an early age and who had their first pregnancy while they were still very young. An increased frequency in women who have had a large number of sexual partners and who have been infected with genital herpes or with genital warts suggests that infection must, in some way, play a part in the development of this type of cancer. For a reason which has yet to be explained adequately, some racial groups are far less prone to develop cervical cancer than others – it is quite rare in Jewish and Muslim women but comparatively common in Puerto Ricans.

In Great Britain, cancer of the cervix is the commonest form of cancer of the genital tract. However, it does not cause as many deaths as cancer of the ovary, which is far less easy to diagnose at an early stage.

# Cervical Smears

Because cervical cancer can be detected at a very early stage in its development using the cervical smear, it is possible to cure it in very many cases. Specialists recommend that all women should have smears, starting either at twenty-five years of age or within two years of the first intercourse, whichever is earlier. Most believe that it should be repeated every three years until the age of about forty-five and then five yearly after that. At the time of writing, the Department of Health still recommends five-yearly intervals between smears. However, most young women will have smears more frequently than this, since they are usually performed at family planning and ante- and post-natal clinics. Unfortunately, the bulk of cases of cervical cancer occur in older women, who may have completed their family and are no longer attending family-planning clinics. It is important that these women arrange to see their own doctors or to attend a well-woman clinic in order to continue to have regular smears.

Not only does the smear show up abnormal cells but it will also indicate if there is any infection present on the cervix, such as thrush. The majority of patients who are recalled after having a smear have either an infection which needs treating or dysplasia – a condition in which the cervical cells show some abnormality although they are not frankly malignant.

# Stages of Cervical Cancer

Cervical cancer is broken down into stages according to how advanced it is, the earliest being CIN, or cervical intra-epithelial neoplasia. CIN I includes all patients with mild dysplasia. Eighty-five per cent of cases of CIN I disappear of their own accord but, because the remaining 15 per cent can progress, it is vital that all patients continue to be followed up until they are told that they are clear. CIN II is moderate dysplasia, while CIN III includes severe dysplasia and carcinoma in situ (cancer that has not started to invade the surrounding tissues). The three CIN stages make up stage 0.

Stages I to IV comprise invasive cancer, which is no longer

confined to the layer of cells on the surface of the cervix in which it arises. In stage I, the cancer is still confined to the cervix itself. Later stages are defined by how far the cancer has spread to adjacent organs such as the rectum or bladder or, via the blood and lymphatic system, to distant parts of the body.

## Symptoms

Stages 0 and Ia (in which the cancer has only just begun to invade the cervix) produce no symptoms, but can be picked up by a cervical smear. Once the cancer has started to invade the cervix and other local tissues, vaginal bleeding may occur after intercourse or between the periods and may also affect post-menopausal women. If the condition is allowed to progress, the patient may develop a foul-smelling watery discharge which may be blood-stained.

A more advanced cancer may obstruct the ureters which lead from the kidneys to the bladder, interrupting the normal flow of urine and causing kidney failure. Pain in the back and pain and swelling of the legs may also occur. Involvement of the bladder may produce pain on passing water and blood-stained urine. Spread to the rectum (back passage) may cause bleeding, pain on defaecation or diarrhoea.

## Investigations

A cervical smear is a quick and easy procedure. It may be slightly uncomfortable for a matter of seconds but this is a small price to pay for a test which can detect cancer at an early enough stage to allow it to be cured.

If an abnormality is found, the patient may be referred for colposcopy. This takes slightly longer than a smear and is usually done in the out-patients' department. The patient lies on her back with her legs apart and a metal instrument is inserted into the vagina so that the doctor can see the cervix. The smear is repeated and a swab is taken to check for infections. The cervix is swabbed with a saline solution and a special microscope is used to inspect it. The saline will cause the blood vessels on the cervix to stand out so that any abnormalities can be seen. Then the cervix is swabbed with dilute acetic acid, which may sting briefly. This shows up abnormal areas of cells as white patches. Finally a swab of iodine is used, which will show normal areas as brown and abnormal areas as white or yellow. A little instrument is inserted into the cervical canal, so that the doctor can also inspect the cells that line it. If any abnormal areas are seen either on the surface of the cervix or in the canal, a biopsy is taken. A tiny piece of tissue, no larger than a grain of rice, is pinched out and any resulting bleeding is stopped by holding a silver nitrate stick against the area for a few minutes. This is not a painful procedure so no anaesthetic is needed.

Depending on the findings of the biopsy and the symptoms of which the patient is complaining, other investigations that may be performed include proctoscopy (inspection of the back passage using a little metal instrument), cystoscopy (inspection of the bladder under general anaesthetic, using a fine telescope), X-ray of the kidneys (intravenous pyelogram) and other X-rays.

# Orthodox Treatment

Patients with CIN can often be treated in a day clinic, without needing admission to hospital. Techniques used include electro-cautery, electrocoagulation diathermy, laser and cryocautery. In other words, the abnormal tissue can be destroyed either by burning or freezing. Diathermy is a painful procedure and there-fore has to be done under a general anaesthetic. All these methods cure the condition in over 90 per cent of patients. However, follow-up is vital to ensure that those few who do not respond are given further treatment.

If the cancer cells seem to be extending up the cervical canal, a cone biopsy is performed. This is done under general an-aesthetic and entails a few days in hospital. A cone of tissue is removed from the cervix, reaching up the canal. This procedure helps confirm the diagnosis and, in many cases, will also cure the condition by removing all the cancerous tissue. The com-monest complication is bleeding. This may occur within twelve hours of the operation, in which case a return to theatre may be necessary, or it may happen a week or so after the operation, when it is often associated with infection and the patient may need to be treated with antibiotics. The bleeding may be heavy but is usually easily controlled. Occasionally, the cervix is damaged so that either it becomes scarred (causing pain at period times and retention of blood in the womb) or it becomes lax (causing miscarriage). In the latter case, a special stitch can be inserted into the cervix once the patient knows she is pregnant to prevent it from opening until the pregnancy has reached full term.

Patients who have had a cone biopsy or treatment with a laser must avoid using tampons and refrain from having sexual intercourse for a month afterwards.

Patients who continue to have abnormal cells on smears taken after a cone biopsy, or who have other gynaecological problems such as fibroids, may be offered a hysterectomy even though their cancer is at a very early stage.

Where the cancer has started to invade the cervix but has progressed no further, surgery may be performed. This usually takes the form of a radical, or Wertheim's, hysterectomy in which the entire womb, the tubes, the upper third of the vagina and the local lymph glands are removed. Some specialists also remove the ovaries but others consider this unnecessary, especially in younger women.

More advanced cases are treated with radiotherapy. However, in some centres, this is used to treat all patients with invasive cancer, whether this is at stage I, II, III or IV. Usually a radioactive implant is inserted into the womb and external radiotherapy is given in addition. Both surgery and radiotherapy have their drawbacks. Surgery, which is only suitable for certain patients, may be followed by bleeding, infection and bladder problems. The shortening of the vagina may be a disadvantage in young, sexually active women. Radiotherapy, however, may cause sickness and diarrhoea at the time of treatment and, later on, shrinking of the vagina (causing sexual difficulties), bladder problems and constipation or diarrhoea. Vaginal shrinkage can be minimized by giving the patient an oestrogen cream to use once radiotherapy has been completed.

Surgery may sometimes be appropriate when the cancer has invaded the bladder or the rectum but seems to involve no other structures. The rectum can be removed and the healthy end of the large intestine brought out to the abdominal surface as a colostomy. If the bladder is removed, the urine flow has to be diverted. This is done by removing a piece of large intestine and forming it into a sac. The ureters, which carry the urine from the kidneys, are inserted into this sac and an exit is formed in the abdominal wall through which the urine can be passed.

## Prognosis

Doctors usually assess the results of treatment for cancer in terms of five-year survival – in other words, how many patients are still alive five years after the original diagnosis was made. For stage I cancer of the cervix, this is around 90 per cent. Since recurrence, if it occurs, is likely to do so within eighteen months of treatment, one can, in this instance, talk about a 90 per cent cure rate. Stage II has about a 75 per cent five-year survival rate. For stage III, it is around 40 per cent. Even in stage IV, the most advanced form, 10 per cent of patients will still be alive in five years. The results for patients treated with surgery and those having radiotherapy are much the same.

## Recent Advances

In 1987, scientists at the department of veterinary pathology at Glasgow University who were investigating tumours caused by the papilloma virus in cows found that they could cure them by injecting them with a preparation made from the same tumours. The virus concerned is identical with the virus that causes genital warts in humans and which is thought to be associated with the development of cervical cancer. This research suggests that, one day, it may be possible to produce a vaccine against some forms of cervical cancer.

In 1988 doctors at the Whittington and Royal Northern Hospitals in London found that smokers were more vulnerable to viral infections of the cervix than others. Smoking seemed to reduce the normal immune response of the cells of the cervix, so that viruses were not readily destroyed. The doctors also found nicotine (known to be a carcinogen) in the cervical secretions. It seems likely, therefore, that smokers have a greater risk of developing cervical cancer than non-smokers.

## Complementary Treatment

Because orthodox treatment of cancer of the cervix is nowadays so effective, it would be extremely foolhardy to rely solely on complementary treatment for this complaint. However, the complementary therapies can be invaluable as an adjunct to orthodox treatment, since their action is to stimulate the patient's immune system, which allows her body to play a greater role in fighting her disease. Naturopaths may recommend a diet consisting mainly of uncooked organically grown fruit and vegetables. Nutritionists are likely to suggest large doses of vitamins and minerals. Vitamins B, C, E and folic acid strengthen the immune system, as does zinc. Vitamins C and E, zinc, manganese and selenium help to defend the body against damage caused by carcinogens, and vitamins C and A detoxify carcinogens, preventing them from causing harm.

Herbal medicine, homoeopathy, acupuncture, radionics and healing can all play a role in strengthening the patient's resistance and raising her level of health.

Visualization is a technique that has been pioneered in the USA by a psychologist, in which the patient pictures her cancer slowly being overcome by her medication and her body getting stronger. It has proved the truth of the old adage of 'mind over matter', since it seems to be remarkably effective in many cases.

## Organizations

The Bristol Cancer Help Centre was one of the first in the country to offer patients a way of combining complementary and self-help methods with orthodox treatment. Its address is Grove House, Cornwallis Grove, Clifton, Bristol, BS8 4PG (tel. 0272 743216).

The British Association of Cancer United Patients (BACUP), 121–3 Charterhouse St, London, ECIM 6AA (tel. 071-608 1785), offers information and support to cancer patients and their families. It publishes booklets as well as a newspaper three times a year and runs a telephone information service on 071-608 1661. For people ringing from outside London there is a Freephone number – 0800 181199.

The Cancer Aftercare and Rehabilitation Society (CARE), 21 Zetland Rd, Redland, Bristol, BS6 7AH (tel. 0272 427419), offers help to patients and anyone whose life has been affected by cancer.

Cancer Contact, 6 Meadows, Hassocks, West Sussex, BN6 8EH (tel. 07918 4754), is an organization for cancer patients or ex-patients who are interested in the 'gentle methods' of treatment.

Cancerlink, 17 Brittania St, London, WCIX 9JN (tel. 071-833 2451), offers information and support to cancer patients, their relatives and friends.

Cancer Relief Macmillan Fund, Anchor House, 15–19 Britten St, London, SW3 3TZ (tel. 071-351 7811), provides nurses who specialize in the care of patients with cancer.

The Marie Curie Memorial Foundation, 28 Belgrave Square, London, SWIX 8QG (tel. 071-235 3325), provides residential care for cancer sufferers.

New Approaches to Cancer (NAC), c/o The Seekers Trust, The Close, Addington Park, nr Maidstone, Kent, MEI9 5BL (tel. 0732 848336), offers support and encouragement to those who have or who are afraid of developing cancer by showing how it can often be reversed.

# Further Reading

_The Bristol Programme_ by Penny Brohn (Century Paperbacks) explains the therapies used at the Bristol Cancer Help Centre and offers valuable advice.

_Cancer and Its Nutritional Therapies_ by Dr Richard A. Passwater (published in the USA by Keats/Pivot but available in the UK) is a straightforward and informative overview of how optimum nutrition is being used to treat malignancy.

*Getting Well Again* is by Carl and Stephanie Simonton and James L. Creighton, all of whom have pioneered the use of self-help techniques, including visualization, in the treatment of patients with cancer. Published by Bantam, it explains the techniques that they have used and contains many interesting case histories.

Other books that concentrate on the self-help theme include *You Can Conquer Cancer* by Ian Gawler (Thorsons) and *A Gentle Way with Cancer* by Brenda Kidman (Century).

# Constipation

## Definition and Causes

Constipation may be defined as a condition in which the patient opens his bowels less than three times a week or in which he passes small or hard stools or needs to strain. It is extremely common and may be a symptom of a number of diseases (one textbook lists thirty-two causes of constipation). The commonest cause is poor bowel habits. These may arise in children as a result of problems with toilet training or may occur later in life for a variety of reasons. Most frequent, perhaps, is a change in daily routine. For example, someone who normally defaecates (opens his bowels) after breakfast each day changes jobs and has to catch an earlier train. He no longer has time to go to the toilet after breakfast and, by the time he reaches work, the urge to defaecate has passed. Similarly, children may become constipated when they go to school because they do not want to use the school toilets. Sometimes a child may find a stool painful to pass and, after that, be unwilling to defaecate in case it should hurt. Often constipation runs in families.

Another common cause of constipation is a poor diet – either inadequate in itself (for example in the case of someone on a strict reducing diet or a patient with anorexia nervosa) or else a diet lacking in roughage. Inadequate fluid intake, or excess fluid loss such as occurs during a fever, also results in the formation of hard stools.

Constipation is frequently a symptom of irritable bowel syndrome and diverticular disease and may be the first symptom of cancer of the bowel. It can also occur in diabetes, myxoedema (hypothyroidism), Parkinson's disease, multiple sclerosis and depression. Certain drugs may cause constipation – such as opiates (morphine, heroin, codeine), aluminium salts (present in many antacids), iron, methotrexate (used in the treatment of various malignant conditions and also in psoriasis and arthritis) and aspirin – as may the toxic mineral lead.

Pregnant women frequently become constipated. This is probably partly due to the pressure of the womb on the bowel and partly to the iron supplements that they take. Sudden changes in diet or physical activity will often cause transient constipation.

Babies not infrequently go a day or two without passing a stool but, as long as the stools remain soft and the baby seems well, there is usually nothing to worry about. However, one condition which starts in childhood is Hirschsprung's disease, in which the nerves leading to the lower part of the large bowel are abnormal. As a result, that part of the bowel remains constricted, making it difficult for stools to pass through, and the normal bowel above it may become distended. It is an uncommon disease, affecting fewer than one in 5000 babies, but it tends to run in families.

## Investigations

It is usual to investigate children who have been constipated since birth and adults who suddenly become constipated because in these cases there may be an underlying physical problem. However, because constipation is so common in older children, they are not usually investigated fully unless they fail to respond to basic treatment.

Initially the doctor will examine the patient's abdomen for any masses, inspect the anal area for any painful conditions which may be making defaecation difficult (such as a split, or fissure, in the skin, or prolapsed piles), and examine the rectum (back passage) with a finger to see whether it is full of stool or empty. In patients whose constipation is due to faulty habits, the rectum is usually clogged up with stool.

If considered necessary, blood tests may be taken to check the patient's thyroid function, a urine test to check for diabetes and a stool specimen to check for intestinal bleeding. If the diagnosis is still in doubt, the patient may need a sigmoidoscopy (inspection of the bowel with a flexible telescope) or a barium enema (X-ray of the bowel). If the cause of the constipation has still not been found, more sophisticated hospital tests may be required. A biopsy of the rectum will indicate whether or not there is a neurological cause for the constipation (that is, whether it is due to a malfunction of the nervous system as in Hirschsprung's disease), and tests that measure the pressures within the bowel will help to assess bowel function.

## Orthodox Treatment

In cases where there is an underlying physical cause for constipation, this must be treated. Sometimes surgery will be necessary to remove an abnormal segment of bowel, for example in patients suffering from cancer of the bowel or babies with Hirschsprung's disease.

However, for those patients whose constipation is due to faulty habits, the treatment consists in changing those habits and, if necessary, giving a gentle laxative. The diet should be changed to include plenty of fresh fruit and vegetables and the amount of red meat (which slows down intestinal activity) should be reduced. Time should be allowed to open the bowels – those people who know that they usually need to go straight after breakfast should make sure that they have time to do so without missing their train or being late for school. Children must be reassured that it is quite acceptable to ask to go to the toilet when the need arises. However, straining to pass a stool when one does not feel the desire to do so may be damaging and should be avoided.

In severe cases, enemas or wash-outs may be necessary, or

even manual removal of the stools under anaesthetic, in order to clear very hard stools and allow other treatments to start working. Patients may also find suppositories (which are pushed up the back passage) helpful and there are enemas that patients can be taught to give themselves.

Normally, however, a change of diet and habits and a gentle laxative is enough. If the use of a laxative can be avoided, so much the better. If one is used, the patient should not buy it over the counter without advice but should first consult his doctor. The best type is a hydrophilic agent – one that absorbs water in the bowel and therefore softens the stool and makes it bulky and easy to pass. These include agar, bran and various proprietary 'bulking agents'. Bran is best avoided since, in large quantities, it has been known to cause blockage of the bowel. Also it is less pleasant to take than some of the other preparations. All of these may cause flatulence but this is usually avoided by starting with a small dose and working upwards until the constipation is relieved.

For those patients who fail to respond to a hydrophilic agent, lactulose may be helpful. This is a synthetic sugar-like substance which, when broken down in the bowel, draws water into the stool, making it softer and bulkier. However, it, too, may cause flatulence and also diarrhoea.

As a last resort, other laxatives include docusate sodium (which softens the stools), anthracine derivatives (such as senna and cascara) or inorganic salts (such as magnesium sulphate, Epsom salts). However, these laxatives irritate the bowel and may cause diarrhoea, colic, dehydration and an imbalance in the body's chemicals.

Many doctors now advise that the old favourites castor oil and liquid paraffin should never be used. Castor oil can cause a severe loss of water and minerals from the body while liquid paraffin can produce irritation round the anus and, more important, can cause pneumonia if it 'goes down the wrong way' and gets into the windpipe. There is also a suspicion that, taken long term, it may encourage the development of cancer.

# Laxative Abuse

Before the current interest in healthy eating, it was common for people (especially the elderly) to dose themselves regularly with laxatives. Patients suffering from anorexia nervosa may also surreptitiously take laxatives as part of their attempt to lose weight.

People who have taken laxatives over a long period of time may develop diarrhoea, abdominal discomfort and bloating, together with tiredness and lethargy. Sometimes they may become dehydrated and their body chemistry may be severely disturbed, resulting in heart or kidney problems. It is therefore very important that laxatives should only be taken over a short period unless absolutely necessary. Patients who need laxatives long term should only take hydrophilic agents, which are unlikely to cause problems.

For those patients who have become 'hooked' on a laxative, it may be very hard to come off. When they do finally manage to stop taking it, the large bowel may no longer work because it has become so used to having its work done for it by stimulants. In such a case, an operation to remove the non-functioning section of bowel may be necessary.

# Complementary Treatment

_Aromatherapy_
An abdominal massage with fennel or rosemary may be recommended.

_Herbalism_
Many orthodox laxatives are derived from herbs, such as senna and cascara. Although herbalists feel that the whole herb is likely to be more effective than an extract from it, as well as having fewer side effects, their policy when prescribing laxatives is much the same as that of an orthodox practitioner. In other words, where necessary, strong laxatives may be given for a short period of time but gentle bulk laxatives such as linseed, ispaghula and psyllium are preferred.

*Homoeopathy*

A patient whose stools are quite soft but who has to strain to pass them may benefit from alumina. For one who has overused laxatives in the past and who, although he frequently desires to go, manages only to pass a small amount each time, nux vomica may be helpful. Opium is used for patients who have no desire to defaecate and who, when they do go, pass small, hard, dry pellets. If the passage of small, hard, dry stools is associated with great effort, pain and burning, especially if the patient also has piles or a distended abdomen, sulphur may be prescribed. If constipation is linked with a great deal of flatulence, lycopodium may be suitable. Other remedies may also be appropriate in individual cases.

*Nutrition*

Figs, liquorice, prunes, raw spinach, strawberries and honey all have gentle laxative properties. A high-fibre diet will be recommended, consisting of plenty of fruit, vegetables and wholegrain products, and a minimum of refined carbohydrates. Unsalted peanut kernels (eaten with their brown fibre coating) are a pleasant way of taking additional fibre.

Vitamin C has a laxative action in high doses and a deficiency of vitamin $B_5$ (pantothenic acid) may cause constipation, so supplements may be prescribed.

# Depression

## Definition

It is only in this century that psychiatry has become a medical speciality in its own right and that diseases such as depression have been recognized as having a physical basis. Older textbooks say that depression can be divided into two main groups – endogenous (arising 'from within') or reactive (resulting from a particular stress or event) – whose symptoms differ from each other. However, in many cases, the symptoms of both endogenous and reactive depression can be found together and most specialists now agree that symptoms vary only according to the severity of the attack and not according to its cause.

What has been called reactive depression is now also called minor depression or depressive neurosis, while endogenous depression is also known as major depression or depressive psychosis. Neurosis and psychosis are two commonly used terms in the field of mental illness. Both may be defined simply as types of mental disorder, the difference between them being that psychotic patients lose touch with reality to a greater or lesser extent, suffering, for example, from delusions or hallucinations, whereas neurotic patients retain contact with reality and have some insight into their condition.

The other end of the scale from depressive psychosis is mania, a state in which there is a very marked elevation of mood and the patient becomes over-active, uninhibited and, even in the face of disaster, inappropriately high-spirited. Manic patients may go out on spending sprees or behave extravagantly in other ways. In manic depressive psychosis, which in some cases may be an inherited condition, patients tend to swing between depression and mania. Patients who never experience mania are said to have 'unipolar' depression, whereas manic depressive psychosis is described as 'bipolar'.

Depression is very common. About 5 per cent of all men and 9 per cent of all women will suffer from major depression at some time during their lives. Many more suffer from minor degrees. Ninety per cent of all cases are unipolar and tend to start in early middle age. Only 10 per cent suffer from manic depressive psychosis, which tends to begin in the early thirties. Some patients will only ever suffer from one attack but others have recurrences. About 15 per cent of those suffering from major depression commit suicide.

Most patients recover fully from their first attack of depression but may later relapse. Eventually 30 to 35 per cent develop persistent symptoms and, of these patients, up to a third may spend long periods in hospital.

No one knows exactly what causes depression, although it would appear to be a malfunction of certain chemicals, known as neurotransmitters, which are responsible for carrying electrical impulses between the millions of cells that make up the brain. It is these electrical impulses that are translated into thoughts and actions by the body. Some of the drugs used in the treatment of depression are known to affect the neurotransmitters in various ways.

In 1988 doctors interested in the effect of diet on depression reported the results of vitamin assays that had been carried out over the course of twelve years on patients admitted to the psychiatric unit at Northwick Park Hospital in Middlesex. They found that those with depression tended to have a deficiency of riboflavin ($B_2$), pyridoxine ($B_6$) and folic acid. In some cases the depression seemed to stem from the deficiency whereas in others

113

the deficiency seemed to result from the reduction in appetite that occurred as part of the illness.

## Symptoms

In most cases the overwhelming symptom is a feeling of depression, which may be described in physical terms – for example, as a great weight pressing down on the shoulders. The world seems grey and the patient becomes incapable of feeling any normal emotion.

In severe cases, patients may develop inappropriate feelings of guilt, may believe that they are being persecuted or may become convinced that they are suffering from some appalling physical disease. They feel unworthy and reproach themselves for all that they have done in the past. They are absent-minded, unable to concentrate or to remember things, and they tend to speak slowly and monotonously. They become very pessimistic and may have recurrent thoughts about suicide or death. A psychotic patient may hear voices telling her how unworthy she is and urging her to kill herself.

Physical symptoms of depression include sleep problems (commonly waking early in the morning), loss of appetite and subsequent loss of weight, constipation, loss of interest in sex, fatigue and lack of energy. Sometimes, however, anxiety is a major symptom, in which case the patient may be agitated and restless. Some patients, while quite willing to speak to a doctor or to relatives about their physical symptoms, are loath to mention the associated mental symptoms and, occasionally, physical symptoms may occur without any associated change in mood.

## Orthodox Treatment

There are three methods of orthodox treatment, which can be used separately or together. Psychotherapy is of most value in the treatment of less severe forms of depression. Drug treatment can be useful in severe depression and mania, as well as in less serious cases. Finally, physical treatment – electroconvulsive

114

therapy (ECT) and psychosurgery (leucotomy) – are reserved for the most severe cases.

Depending on the severity of the symptoms, patients may need to be admitted to hospital or may be treatable by the GP.

### Psychotherapy

Supportive psychotherapy, consisting of sympathy, reassurance and explanation about the illness, may be all that some patients need. Cognitive psychotherapy is a more active treatment which is based on the fact that depressed patients tend to develop negative attitudes very readily. The patient is shown how to overcome these attitudes which are likely to prolong the depression. She is helped to look objectively at her ideas and feelings about herself and the world around her and to assess whether she is seeing things in their true light. She is also encouraged to start doing things that she used to do before she became ill. Although helpful, this treatment is time-consuming, requiring about one hour a week for a period of approximately three months.

### Drugs

Antidepressant drugs can be broken down into three main groups – tricyclics and related drugs, monoamine oxidase inhibitors (MAOIs) and other, newer, drugs. None of these drugs is a tranquillizer, like Valium, and none is addictive. It is important that, at the start of treatment, both patient and doctor persevere with the chosen drug for several weeks even if it seems to be ineffective. Sometimes the patient may start to sleep better (a good sign that the drug is working) some weeks before she begins to feel any improvement in herself. Once an antidepressant has started to work, it usually needs to be taken for several months and it is recommended that a patient with moderate or severe depression should continue to take her medication for at least four months after she has fully recovered in order to avoid risking a relapse. Someone who has recurrent depression may need to take drugs for several years. When treatment is completed, the antidepressant must be tailed off since stopping suddenly may also precipitate a relapse.

TRICYCLICS

The tricyclic drugs include imipramine and amitriptyline (the two most commonly used), nortriptyline, doxepin, mianserin and trazodone. Although very effective, particularly in cases where the patient has noticeable physical symptoms, they do have drawbacks. Not only may they take two weeks before they start to work, but the full effect may take up to six weeks. Side effects include drowsiness, a dry mouth, constipation, trembling, blurred vision and weight gain. Tricyclics can also cause abnormalities in the heart's rhythm or an abnormally fast heart rate. Mianserin, one of the newer drugs in this range, is safer in this respect and can be used if a patient with heart trouble needs an antidepressant. However, it can cause a reduction in the number of white cells in the blood, lowering the patient's resistance to infection. For this reason, people who are taking this drug have their blood tested after they have been on it for six weeks. If there is any sign of trouble, the drug is withdrawn, allowing the blood to return to normal. Viloxazine, another fairly new drug, causes nausea in about 20 per cent of those who take it.

Because the mechanics of depression are not fully understood, the way in which antidepressants work can only be suggested. However, it is known that the tricyclic antidepressants reinforce the action of the neurotransmitters noradrenaline and serotonin.

MONOAMINE OXIDASE INHIBITORS (MAOIs)

Monoamine oxidase is an enzyme (a substance that speeds a chemical reaction within the body) whose function is to break down certain neurotransmitters (noradrenaline, dopamine and 5-hydroxytryptamine). By inhibiting its action, MAOIs allow the neurotransmitters a longer life span so that they can be more active.

The MAOIs are very effective in the treatment of depression but have a major drawback, in that the patient has to restrict her diet in order to avoid two chemically active substances – dopamine (which is found in broad beans) and tyramine (which is found in cheese, pickled herrings, yeast or meat extracts, some red wines and any food such as game that has undergone partial decomposition). Both tyramine and dopamine are normally broken down in the wall of the intestine by monoamine oxidases. If,

116

under the influence of MAOIs, they are not broken down but are absorbed unchanged into the bloodstream they can cause the blood pressure to rise suddenly and dramatically causing, at best, a severe headache and, at worst, a stroke. Some over-the-counter cold cures and cough linctuses also contain substances that may do this and so must be avoided by the patient on MAOIs.

This class of antidepressants has the advantage of starting to work within 24–48 hours and, if the restricted diet is kept to, has few side effects.

OTHER DRUGS

In recent years a number of new drugs have been brought out which are unrelated to either tricyclics or MAOIs. One of these is flupenthixol, a medication which is used in the treatment of schizophrenia but which, in considerably lower doses, is very effective in the treatment of depression when it is associated with anxiety.

L-tryptophan is an amino acid and therefore a natural constituent of the diet. Given in tablet form, it has been found to enhance the action of antidepressants. The main side effects are nausea and drowsiness.

Lithium carbonate is a drug which has been in use for many years in the treatment of manic depression, where long-term medication seems to prevent the patient from relapsing. It is also useful in the prevention of recurrent unipolar depression. Patients who have failed to respond to tricyclics sometimes improve dramatically within two weeks when lithium is given in addition. However, because it can be toxic in overdose, blood tests must be taken every few months to ensure that just the right amount is being absorbed. Side effects include thirst, trembling, weight gain, diarrhoea, nausea, and swelling of the face, hands and feet, while overdosage causes confusion and staggering. For manic depressive patients who do not respond to lithium, carbamazepine (a drug used in the treatment of epilepsy) has recently been found helpful in preventing huge swings of mood.

*Physical Treatment*

ECT is the treatment of first choice for any patient in whom an immediate improvement of mood is essential – for example, one who is seriously contemplating suicide or one who is refusing to eat or drink. It is also used for patients who have failed to respond to drug therapy and can be extremely effective when depression is associated with severe anxiety. It works rapidly and has remarkably few side effects, although some patients complain of problems with memory for a short period after the treatment. The patient is anaesthetized and is given a muscle relaxant, then an electric current of about 80 volts is passed, for a fraction of a second, between two electrodes placed on either side of the head. How ECT works is unclear, but results are sometimes quite dramatic.

Psychosurgery is rarely used, and then only for patients whose illness is severely disabling and who have failed to respond to all other forms of treatment. A minute portion of the brain is destroyed, resulting, in over 50 per cent of cases, in a marked improvement in mental condition. This technique has now become highly skilled so that those patients who do not benefit from it rarely end up any worse.

# Post-natal Depression

Like depression that occurs at other times, depression occurring after childbirth can be mild or severe, neurotic or psychotic. Sixty per cent or more of women become weepy and irritable two or three days after the birth of a child but this usually resolves in a matter of days; 10–20 per cent develop a mild depression during the first year of their baby's life, usually recovering after a few months. This is often associated with additional stresses such as financial problems, poor family relationships or being a one-parent family. Support and help from the doctor and other professionals is usually all that is needed and medication is best avoided.

Five per cent of mothers develop severe depression during the first three months after the birth. Symptoms usually begin in the first two weeks and gradually get worse. The patient often feels guilty and worthless and worries about her fitness as a mother and about the health and safety of her baby. She may think that her child is ill or deformed in some way or may believe that it is evil, leading her to try to kill it. There is also a danger that she may try to commit suicide. Often a mother says that she is unable to feel love for her baby while, at the same time, handling the baby in an obviously loving and caring way. If untreated, some two thirds of patients get better in about six months but the rest may continue to have symptoms for a further six months or more.

Many psychiatric units now have facilities for mothers and babies to be admitted together and often this is the best course. The most severe cases may need to be treated with ECT, to which the response is generally very good. Less seriously ill patients can be given tricyclic antidepressants, on which they usually start to recover within two weeks, feeling fully well again after about six weeks. However, treatment must be continued for at least six months to avoid a relapse.

Post-partum psychosis occurs once after every 500 or so births. The patient usually becomes ill during the first two weeks after the birth. The initial symptoms are those of confusion, fear, distress, restlessness and insomnia, followed by hallucinations and delusions. Then the condition will resolve into a severe depression, mania or a schizophrenia-like illness. Fears about the baby are very common – that it has died or is about to, or that another baby has been substituted. One third of these patients have relatives who have suffered from manic depression or schizophrenia.

Treatment of post-partum psychosis involves admission to hospital where the patient is given a phenothiazine drug (such as is used to treat schizophrenia) to reduce her fear, delusions and any hallucinations that may occur. ECT is usually the treatment of choice, since it works so quickly, although antidepressant drugs may be used. Unfortunately, the use of drugs usually means that the mother cannot breast-feed.

Most women recover rapidly (mania normally resolving within two weeks, depression within six weeks and schizophrenia-like conditions within eight weeks). However, because there is the risk of relapse, patients need to continue to take a reduced dose of a phenothiazine drug until the baby is about three months old. Lithium is useful for patients who suffer from mania, but may have to be taken for a year or more.

One third of patients who have a previous history of a major psychiatric illness and one fifth of those whose only mental problems have occurred as the result of a previous pregnancy will have another attack after the birth of their next child. This second attack is usually of the same type as the first and is likely to last as long and respond to treatment in the same way. Sometimes lithium started immediately after the birth, may prevent a recurrence of post-partum psychosis in a susceptible patient.

Why some women and not others should suffer from post-natal depression is unknown. It used to be thought that it had to do with the hormonal changes that occur at the time of delivery, but affected women have hormone levels that are no different from those in patients who are unaffected. It seems probable that some people are just more susceptible to depression than others, and that an attack may be sparked off by any major life event, of which childbirth is one.

# Complementary Treatment

_Acupuncture_
The mind and spirit are, in traditional Chinese theory, aspects of the energy of the heart. Treatment of mental problems involves the use of points that will restore the normal flow of energy to the heart and will calm and strengthen the mind and the spirit.

_Aromatherapy_
Basil, clary sage, jasmine, rose and chamomile are among the essences that may be beneficial.

_Bach Flower Remedies_
Cherry plum may help patients who feel desperate and are afraid of going mad, as well as those who are suicidal. Sweet chestnut may be useful for those who suffer from despair and are extremely negative in their feelings.

Mustard is helpful in the treatment of depression that has developed for no apparent reason.

Olive may be beneficial in post-natal depression since it is for those suffering from mental and physical exhaustion.

### Herbalism
Certain herbs are known as nervous restoratives which slowly and steadily improve nervous and mental conditions. They include wild oat, St John's wort, vervain, scullcap and lady's slipper. As in the case of orthodox treatment, it may be weeks or months before the patient recovers fully.

### Homoeopathy
Any number of remedies may be appropriate, depending upon the individual patient. Aurum may help someone who is suicidal.

### Hypnotherapy
In most cases, hypnotherapy is *not* effective in the treatment of depression. In addition, there is a risk that it may lower the patient's mood still further by removing any associated anxiety, which acts as a positive, active factor against the negative, passive depression. Patients who wish to try complementary treatment for depression, therefore, should choose one of the other therapies.

### Nutrition
Dr Carl Pfeiffer of the Brain Bio Centre in Princeton, New Jersey, classifies most psychoses into histadelia and histapenia, where the function of the nervous system is impaired, respectively, by excessive or inadequate amounts of histamine. Suicidal depression, blank mind, obsessions and phobias seem to be associated with histadelia. Such patients also tend to have low pain thresholds, few fillings in their teeth (thanks to a good flow of saliva), frequent headaches and allergies. Supplements of calcium, zinc, manganese and the amino acid methionine help to bring the histamine levels down and thus relieve the patient's symptoms.

Post-natal depression may be associated with the rise in copper levels that occurs during pregnancy, because the raised levels of oestrogen increase its rate of absorption from the intestines. Copper levels can be lowered by taking supplements of vitamins C, E and A, and zinc, and by eating apples, which contain pectin. Patients who have post-natal depression should not have copper IUCDs (intra-uterine contraceptive devices) fitted, as this may delay recovery. Vitamin $B_6$ may be helpful but should always be taken together with zinc.

Various amino acids may be beneficial in the treatment of depression. They include phenylalanine, tryptophan (which should be taken with vitamin $B_3$) and tyrosine. However, neither phenylalanine nor tryptophan should be taken by patients who are taking MAOIs, tryptophan should not be taken before or during pregnancy and tyrosine should be avoided by anyone who has suffered from a melanoma (a type of skin cancer).

## Organizations

Depressives Associated, PO Box 5, Castle Town, Portland, Dorset, DT5 1BQ, offers information and support to patients with depression and their families.

The Fellowship of Depressives Anonymous, 36 Chestnut Avenue, Beverley, North Humberside, HU17 9QU, is a national self-help organization.

The Manic Depression Fellowship, c/o Council for Voluntary Service, 51 Sheen Rd, Richmond, TW9 1YO (tel. 081-332 1078), provides a central contact point for manic depressive patients and their families.

The Association for Postnatal Illness, 7 Gowan Ave., Fulham, London, SW6, has a nationwide network of volunteer counsellors, all of whom have suffered from the condition themselves.

# Diabetes

## Definition and Incidence

Diabetes is a condition in which the body's use of carbohydrate is disturbed. Carbohydrate – made up of starches and sugars – is a vital energy source and without it the body cannot function. But in order for dietary carbohydrate to be used by the body tissues, it has to be broken down in the small intestine into glucose, which is then absorbed into the bloodstream. From the blood, under the influence of insulin, the glucose enters all the cells of the body, where it is broken down still further to provide energy. Normally, insulin is secreted by one section of the pancreas – the beta cells – whenever carbohydrate is eaten. Diabetes can be due to a failure of the pancreas to produce this hormone or a failure of the body cells to respond to it in the normal way.

Diabetes is therefore divided into two classes known either as type I and type II, or as insulin-dependent diabetes mellitus (IDDM) and non-insulin-dependent diabetes mellitus (NIDDM), or as juvenile onset and maturity onset. The last of these descriptions has rather dropped out of favour since, although most cases of type I or IDDM occur in young patients and type II or NIDDM in older patients, IDDM can occur at any age.

In IDDM, the patient's pancreas does not function normally

and he has to have regular injections of insulin. In NIDDM, the patient continues to produce some insulin and the condition can be controlled by dietary measures or by tablets.

It is estimated that there are some 200 million diabetics in the world of whom three quarters have NIDDM and are middle-aged or elderly. In Britain and other developed countries diabetes affects 1–2 per cent of the population, well over half of whom are overweight. Obesity is considered to be a very important risk factor in the development of NIDDM and during both world wars, when there was food rationing, the incidence of this type of diabetes fell.

Diabetes seems to run in families and, although it is not inherited as such, it is suggested that patients inherit a susceptibility to it, the disease itself being triggered off by other factors such as obesity, pregnancy, surgery or infection. If one identical twin develops NIDDM when over the age of forty-five, then the other one is likely to as well. In young patients, it is thought that IDDM may be an auto-immune disease in which the immune system attacks the body as it would an invasion by bacteria or viruses. Possibly, an inherited susceptibility allows a viral infection somehow to spark off the body's destruction of the pancreatic beta cells.

Although IDDM tends to develop at an earlier age than NIDDM, it is quite uncommon in the very young, affecting only one child per thousand in the under-sixteen age group. Most cases of NIDDM begin when the patient is in his sixties or older but, in Asians, in whom the disease is four times more common than in Caucasians, the onset is more often between the ages of thirty and sixty.

## Insulin-dependent Diabetes Mellitus

The onset of symptoms is often quite sudden, with the patient complaining of excessive thirst and weight loss and passing large amounts of urine. In some cases, however, he may just feel increasingly weak and tired and the weight loss and thirst may be only slight. Occasionally, in children, the illness may start with a chest infection that seems to go on for a very long time, or the first symptom may be constipation due to increasing loss of water from the body through an excessive output of urine. If glucose builds up in the bloodstream, the only way in which the body can break it down is to turn it into ketones – acidic chemical compounds smelling of acetone. The effect of ketones on the body is dramatic and, if the condition is untreated, the patient can start to vomit, develop severe abdominal pain and kidney failure and, ultimately, will lapse into coma and die. Occasionally, vomiting and abdominal pain may be the first signs of diabetes in a child who previously appeared healthy.

Sometimes the symptoms may come and go for a period of days or weeks before they become constant and, in up to a third of young diabetics, may disappear completely, usually within three months of the first signs of the disease. Unfortunately this remission is short-lived, sometimes lasting only days but occasionally up to a year. During this period, the patient needs no insulin and may appear to be perfectly healthy.

## Non-insulin-dependent Diabetes Mellitus

Patients who develop this type of diabetes are usually middle-aged or older and overweight. The condition may be asymptomatic at first and only be diagnosed through a routine urine test. Such patients often go on to develop symptoms unless their diet is controlled. First symptoms in NIDDM may include weakness, especially in the elderly, unexplained weight loss, skin problems such as ulcers on the feet or boils, itching of the vulva, visual problems such as the development of cataracts, or numbness, tingling or pain in the feet and hands.

Although, by definition, NIDDM patients can have their disease controlled by tablets or diet, occasionally an infection or other illness (such as a heart attack) can make their diabetes harder to control and necessitate them having insulin injections. Sometimes this is only a temporary condition, the patient being able to revert to tablets in due course.

# Complications of Diabetes

Until the discovery of insulin in the 1920s, type I diabetes was a rapidly fatal disease. Nowadays, patients can live long and active lives. However, as they live longer, it has become apparent that, even though their blood sugar levels are controlled by injections of insulin, complications can occur. These are probably more common in those patients (known as 'brittle diabetics') who have difficulty in keeping their blood sugar to normal levels, so doctors put great emphasis on maintaining as good a control as possible. There are seven important conditions which the diabetic patient risks developing. These are excess sugar in the blood (hyperglycaemia), excess insulin or inadequate sugar in the blood (hypoglycaemia) and problems affecting the heart and circulatory system, the nervous system (neuropathy), the feet, the eyes (retinopathy) and the kidneys (nephropathy). The complications that affect individual parts of the body will be dealt with first.

## CONDITIONS AFFECTING THE CIRCULATORY SYSTEM

Furring up of the coronary arteries that supply the heart causes angina and heart attacks and is twice as common in diabetics as in non-diabetics. It affects both men and women equally. The arteries supplying the legs may also become involved, causing poor circulation and resulting in intermittent claudication (inability to walk very far because of pain in the legs due to lack of blood), chronic ulcers and, occasionally, gangrene.

## NEUROPATHY

Around 40–60 per cent of diabetics have a mild neuropathy, while 5–10 per cent have severe symptoms. For 50 per cent of patients with NIDDM, the first symptoms they experience are those of neuropathy, pain in the feet being particularly common. Other symptoms may include numbness, tingling, weakness, paralysis and shaking muscles. The nerves that supply the digestive system may be involved, so that the stomach takes longer than normal to empty, the gallbladder stops functioning normally or the patient suffers from diarrhoea, particularly at night, this often alternating with periods of constipation. Involvement of other body systems may result in impotence or problems with ejaculation, low blood pressure on lying down (causing giddiness), damaged and swollen but painless joints, and inability to empty the bladder. The commonest form of neuropathy consists of a slight numbness and tingling in the toes and feet and, less often, the fingers, affecting both sides equally and sometimes associated with aching or shooting pains in the feet and legs, especially at night.

One form of neuropathy, in which the patient develops pain and weakness in the legs but no loss of sensation, may progress for weeks or even months before recovering, sometimes completely.

## CONDITIONS AFFECTING THE FEET
Normally an injury to the foot is painful, but in patients suffering from diabetic neuropathy sensation is dulled and minor injuries may go unnoticed. Areas with poor circulation heal poorly and, if left unattended, such injuries may develop into ulcers or become gangrenous. However, an ulcer affecting a patient who has circulatory problems but no neuropathy may be very painful.

It is the older male diabetic who is particularly at risk of developing foot ulcers. Ultimately, a gangrenous ulcer may mean amputation but some specialists believe that 50 per cent or more of amputations in diabetics could be avoided if patients followed simple guidelines on foot care (see below) and attended a chiropody clinic regularly.

## RETINOPATHY
Of those patients who have been diabetic for thirty years, 10 per cent will have lost their sight as a result of retinopathy. This is a condition which, in the long term, affects most patients to a greater or lesser extent but, fortunately, only in a small proportion does it cause total blindness.

The initial abnormality is in the tiny blood vessels that supply the light-sensitive retina at the back of the eye. These become swollen and ultimately leak, producing haemorrhages within the retina itself. As well as blood, fluid that is rich in fats and protein leaks out, forming little patches known as exudates. These may impair vision by preventing light from reaching the retina. In addition, new blood vessels tend to form across the retina. These are often fragile and bleed easily, resulting in the formation of fibrous tissue around them. This, too, obscures the vision and may ultimately pull the retina away from its moorings (retinal detachment) so that the sight is suddenly lost in one eye. Sometimes the earliest symptom of retinopathy is abnormality of colour vision. When total blindness occurs it is usually due to retinal detachment, often as the result of a sudden massive haemorrhage into the eye. However, loss of vision rarely happens rapidly and in most cases is a slowly progressive process. Diabetic patients also have a higher than average risk of developing cataracts (opacities in the lens at the front of the eye).

NEPHROPATHY

The function of the kidneys is to extract waste products and excess water from the bloodstream so that they can be expelled from the body as urine. This is carried out by a tiny system of tubes and blood vessels known as a nephron, of which there are about a million in each kidney. One of the most important structures in the nephron is a group of blood vessels known as the glomerular tuft. For some reason, in diabetes, a structureless material is laid down at the edge of the glomerular tuft, interfering with its function. When enough of the tufts have been affected, kidney failure results. Some 40 per cent of IDDM patients have some degree of kidney failure and, of these, about half are severe enough to need to go on a kidney machine or to have a transplant in order to survive.

The interference with kidney function can also cause high blood pressure (see separate section) and puffy swelling of the body tissues (especially the legs). The urine of most affected patients contains protein. However, not all diabetics with protein in their urine go on to develop renal failure, which is commoner in IDDM than in NIDDM.

Patients who develop nephropathy are usually middle-aged or

older and have had diabetes for at least ten years. Frequently, other complications have already occurred, notably retinopathy and problems with the circulatory system. Women are more often affected than men.

## HYPERGLYCAEMIA

If a patient with IDDM fails to take insulin regularly, he will become hyperglycaemic, develop ketoacidosis (ketones in the blood), as described above, and lapse into coma. Such a coma (termed ketoacidotic, hyperglycaemic or diabetic) may take hours or days to develop and during this time the patient will be thirsty and pass a lot of urine; he may vomit and have abdominal pain and his breathing will become heavy and laboured, his breath smelling strongly of acetone. Untreated, he will die. However, some patients whose diabetes is hard to control may have a mild degree of hyperglycaemia from time to time without becoming ketoacidotic. This may make them more susceptible to infections and to ulceration of the feet.

Patients with NIDDM rarely develop ketoacidosis since they are usually able to produce some insulin of their own.

Hyperglycaemia sometimes occurs when patients develop an infection (which may increase the need for insulin) and think that, because they are eating very little, they have to omit their injections.

## HYPOGLYCAEMIA

Too much insulin and too little glucose in the blood can also cause coma, which may come on very much more rapidly than a ketoacidotic coma. Usually when patients are newly diagnosed as having IDDM, they are allowed to go slightly 'hypo' in order to know how it feels. They are then instructed that if ever they are aware of such symptoms arising – weakness, hunger, nausea, sweating and trembling – they must take steps to treat them immediately by eating some rapidly absorbable carbohydrate, for example a sugar lump or a piece of chocolate.

Hypoglycaemia may occur if the patient accidentally gives himself too much insulin or injects it into a vein instead of muscle, or if he misses a meal or takes a lot of exercise to which he is unaccustomed.

Other symptoms of hypoglycaemia include mental confusion and abnormal behaviour, such as aggressiveness or emotional instability. Because the speech is often slurred, such patients may appear to be drunk. The wearing of a Medicalert bracelet proclaiming him to be diabetic will avoid the potential tragedy of a hypoglycaemic patient being arrested for drunkenness and, later, being found in a coma in a police cell.

During a hypoglycaemic coma a patient may have convulsions, so there is a risk that, even if he recovers following treatment, brain damage may have occurred.

## Investigations

Diabetes is usually easily diagnosed. Two to three hours after eating, the patient is asked to empty the bladder and then, half an hour later, to pass a specimen of urine for testing. Blood can also be taken at this time or first thing in the morning, before the patient has had breakfast. Sugar in the urine and a higher than normal blood sugar level is diagnostic of diabetes.

However, if a routine test of the urine in someone with no symptoms contains sugar and the blood sugar is apparently normal, a glucose tolerance test may be needed. In this, the fasting patient has blood taken, then has a drink containing a measured amount of glucose. Further samples of blood are taken at half hourly intervals until two hours have elapsed. The results will enable the patient with diabetes to be distinguished from someone who has a low renal threshold – a condition in which the kidneys allow some sugar to pass into the urine, although the patient is perfectly healthy.

All patients who develop diabetic symptoms will have their eyes examined, since many middle-aged diabetics have already developed a degree of retinopathy by the time symptoms appear.

Because the onset of diabetes may be precipitated by an infection, it is usual to do a chest X-ray and to send a urine specimen for culture when the condition is first diagnosed.

When complications occur, special investigations may be necessary to determine the extent of the problem. For example, ultrasound may be used to investigate the kidneys in nephropathy, and blood tests and twenty-four-hour urine collections may be taken to assess how well the kidneys are functioning. For patients with retinopathy, a fluorescein angiogram may be necessary – a fluorescent dye is injected into a vein in the arm and is photographed as it travels through the blood vessels in the back of the eye. The investigations described in the section on ischaemic heart disease may be appropriate for diabetic patients whose heart and blood vessels are affected.

# Orthodox Treatment

INSULIN-DEPENDENT DIABETES MELLITUS (IDDM)
Patients with IDDM will need regular injections of insulin for the rest of their lives. These are given at least twice a day. Either a base level of insulin is provided by a very slow-acting preparation while a more rapidly acting type (known as soluble insulin) is used to coincide with the patient's main meals, or a mixture of a moderately slow-acting preparation and soluble insulin is given twenty minutes before breakfast and again before the evening meal.

It is very important that the patient should regulate his diet, avoiding sugars which are rapidly absorbed into the bloodstream. Although about half his calorie intake should be taken as carbohydrate, this should be in the form of starchy foods, preferably unrefined, such as brown bread, high-fibre cereals, and fruit and root vegetables, because these are slowly digested and absorbed. A high level of fibre in the diet may make the diabetes easier to control. Regular meals are very important. Overweight patients should not drink alcohol, which is very fattening, but others can usually have an occasional drink, although they should avoid sweet sherries, liqueurs and mixers that have sugar in them. Obese patients should also reduce their calorie intake, since diabetes is much easier to control in those who are not overweight.

Any patient who has ketoacidosis requires urgent hospital admission. Treatment consists of fluid given through an intravenous drip to replace that which has been lost, insulin injections and treatment of any infection which may have precipitated the onset of the condition.

Occasionally, patients who are on insulin react to it, developing painful, red, itching bumps at the injection site, which last about thirty-six hours before disappearing. Usually this can be cured by changing to a different brand or type of insulin but, rarely, desensitization may be necessary.

Insulin can also cause fat to break down in the area into which it is injected and may therefore produce unsightly hollows in the skin. Most cases occur in women and children, men rarely being affected. However, patients can be taught to inject into their lower abdomen or buttocks where the fat loss will not be seen, or where it may even be welcome.

NON-INSULIN-DEPENDENT DIABETES (NIDDM)
Many patients with NIDDM can control their diabetes simply by following a suitable diet, similar to that outlined above for IDDM. Those who are overweight will also need to go on a reducing diet, since obesity makes diabetes harder to control.

Various types of tablet are available for those patients who, despite dietary control, continue to have glucose in their urine. These drugs are divided into two main groups, the sulphonyl-ureas and the biguanides.

The sulphonylureas, which include tolbutamide, glibenclam-ide, acetohexamide, chlorpropamide and tolazamide, are the most frequently used. They act by stimulating the secretion of insulin by the under-functioning pancreatic cells. Chlor-propamide and glibenclamide may cause hypoglycaemia in thin patients, who should always have some food available with which to relieve the symptoms and who should report any such occurrences to their GPs. In a few patients, the sulphonylureas may cause weight gain, in which case the addition or substitution of a biguanide, may be helpful.

For some time it was unclear how the biguanides worked but now research has revealed that they inhibit the absorption of glucose from the intestines into the bloodstream, stimulate the passage of insulin into the muscle cells so that it can work normally and inhibit the body from producing glucose from other forms of food. The only biguanide now in use is metformin. In those cases where diabetes is due to a reduced output of

132

insulin by the pancreas, a sulphonylurea is likely to be most helpful, whereas patients who have developed a resistance to insulin (and whose insulin output may well be normal) are likely to respond to metformin. Unfortunately, the latter may cause nausea, vomiting, loss of appetite and diarrhoea, but these can often be controlled by a slight adjustment in the dose.

TREATMENT OF COMPLICATIONS
Renal failure that results from diabetic nephropathy may need treatment on a kidney machine or a transplant.

Infection or ulcers on the feet need urgent and vigorous treatment to try to prevent them from progressing to gangrene. This includes the use of antibiotics and frequent cleansing of the affected area, with removal of any dead tissue.

Gangrene in the foot may require amputation. The level of the amputation will depend on the severity of the arterial disease. The surgeon will wish to remove all the tissue which has an inadequate circulation and in which there is the possibility of gangrene recurring. This may mean, for example, that the amputation is performed at knee level, even though the gangrenous area appears to be confined to the foot.

In recent years, the laser has proved useful in the treatment of progressive diabetic retinopathy. By sealing off the leaking retinal vessels (a technique known as photocoagulation) it can reduce the risk of visual loss by about 50 per cent. If cataracts develop in the lens, these can be removed surgically and the sight corrected with spectacles.

It is sometimes difficult to distinguish between a hypoglycaemic and a ketoacidotic (hyperglycaemic) coma but the differentiation is vital since hypoglycaemic patients must be given glucose while those who are ketoacidotic must be given insulin. However, as a first-aid measure, it is safe to administer a small amount of sugar. This is unlikely to do much harm to a ketoacidotic patient and may be life-saving for someone who is hypoglycaemic. Insulin, on the other hand, must never be given until it is certain that the coma is ketoacidotic, since it could greatly reduce the hypoglycaemic patient's chances of recovery. Normally the ketoacidotic patient is dehydrated (dry), flushed and breathing heavily, and the breath smells strongly of acetone, whereas the hypoglycaemic is usually pale, sweating and restless with dilated pupils and a fast heart rate. Once the patient has reached hospital, a blood sugar estimation will confirm the diagnosis. A ketoacidotic coma is treated with insulin, usually given both intravenously and intramuscularly to begin with, plus intravenous fluids, while a hypoglycaemic patient is given glucose solution by means of an intravenous drip.

## Diabetes in Pregnancy

Occasionally, a previously healthy woman may become diabetic during pregnancy. Normally, in such cases, the diabetes disappears once the baby has been born although it may recur many years later. Rarely, it persists once the pregnancy has ended.

For those women who are already diabetic, pregnancy can have an adverse effect, causing a worsening of retinopathy, nephropathy and neuropathy. Conversely, diabetes may affect the pregnancy, increasing the risks for both the mother and her baby. It is therefore essential that all diabetic women, whether long-standing diabetics or 'pregnancy diabetics', ensure that they have adequate antenatal care and that their diabetes remains well controlled throughout the pregnancy in order to minimize the risks and complications.

Maternal problems include an increased risk of premature labour and pre-eclamptic toxaemia (rapidly rising blood pressure towards the end of pregnancy) and an increased likelihood of developing cystitis, thrush or other infections. For the baby, the risks of congenital malformations, breathing problems and jaundice are higher.

Babies born to diabetic mothers are often much larger than the average and may therefore cause difficult deliveries. A vivid description of the newborn babies of diabetic mothers was given in *The Child of the Diabetic Woman* by J. W. Farquhar (Archives of Disease in Childhood, 1959):

They resemble one another so closely that they might well be related. They are plump, sleek, full faced . . . During their first twenty-four or more extra-uterine hours they lie on their backs bloated and flushed . . . their lightly closed hands on each side of the head, the abdomen prominent and their respiration sighing. They convey a distinct impression of having had such a surfeit of both food and fluid pressed upon them by an insistent hostess that they desire only peace so that they may recover from their excesses.

Because of the size of the babies, and because there is a slightly increased risk of stillbirth in the last few weeks of pregnancy, diabetic mothers often have labour induced slightly before they reach full term.

However, although the babies tend to be large at birth, they are also likely to grow very slowly during their first three months in the womb. Recent research in Denmark has shown that those children of diabetic mothers who did, indeed, grow slowly at first had impaired abilities in social skills and the use of language by the time they were four years old, compared with other children who grew normally, whether their mothers were diabetic or not. This is another reason, therefore, why strict control of diabetes is so important during pregnancy.

## Preventive Measures

All diabetics must monitor their glucose levels, by testing either their urine or their blood regularly. For NIDDM patients, urine testing is usually all that is necessary. As soon as they get up in the morning, they should empty the bladder. Half an hour later another specimen of urine is passed and this one is tested. They should not, of course, eat until after they have passed this specimen. Again, two hours after the main meal, they should empty the bladder, wait half an hour without eating and then pass a specimen for testing. When the diagnosis has first been made, the patient will need to test his urine every day but, once his diabetes is well controlled (with at least seven out of every ten specimens showing no evidence of sugar) he may be allowed to reduce his testing to once or twice a week.

About three times a year, the NIDDM patient will need to have his blood tested by his doctor. However, the IDDM patient will be taught to test his own blood, since this more accurate assessment of glucose levels is needed in order to calculate the dose of insulin required. Meters are now available which will measure the amount of glucose in a drop of blood placed on a paper test strip. The most recent, at the time of writing, is very small and takes only thirty seconds to give a reading.

As well as checking his urine or blood regularly, it is very important that the diabetic checks his feet frequently so that minor injuries or infections do not go unnoticed. This is especially important for older diabetics, among whom the risks of gangrene are greater. The patient should wash his feet with warm (not hot) water every evening and apply an emollient to soften the skin if it becomes dry. He should put a pad of lamb's wool between toes that overlap in order to stop them rubbing on each other and should never go barefoot. Patients whose eyesight is poor should never cut their own toenails and all should attend a chiropodist if they develop corns or areas of hard skin.

Plastic shoes, which do not allow sweat to evaporate, should be avoided, particularly as, early on in the disease, patients' feet tend to sweat excessively. Absorbent socks or stockings, made of wool or cotton, should be worn in preference to nylon.

According to doctors at the foot clinic of King's College Hospital, patients are at greatest risk of developing foot problems when they are on holiday, but this risk can be avoided by taking simple precautions. On long journeys, whether by plane, train or car, the patient should walk around for a few minutes every half hour. This will prevent or minimize swelling in the feet and ankles. New shoes, which may rub the feet, should not be worn on holiday when the patient may be walking more than usual. When sitting in the sun, a good-quality sunscreen cream should be applied to the feet and legs or they should be kept covered. If the feet become dry an emollient should be used, especially on the heels; if they become moist, they should be dabbed with surgical spirit. The normal routine of not going barefoot and of inspecting the feet every day for swelling, sores or changes in colour should be adhered to and any problems reported immediately to a state-registered chiropodist (in Britain) or a doctor (in Britain or abroad).

# Recent Advances

A new class of antidiabetic drugs has been developed which reduce the absorption of sugar from the intestine. They do this by inhibiting the breakdown of the 85 per cent of sugars in the diet which need to be turned into simpler substances before they can be absorbed. Known as alpha glucosidase inhibitors, these drugs include acarbose, miglitol and emiglitate and may be used alone or in combination with a sulphonylurea. They may also be given to patients with IDDM so that the dose of insulin can be reduced. The main side effects seem to be flatulence and diarrhoea, caused by sugars reaching the large bowel where they ferment. However, it seems that the side effects are usually bad only when the drug has just been started and disappear after a while.

It is possible that within the next few years injections of insulin may be used less and less, as new ways of administering it are developed. The insulin pump, which is about the size of a cigarette packet, delivers a constant amount of insulin into the tissues just below the skin, from where it is absorbed into the bloodstream. This is equivalent to the long-acting insulin which has to be injected each morning. And instead of an injection before mealtimes, the patient presses a button on the pump which then gives him the required dose. However, frequent blood tests are necessary in order to monitor the dosages – at least four a day on at least two days a week. But now specialists are working on a new model which will incorporate a glucose monitor, so that the pump itself will adjust the dose of insulin according to the patient's blood sugar levels.

The reason why insulin has to be injected is because it is digested in the stomach and therefore is destroyed if taken by mouth. However, doctors at the Medical College of Ohio have developed a plastic-coated capsule that will pass intact through the stomach and the small intestine. On reaching the large intestine, where there is no longer any risk of digestion, the capsule is broken down by the bacteria that reside there and the insulin is absorbed. At present this method seems to be less efficient than injections but it is still only in its early stages of development. Reports of the initial trials were published in the spring of 1987 and the capsule was not expected to be tried on humans until later that year. Further development, testing and approval could take several years.

However, insulin in the form of a nasal spray, which has been tested in Australia and the USA, may be available by 1990. It has been found to be very much more convenient than injected insulin since it is absorbed within ten minutes and has disappeared from the bloodstream within an hour. This means that mealtimes don't have to be carefully planned in advance. However, nasal insulin would only replace the mealtime doses and not the morning injection which gives a long-acting base level. Long-term trials of this method of treatment were to start in the summer of 1987 but the major drawback seems to be its expense. Because only 10 per cent of each puff is absorbed, ten times the normal dose has to be given.

The development of another nasal spray was reported in the summer of 1988. This contains glucagon, a hormone that stimulates the breakdown of glycogen (which is stored in liver and muscle) to glucose, which is released into the bloodstream. The glucagon nasal spray was found to revive hypoglycaemic patients within about seven minutes and could prove to be a piece of lifesaving first-aid equipment. Unfortunately, at present, it is very expensive to produce and lasts only a short time before deteriorating. However, scientists are looking for ways of making it more stable and more absorbable.

The prevention of diabetes and its complications is occupying many researchers around the world. ICI has developed a drug called ponalrestat which may be able to prevent diabetic neuropathy, retinopathy and nephropathy by stopping the deposition of certain abnormal substances in the nerves, eyes and kidneys. At the time of writing, a licence has not yet been granted to allow marketing of this drug.

Several specialists have been trying out immunosuppressant drugs on newly diagnosed diabetics, based on the widely held theory that diabetes is an auto-immune disease in which the patient's immune system attacks his own body – in this case, the pancreas. In Canada and Europe, trials showed that patients who were given cyclosporin lost most of their symptoms, although not reverting completely to normal. However, once the drug was stopped, they all eventually relapsed. Some doctors believe that antibodies to the pancreas can be detected up to thirteen years before the patient actually develops diabetes so that, in the future, it might be possible to screen people and then give immunosuppressive therapy to those who seem to be developing diabetes.

Meanwhile, for those patients who suffer from IDDM, surgical treatment is also beginning to offer a complete recovery. Pancreatic transplants seem to be successful, particularly when given to patients before they develop complications of their disease. At the time of writing over a thousand have been done world-wide. And at the Hospital of the University of Pennsylvania, transplants of just the insulin-secreting beta cells have been performed. This treatment is in its early stages but it seems that the transplanted cells begin to function in the recipient within forty-eight hours of the operation.

## Complementary Treatment

Treatment by a herbalist, homoeopath or acupuncturist may reduce the diabetic patient's need for medication, either insulin or tablets, and, for the brittle diabetic, may make the disease easier to control.

Nutrition therapy may also be of value. Insulin is more potent when adequate amounts of the hormone-like glucose tolerance factor (GTF) are produced. Some diabetics who secrete normal amounts of insulin seem to lack GTF, which contains chromium, vitamin $B_3$ (niacin) and two amino acids. Supplements of chromium and $B_3$ may be beneficial, together with manganese, which is essential for the correct functioning of the beta cells in the pancreas.

## Organizations

The British Diabetic Association, 10 Queen Anne St, London, WIM OBD (tel. 071-323 1531), has local branches in most towns, through which patients can obtain advice and information.

# Further Reading

The publishers Martin Dunitz have produced a series of books about diabetes which include *Diabetes: A Practical New Guide to Healthy Living* by Dr James W. Anderson and *The Diabetics' Get Fit Book* by Jacki Winter, a keep-fit and relaxation teacher who is herself a diabetic. Other titles are *The Diabetics' Diet Book* by Jim Mann and *The Diabetics' Cook Book*, by Jim Mann and Roberta Longstaff.

*Diabetes in the News* is a quarterly magazine giving information and news on topics of interest to diabetics. It is published by the pharmaceutical company Ames, and is available from DITN, The Three Pines, Church Rd, Penn, Bucks., HP10 8EG.

# Diverticular Disease

## Incidence

Diverticular disease is an extremely common condition of the colon (large bowel) which, in 80–90 per cent of cases, causes no symptoms at all. It occurs in people over the age of forty, men and women being affected equally. At post mortem, it is found in over 50 per cent of those over the age of sixty and two thirds of those over seventy. In about 95 per cent of cases, it is the lowest part of the colon (the sigmoid) that is affected. (See diagram of the colon on p. 257.)

## Diverticulosis

Diverticula, or pouches, in the colon arise at points where the bowel wall is weak and result from increased pressure in the bowel itself, due to over-development of the muscles within its walls. It is thought that a major factor leading to the development of diverticulosis is inadequate roughage in the diet and this seems to be borne out by the fact that it is rare in those parts of the world where people eat a large amount of raw food and that it has been produced experimentally in animals by feeding them a diet low in fibre.

When symptoms occur, they may be very similar to those of

irritable bowel syndrome, the commonest being left-sided cramp-like abdominal pain associated with diarrhoea or constipation. The diverticula tend to get filled up with faecal material and the pain is due to muscle spasm within the bowel wall as an attempt is made to empty them. Patients who tend to be constipated are more likely to develop symptoms than those who have regular bowel movements.

# Acute Diverticulitis

If faecal material remains for any time within a diverticulum, infection may occur. This is known as diverticulitis. Symptoms develop suddenly and consist of severe central abdominal pain that moves over to the left, associated with diarrhoea, vomiting and fever. It may be possible to feel a vague mass in the left-hand side of the abdomen, which is due to thickening of the colonic wall. Occasionally, the bowel haemorrhages and the patient passes large amounts of blood. Some patients have only a single attack of acute diverticulitis. Others may have repeated attacks at intervals of months or years, or may develop chronic diverticulitis.

# Chronic Diverticulitis

Symptoms of chronic diverticulitis may include diarrhoea alternating with constipation, wind, indigestion, the passage of bright red blood, mucus or melaena (stools that are black and sticky because they contain digested blood), and left-sided abdominal pain which is worse on movement but relieved by passing wind. Continual loss of small amounts of blood may lead to anaemia. A thickened mass is often felt in the left side of the abdomen.

# Complications of Diverticulitis

The outer surface of the inflamed diverticulum becomes sticky and may adhere to the small bowel, choking it off and causing an obstruction, past which the bowel contents cannot flow. Obstruction of the large bowel may also occur. In either case, the patient develops severe abdominal pain, constipation, swelling of the abdomen and vomiting. Partial obstruction may occur in which the symptoms are less severe, with some faecal material getting through.

An inflamed diverticulum may rupture, causing peritonitis or producing a localized abscess. It may also perforate into an adjoining structure producing a fistula, or hole, between the two. The commonest is a vesico-colic fistula (between the bladder and colon). The patient may have symptoms of bladder irritation, such as frequency, and then begin to pass faecal material and gas in the urine. The main danger of this is that the kidneys will become infected.

Diverticulitis is also the commonest cause of massive bleeding through the rectum (back passage).

# Investigations

In older patients, it is very important to exclude the presence of cancer, which may occasionally produce the same symptoms as diverticular disease. Therefore full investigations of the bowel will be performed. The first is a barium enema in which a barium-containing substance (that appears white on an X-ray) is gently pumped up the back passage and a series of X-rays is taken enabling the doctor to see the outline of the large bowel. Sigmoidoscopy is also necessary, in which the colon is inspected through a flexible telescope. Sometimes a tiny piece of tissue is removed through the sigmoidoscope to be examined under a microscope.

Occasionally it is necessary to perform an endoscopy in which a flexible telescope is passed into the stomach and duodenum in order to ensure that haemorrhage is not due to a peptic ulcer.

# Orthodox Treatment

If the symptoms of diverticular disease are mild, they can be relieved by a high fibre diet which keeps things moving within the bowel and thus lowers the pressure and spasm. The amount of fibre is slowly increased over a period of about six weeks. A 'bulking agent' which absorbs water in the bowel, swells up and thus helps the patient to pass large soft stools may also be helpful. Anti-spasmodic drugs may be necessary in the short term. These include atropine, belladonna, dicyclomine hydrochloride, hyoscine and propantheline bromide.

In acute diverticulitis, treatment consists of bed rest, pain-killers, antibiotics and plenty of fluids. Solid food is withheld until the patient feels better. In severe cases, the patient may need admission to hospital and intravenous fluids. Admission is also necessary if complications supervene. An abscess is treated with antibiotics and, in most cases, will respond. However, sometimes it is necessary to drain the abscess surgically. Small bowel obstruction which is due to inflammation may settle on a regime of intravenous fluids and suction through a tube inserted into the stomach through the nose, which keeps the digestive system empty. Large bowel obstruction, however, warrants an emergency operation to relieve the blockage.

Peritonitis is also a surgical emergency and, like obstruction, requires removal of the affected part of the bowel (usually the sigmoid colon) and a colostomy, in which the end of the bowel is brought out through an incision in the abdominal wall. Patients with peritonitis are also given antibiotics. After the inflammation has died down, usually within two months, another operation is performed in which the end of the colon is brought down and attached to the remaining section of the back passage, and the abdominal opening is closed.

A fistula is treated in a similar way, with removal of the affected section of the colon, closure of the fistula and a temporary colostomy. Surgery is also necessary for partial obstruction, persistent or recurrent bleeding, and, sometimes, for recurrent disabling attacks of diverticulitis. However, none of these cases needs treatment as an emergency.

Haemorrhage, when it occurs, is treated with a blood transfusion and most patients stop bleeding spontaneously. Very occasionally it may be necessary to operate to remove the bleeding section of colon.

# Complementary Treatment

*Herbalism*

Slippery elm may be used to reduce inflammation, peppermint to reduce pain, diarrhoea and flatulence, and comfrey to heal any damage in the intestinal wall. Chamomile also has anti-inflammatory and anti-spasmodic properties.

# Self-help

Patients with diverticular disease may feel better if they eat a diet that is high in fibre, low in fat and low in sugar. The fibre prevents constipation and stagnation. Fat slows down the passage of food through the intestine and sugar may result in the production of excessive amounts of wind, so reduction in both of these will relieve some of the symptoms of diverticular disease. It may also be necessary to avoid red meat (which also tends to slow down the passage of food), and alcohol, coffee and strong tea, which may irritate the lining of the digestive tract.

# Ear
# Infections

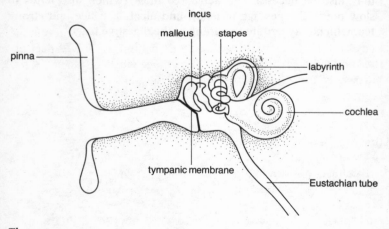

*The ear*

## Mechanics of the Ear

The ear is a complex piece of machinery which is made up of three separate compartments known as the outer, middle and inner ears. The large flaps of skin and cartilage (gristle) which we refer to as our ears are, in fact, the least important part, since we can no longer move them around, as animals can, to pick up the direction of a sound. The flap, which is called the pinna, and the external auditory canal, which leads from it into the ear proper, make up the external ear. The canal ends at the ear-drum, or tympanic membrane, which stretches across, dividing it from the middle ear. Sound causes the membrane to vibrate and these vibrations are transferred to a tiny piece of bone, called the malleus, which is attached to it inside the middle ear. The malleus is the first in a chain of three bones, or ossicles, the others being the incus and the stapes. The vibrations travel down this chain and are transferred by the stapes to the fluid-filled inner ear, which contains a complex mechanism control-ling balance (the labyrinth) as well as the nerve endings con-cerned with hearing. Here the vibrations are picked up by the nerves which translate them into electrical impulses and relay them to the brain, where they are interpreted into recognizable sounds.

The middle ear also communicates with the mastoid process, a bony section of the skull situated just behind the lower part of the pinna, and, via the Eustachian tube, with the throat. The purpose of the Eustachian tube is to allow the air pressure on both sides of the ear-drum to remain equal. That is why, when the air pressure changes, for example in a descending plane, one's ears feel uncomfortable, but if one swallows, thus opening the tube and allowing air to pass through, the discomfort is relieved.

Ear infections, known as otitis (from the Greek *otos*, meaning 'ear') affect either the outer or middle ears. An infection of the inner ear – known as labyrinthitis – is usually due to a virus and often occurs in epidemics. It causes giddiness and vomiting but normally clears up by itself after about ten days. Bacterial laby-rinthitis is rare and is a complication of a middle-ear infection.

## Infection of the Outer Ear (Otitis Externa)

This may be diffuse, involving one or both ears, or may be localized, in the form of a boil in the external canal. A boil in this position causes severe earache which is made worse if the pinna is moved or even touched. The area around the boil becomes red and swollen and this may even extend to the skin behind the ear.

Diffuse otitis externa may be caused by bacteria, fungi, chemical irritants or a generalized skin disorder such as eczema. Sometimes it can be provoked by cleaning out ear wax with an inappropriate instrument (such as a hair pin) which scratches the canal and allows bacteria to enter the skin. The area becomes red, swollen and very itchy. Pus forms and discharges from the ear and, because it blocks the canal, the patient often becomes temporarily deaf in that ear.

## INVESTIGATIONS

Recurrent boils in the ears may be the result of infection from bacteria harboured in the patient's nose. A nose swab will detect any bacteria that may be causing the boils and an antiseptic cream can be used to eliminate them. A urine sample may also be taken to test for sugar, since recurrent boils are sometimes the first sign of diabetes.

## ORTHODOX TREATMENT

Patients suffering from boils in the ear are usually given aspirin or paracetamol to control the pain and an antibiotic (which may be given intramuscularly as an injection) to kill the infection. A small piece of gauze soaked in glycerine and magnesium sulphate paste is put into the ear to draw out the infection. This is changed every day.

The first step in the treatment of diffuse otitis externa is to clean out the external canal. This is done daily until the infection has cleared up. In addition, a piece of gauze soaked in mercurochrome, glycerol and ichthammol or aluminium acetate may be put in the ear, these preparations all acting to reduce inflammation. Antibiotic drops or creams are not normally used as these may cause an allergic reaction. Painkillers may be taken if required.

# Acute Otitis Media

This is a common complaint in young children, especially during the winter months and among those living in industrial areas. It usually occurs as a result of an infection in the nose or throat. Bacteria may be forced up the Eustachian tube if the nose is blown vigorously, infected mucus from the sinuses may flow into the nose and up the Eustachian tube, or bacteria may travel up the tube from infected adenoids. Sometimes otitis media follows an attack of measles, scarlet fever or other infection.

The cells lining the middle ear and the ear-drum become inflamed. Pus forms, causing the drum to bulge and then rupture, which releases the pus into the external canal. With treatment, the drum heals, the inflammation subsides, the Eustachian tube opens up again and the middle ear returns to normal.

The first symptom is usually pain. The child may wake in the middle of the night, screaming. A young baby may just seem unwell without giving any indication of the site of the problem, but may bang his head against the side of his cot or pull at his ear. Usually the patient is feverish and may vomit and have diarrhoea. When the drum bursts, there is immediate relief from pain. Sometimes the discharge this causes is the first symptom.

The doctor will look through an instrument (an auroscope) at the patient's ear-drum to confirm the diagnosis and, if the drum has burst, may take a swab of the pus.

ORTHODOX TREATMENT

The external canal is cleaned out daily until there is no longer any discharge. The patient is given aspirin or paracetamol and antibiotics, which should be taken until the ear-drum looks normal again and there is no longer any evidence of deafness in that ear.

Occasionally the infection fails to resolve and it may be necessary to try a different antibiotic or a longer course of treatment.

Sometimes the condition may recur soon after treatment has

been stopped, or deafness, due to mucus or pus in the middle ear, may persist. In such cases, a myringotomy may be performed, in which a small incision is made in the ear-drum and the fluid is sucked out.

Rapid recurrence may be due to infected adenoids or sinusitis. In such a case, the adenoids may have to be removed or the sinuses washed out.

COMPLICATIONS

Permanent deafness may occasionally follow repeated attacks of otitis media or a single very severe infection. This results from damage to the ossicles which are no longer able to transmit vibrations to the inner ear. Affected patients will need hearing-aids.

Very occasionally, the infection may spread to the mastoid and the area behind the ear becomes inflamed, swollen and painful. This has to be treated surgically, the bone being opened and the accumulated pus cleaned out.

The facial nerve runs through the middle ear protected by a bony wall in 90 per cent of people. However, if someone whose facial nerve is unprotected develops otitis media, there is the chance that the nerve may become temporarily paralysed. This results in weakness of the muscles on the same side of the face as the infection but they gradually recover as the otitis media resolves.

Rarely, infection may spread to the inner ear, causing labyrinthitis, with symptoms of giddiness and vomiting.


# Secretory Otitis Media (Glue Ear)

This is a very common cause of deafness in children and one paediatrician has suggested that it may affect up to a third of all children. What causes it is not known but it may result from a combination of factors such as enlarged adenoids, recurrent respiratory infections, repeated attacks of acute otitis media or allergies. The mechanism seems to be that the Eustachian tubes become blocked so that the air pressure on the two sides of the ear-drum can no longer be balanced. Some of the air in the middle ear is absorbed into the surrounding tissues and this creates a vacuum which is resolved by fluid being secreted into the cavity and the ear-drum being sucked inwards.

Glue ear commonly affects children between the ages of five and eight and, usually, there are no symptoms other than deafness.

## INVESTIGATIONS

A hearing test is done to assess the loss of hearing and a tuning-fork is used to diagnose the type of deafness from which the child is suffering – this is known as a Rinne test. The tuning-fork is placed first in front of the ear and then touching the mastoid behind the ear. If deafness has been caused by the inability of the ossicles or the ear-drum to transmit vibrations (as occurs in secretory otitis media) the fork will sound louder when it is on the mastoid than when it is in front of the ear.

The doctor will probably also wish to examine the patient's nose and throat to try to determine whether there is any underlying cause for the condition.

## ORTHODOX TREATMENT

If the patient has enlarged adenoids or sinusitis these will be treated by adenoidectomy or sinus wash-out. A myringotomy is performed in which the drum is incised and the fluid sucked out. If the condition recurs, a tiny plastic tube (a grommet) is inserted into a hole in the ear-drum for about six months in order to keep the air pressure in the middle ear normal while the Eustachian tube recovers its function.

# Simple Chronic Otitis Media

If patients have repeated attacks of otitis media, the ossicles and part of the ear-drum may eventually be destroyed, resulting in deafness. Each time reinfection occurs there will be a discharge, but pain is uncommon unless water gets into the ear.

INVESTIGATIONS

When the doctor looks into the ear through an auroscope, he will see a perforation of the ear-drum. A hearing test will show the degree of deafness. A normal X-ray of the mastoid looks dark, since the bone is full of little pockets of air, but in a patient suffering from chronic otitis media, the X-ray may appear denser (whiter) than normal as a result of the inflammation.

ORTHODOX TREATMENT

While the ear is discharging, it needs to be cleaned out daily and a piece of gauze soaked in a mild antiseptic solution inserted. Drops containing a combination of antibiotic and steroid may be prescribed for a period of four weeks or so.

Surgery may be necessary. If deafness is slight, the perforation may be repaired. However, if the damage is greater and the deafness more severe, it may be necessary to reconstruct the ear-drum and the ossicles. But before an operation can be performed, the patient must have been free of infection for at least three months.

# Chronic Suppurative Otitis Media

If the Eustachian tube fails to open properly as it develops during childhood, the air pressure in the middle ear will be constantly lower than that in the external canal. As a result, the softest part of the ear-drum can become distorted and form a pouch. Superficial skin cells are constantly dying and being replaced and this same process occurs in the ear-drum. However, if there is a pouch in the drum, these dead cells accumulate there, forming a mass known as a cholesteatoma. As this enlarges it presses outwards through the bone above the ear-drum. Infection then occurs. The cholesteatoma gets larger and destroys the ossicles. It may also erode the bone around the middle ear so that the infection spreads further. As a reaction to the chronic inflammation, a polyp may grow.

The patient has a persistent foul discharge from the ear and, if there is a polyp, it may bleed. Earache or giddiness may occur, especially if complications set in.

## INVESTIGATIONS

A hearing test demonstrates that the patient is deaf. An X-ray shows abnormal density in the mastoid bone and, sometimes, a cavity in the bone surrounding the cholesteatoma, where it has been worn away.

## ORTHODOX TREATMENT

The patient is given a general anaesthetic and the cholesteatoma is removed. A mastoid operation is also performed. In a radical mastoid operation (performed if the hearing loss is profound) the damaged remnants of the ossicles are removed together with the ear-drum and all the infected tissue within the mastoid. In a modified radical operation (for patients who have been less severely affected) the mastoid is cleaned out but the ossicles are left intact. After a radical operation, the patient no longer has an outer ear and a middle ear but just one large cavity. He must be seen every week by the ear specialist until the cavity has healed and then every six months to have wax removed from the ear, since a build-up of wax will result in pressure on, and irritation of, the labyrinth, causing giddiness.

## COMPLICATIONS

The infection may spread, producing an abscess in the brain or in the layers of membranes that surround it. The patient develops severe headaches and, in the case of a brain abscess, vomiting and drowsiness. The abscess is drained as an emergency operation and the patient is given large doses of antibiotics. When the abscess has resolved, a radical mastoid operation is performed.

Meningitis may also occur. The patient suddenly becomes very ill with a severe headache, vomiting and fever, and soon lapses into a coma. A lumbar puncture (in which a needle is slipped between two of the bones of the spine and a small amount of fluid is withdrawn from the spinal canal) confirms the diagnosis. Large doses of antibiotics are given as well as intravenous fluids, and a radical mastoid operation is done once the patient is better.

Labyrinthitis is the commonest complication of chronic suppurative otitis media and is due to a spread of the infection into the inner ear. The patient becomes feverish, vomits and develops severe giddiness which is made worse if he moves his head. This, too, warrants emergency hospital admission and treatment with large doses of antibiotics. A radical mastoid operation and removal of the cholesteatoma is performed as soon as possible.

A cholesteatoma may also damage the facial nerve, causing weakness or paralysis of the muscles that it supplies. In such a case, an immediate radical mastoid operation is necessary.

# Complementary Treatment

*Aromatherapy*
Lavender essence may help to relieve pain and reduce inflammation in ear infections. Cajuput, chamomile and other oils may also be used.

*Herbalism*
Several herbs which are anti-inflammatory or antiseptic may be used to treat ear infections. These include chamomile, echinacea, garlic oil and marigold. Marigold also promotes healing, as does comfrey. Mullein oil can soothe pain in the ear.

*Homoeopathy*
Glue ear may respond very well to treatment with pulsatilla. Hepar sulph. may be prescribed if the pain is sharp and associated with yellow pus and if the patient wants to be well wrapped up and away from draughts. Aconite is helpful for earache which starts suddenly and which is worse at night. Patients who have a throbbing pain in the ear, headache and pain in the throat and whose skin is hot and dry may find belladonna beneficial. Chamomilla may be prescribed if the pain is stabbing and severe and worse for heat and if the patient is irritable and restless. Sulphur is useful in the treatment of chronic or recurrent infections and merc. sol. is used for patients who have throbbing pain which extends into the teeth, and enlarged glands in the neck. Many other remedies are also available for treating patients with earache.

# Eczema

## Definition

The word eczema is derived from the Greek *ekzein*, which means to break out or boil over and is used to describe a number of conditions in which the skin becomes red, swollen, thickened or scaly, and may weep, split or develop blisters. In people with dark skins, the most obvious sign of eczema may be a lightening or darkening of the skin in the affected areas. Eczema is often very itchy and excessive scratching may cause thickening of the skin associated with more pronounced surface markings – a condition known as lichenification. Continual scratching may also cause bleeding into the skin, especially of the legs, although this is uncommon.

Eczema is usually divided into various types, all with similar symptoms but with different causes. These types are exogenous (where the condition is caused by an external agent such as a chemical), endogenous or atopic (the type commonly seen in children), varicose (occurring on the legs, usually in elderly patients whose circulation is poor), seborrhoeic (a greasy-looking condition which affects the scalp and other hairy areas), nummular (producing small patches, usually in adults), pompholyx (affecting the hands and feet) and nappy dermatitis.

# Exogenous Eczema

Here the position of the rash will always be related to the causative agent. For example, it may occur under a watch strap (reaction to leather), under jewellery (reaction to metal), or may cover the whole of the hands or the feet if the reaction is to rubber gloves or to shoes. Before the days of tights, 'suspender dermatitis' was quite common and was caused by a reaction to nickel, of which most suspenders were made. It took the form of small red patches on the thighs where the suspenders made contact with the skin. Affected women were also likely to have patches of eczema under the metal clips on their bras and were unable to wear nickel jewellery without developing a rash.

Exogenous eczema takes two forms. One is a true allergic reaction whereas the other is purely an irritant reaction in which the chemical in question damages the skin directly (contact dermatitis).

ALLERGIC CONTACT ECZEMA
Before an allergic reaction can occur, the causative factor has to be absorbed through the skin, so areas where absorption is easier are more likely to be affected. Such areas include places where the skin is comparatively thin, such as the back of the hands, and where the moisture from sweat increases absorption of foreign substances, such as in the armpits and groins. If contact with the causative agent continues, the rash may later spread to other areas which are not in touch with it – for example, patients with a reaction to nickel often develop eczema round their eyes and in the bend of the elbows. Such a spread may occur days, months or years after the appearance of the original rash.

The commonest causes of allergic contact eczema are rubber, elastic, metals, dyes, cosmetics, leather, sticking plasters and a variety of ointments including those containing anaesthetics, antihistamines, antibiotics, antiseptics or lanolin.

CONTACT DERMATITIS
Strong irritants may produce a reaction after one or two exposures but weak irritants require prolonged or repeated

exposure. The former include some industrial chemicals while among the latter are household detergents and disinfectants. The resulting rash most commonly appears on the hands; in mild cases it may take the form of redness, dry skin and scaling; more severely affected patients may have thickening of the skin with painful splits. The palms tend to be affected as well as the backs of the hands.

## DIAGNOSIS
Often the diagnosis is obvious from the distribution of the rash and the history given by the patient of contact with an irritant substance. However, if confirmation of an allergic reaction is necessary or if the diagnosis is uncertain, patch tests can be done. The suspected substances are diluted to a concentration at which they will not act as irritants and are then applied to the skin of the back under specially designed aluminium cups which are taped down with hypoallergenic tape. The cups are left in place for two days, after which time they are removed and the results inspected. A rash appearing within these two days or up to two days after the cups have been removed suggests that the patient has an allergy to the substance that was applied at that site.

## ORTHODOX TREATMENT
The most important treatment is, wherever possible, to ensure that the patient no longer comes into contact with the substance that has caused the rash. If this is impractical – for example where the substance forms an integral part of his work – methods must be devised to prevent it from touching the skin. This usually means that the patient must wear some form of protective clothing. For those who have developed a rash on the hands from repeated contact with detergents, the answer is usually to wear rubber gloves, with a pair of cotton gloves inside them to prevent the skin from reacting to the rubber.

The use of soap on the skin should be avoided and an emollient soap substitute used instead. If the hands or feet are affected with a rash which is weeping or blistered, it is helpful to soak them three or four times a day for about ten minutes in a dilute solution of potassium permanganate. When parts of the body are affected that cannot be soaked, compresses of salt solution may be used instead.

The GP may prescribe steroid preparations – a lotion when the rash is still moist, followed by a cream, used three or four times a day, once it has started to dry up. If there is any evidence that the rash has become infected, an antibiotic may be necessary. Antihistamines may be prescribed to control severe itching.

## Atopic Eczema

Atopic eczema is a fairly common condition which affects 3 per cent or more of children under five. Although it rarely appears before the age of three months, 80 per cent of patients develop symptoms before their first birthday; 90 per cent of cases occur before the child reaches the age of five. The condition tends to run in families, together with hay fever and asthma; in cases where one parent has suffered from eczema a child has a 30 per cent chance of developing it but if both parents have been affected the figure rises to 50 per cent. Around 30 per cent of children with eczema will go on to develop hay fever or asthma.

The rash usually appears first on the face or scalp and spreads to other parts of the body. The commonest sites are the bends of the elbows, behind the knees, the wrists and the area behind the ears. The skin becomes red and rough, and may blister and weep. It is usually very itchy and this may prevent the child from sleeping at night and distract him from his daytime activities. This can be a particular problem for children of school age, whose work may suffer. Scratching the rash can make it very sore and may introduce infection to the already damaged skin whose susceptibility to both bacterial and viral infections is increased. The herpes virus can produce a particularly severe infection known as Kaposi's varicelliform eruption and it is therefore advisable to keep children with active eczema away from people suffering from cold sores.

The rash may be made worse by excessive bathing, rubbing by clothes (especially wool), a warm dry atmosphere or stress.

In most cases atopic eczema comes and goes; some patients are affected for only a few years and probably half have outgrown it by the time they reach puberty. The vast majority are free from eczema by the time they reach adulthood but some 2–3 per cent continue to suffer from the condition for the rest of their lives.

## ORTHODOX TREATMENT

Emollient preparations may be prescribed which soften the skin and alleviate the dryness associated with eczema.

Acute cases may need steroid creams but these are not used long term because there are considerable risks of side effects (such as stunting of growth) as a result of the steroid being absorbed into the bloodstream. Very rarely, if the condition becomes extremely widespread and severe, steroids may be given by mouth for a period of not more than two weeks. However, although they may be very effective in treating the acute case, they are not curative but suppressive.

Patches of skin which have become lichenified (thickened) may be treated by wrapping them in bandages impregnated with steroids or with tar and zinc ointment. This is particularly useful for treating the legs.

Antihistamines may be needed to relieve itching but, unfortunately, do not work in all cases. Weeping areas can be treated with potassium permanganate or salt solution soaks, as in the case of exogenous eczema. Wet dressings of lead and zinc lotion may also be helpful.

## RECENT ADVANCES

A concentrate of evening primrose oil, Epogam, is now available for the treatment of eczema. In one study, over 70 per cent of patients were able to reduce their dose of oral steroids, nearly 60 per cent reduced their use of topical steroids, and over 70 per cent were able to stop taking antihistamines when given Epogam. It was found that patients needed to take it for eight to twelve weeks before an improvement was seen and, after that, had to carry on with it in order to prevent a relapse.

SELF-HELP

Extremes of temperatures and wool worn next to the skin may make itching worse and should be avoided.

Bathing should be regular but the patient should not remain in the water for too long, and a soap substitute should be used. After bathing, an emollient should be applied to the skin.

Many young children with eczema seem to be allergic to components of their diet, such as eggs or milk. Excluding eggs from the diet or changing from cows' milk to goats' milk may make a considerable difference. Sometimes a particular type of fruit (such as pineapple) may be responsible.

# Varicose Eczema

Also known as hypostatic eczema, this condition affects the lower part of the leg and tends to occur when the blood from that region is not returned efficiently to the heart. Blood travels to the body tissues through the arteries, which have elastic walls to help potentiate the pumping action of the heart. (This can be felt, in arteries that run close to the body surface, as a pulse.) However, once the blood has been through the tissues, it is collected into veins which are not elastic and whose job it is to carry it back to the heart and then the lungs. (See the diagram of the heart and major blood vessels on p. 262.) Not only does the venous blood have to return to the heart unaided by any pumping action but the blood returning from the lower part of the body has to flow against gravity. To prevent it from flowing backwards, there is a series of valves within the veins and, in the legs, the flow is aided by the pressure exerted by the leg muscles. If these muscles are not used very much – if the patient is inactive or stands still for long periods – it is more difficult for the blood to return along the veins. The long-term effect of this is that the fluid part of the blood leaks out into the tissues, which become swollen and susceptible to damage.

The commonest site for varicose eczema is the inside of the leg just above the ankle, but it may spread to affect the foot and the whole of the leg. The skin is scaly and, in chronic cases, may become darkened and look greasy. Sometimes the skin breaks down and ulcers form. These are dealt with more fully in the section on varicose veins.

ORTHODOX TREATMENT
Support stockings should be worn to assist the flow of blood upwards through the veins.

Ulcers and eczema may be treated by covering them with a bandage impregnated with tar or zinc paste and then applying a firm elastic bandage on top and leaving it in place for one to two weeks. The bandaging is a specialist technique and needs to be done by a nurse.

For acute varicose eczema, bed rest may be necessary, in order to help to reduce some of the pooling in the leg. Compresses of potassium permanganate solution may be helpful, followed, once the condition has started to subside, by a steroid cream and firm bandaging. Steroids are not used for treating ulcers as they can delay healing.

Antibiotics may be necessary if the eczema becomes infected.

SELF-HELP
Avoiding long periods of standing, wearing support stockings, lying down with the feet raised for at least half an hour a day and raising the foot of the bed by about nine inches will all help to get the blood flowing back from the legs.

# Seborrhoeic Eczema

This type of eczema often begins on the scalp with itching and scaling, and spreads to the eyebrows, face, ears and the upper part of the chest. It takes the form of dull red, greasy-looking, scaly plaques and tends to spread to the skin folds, especially in obese patients, where it may become infected with bacteria or monilia (the thrush organism). The condition is commoner in men and tends to run in families.

On the scalp, seborrhoeic eczema may remain mild, causing scaling (dandruff) or may become severe with redness, weeping and crusting. If it is very itchy, continual scratching may cause hair loss, but the hair will grow again once the condition has been treated.

In some patients, seborrhoeic eczema comes and goes and attacks may be brought on by stress.

## ORTHODOX TREATMENT

When the scalp is affected, medications can be applied in the form of shampoo. Tar shampoos used every two to three days may be helpful but more severe cases may need the application of a steroid lotion.

Keratolytics such as salicylic acid remove thick scales and smooth the skin. They are usually applied in the form of a cream two or three times a week at night and shampooed off the next morning.

Steroids, used twice a day, may help to resolve the rash on the face and body but must not be used long term.

Where the skin folds are affected, it is important to keep them as dry as possible in order to avoid infection. Steroid preparations can only be used for a short time as they are more likely to be absorbed into the body through damp skin. Obese patients may be advised to lose weight in order to reduce the area of overlapping skin involved in their skin folds. Antibiotics and anti-fungal creams may be necessary.

# Nummular Eczema

Nummular means coin-like and describes a rash that consists of round patches, usually about 2–4 cm in diameter, although sometimes larger than this where several small patches have merged together. Also known as discoid eczema, it is rare under the age of twenty and occurs most commonly in young and middle-aged adults, especially those who have had atopic eczema in the past. It usually affects the back of the arms, the front of the legs, the shoulders and the back. It can be flat or raised and scaly and may blister, weep or become infected. The rash may persist for several months but tends to clear up of its own accord. However, it may recur from time to time, often in the same place as before.

## ORTHODOX TREATMENT

Small uninfected patches may safely be left without treatment. If there is blistering and weeping, potassium permanganate or salt solution soaks may help to dry the skin and a steroid cream can then be used to reduce the inflammation. Infections will need to be treated with an antibiotic, either in a cream, or taken by mouth if the infection is widespread.

SELF-HELP
An emollient (bath oil) may help to soften the rough patches of skin. Antiseptics and bath salts should be avoided as these may irritate the rash.

# Pompholyx Eczema

The word pompholyx, which is derived from the Greek word for 'bubble', has been given to this type of eczema because it is characterized by many blisters on either the hands or feet or both. The hands are more frequently affected – usually the palms and the sides and backs of the fingers. On the feet, the soles and the sides of the toes are most likely to be involved. However, the rash, which seems to be made worse by excessive sweating, may spread across the hands or feet and up the arms or legs.

Usually the blisters are quite small (only a few millimetres in diameter), appearing like little white spots because of the thickness of the skin on the palms and soles. There may be just a few or quite a large number. Eventually they may burst or the fluid may be reabsorbed and the blister subside. In chronic forms, there may be no blisters but just scaling and splitting of the palms and soles which may be hard to heal.

Pompholyx eczema can occur at any age although it is rare in young children. Usually it is self-limiting, resolving within about four weeks of its first appearance but, occasionally, it becomes chronic, with new blisters arising as the old ones vanish. Attacks may be recurrent, but the intervals between them may vary from a few months to a few years. Often they seem to be brought on by warm weather or by stress.

ORTHODOX TREATMENT
Pompholyx eczema is usually very itchy in the early stages and antihistamine tablets may be needed to control the irritation.

Potassium permanganate soaks will help to dry the rash if the blisters burst. Steroid creams may be useful in chronic cases. If the skin becomes infected antibiotics will be necessary, either in the form of a cream or taken by mouth.

SELF-HELP
When the feet are affected, cotton socks will help to prevent the excessive sweating which can make the rash worse.

# Napkin Dermatitis (Nappy Rash)

There are two types of nappy rash which come under this heading. One, which is probably a reaction to the ammonia produced in a soiled nappy, is a typical irritant contact dermatitis. This takes the form of redness and scaling and may affect all the skin covered by the nappy or just the buttocks, where the contact is greatest. The other type looks similar to seborrhoeic dermatitis, with a dull red rash on which there may be large silvery scales. Both types tend to spread, the contact dermatitic type often affecting the trunk, body folds and scalp. The seborrhoeic type responds quickly to treatment and doesn't tend to recur.

ORTHODOX TREATMENT
If the skin can be kept as dry as possible, by using nappy liners and changing the nappy frequently, all that may be needed is an emollient cleanser to use instead of soap and an emollient to apply to the skin to keep it soft. In severe cases a steroid cream may be prescribed. Infections will need to be treated with antibiotics or anti-fungal preparations.

SELF-HELP
The baby should be left out of nappies for as much of the day as is practicable, in order to keep the skin dry. Nappies should be changed at least once during the night. Rubber or plastic pants should be avoided as these make the area even more moist. Disposable paper nappies or coarse towelling ones may irritate the skin and should not be used. Talcum powder should not be

used as this, too, may cause irritation. Sometimes nappy rash will respond well if beaten egg white is spread over it and left to dry.

When contact dermatitis occurs as a response to the alkaline ammonia in a soiled nappy, it may help if the nappies are made slightly acidic. After they have been washed, they should be soaked for several hours in a bucket of water containing two or three tablespoons of vinegar. They should then be wrung out and dried without rinsing.

# Complementary Treatment

*Aromatherapy*
For dry eczema, geranium or lavender may be recommended, and for a weeping rash juniper or bergamot. Other oils that are used in the treatment of eczema include chamomile, hyssop and sage.

*Herbalism*
Large numbers of herbs are used in the treatment of eczema. Among these are chamomile (which helps to heal the skin and relieve any stress that may be exacerbating the condition), burdock (which is particularly effective in the treatment of dry scaly rashes), chickweed (which is used as a lotion or ointment to soothe, heal and relieve itching), heartsease (which is used for weeping eczema), red clover (which clears toxins from the skin and helps to restore normal function), and nettle (which is particularly useful for atopic and allergic types of eczema).

*Homoeopathy*
The choice of remedy will depend on the patient's symptoms and the distribution of the rash. Commonly used remedies include graphites (for chronic itchy, moist rashes, especially when in the skin folds or on the head, face and behind the ears), rhus tox. (for a dry red rash, particularly on the hands, wrists and in the bends of joints, which is better for warmth, worse for cold and damp, and very itchy especially at night), and sulphur (for a very itchy rash which is rough, worse for heat and for contact with water and often infected).

*Hypnotherapy*

This can be very helpful in the treatment of atopic eczema. However, it is not suitable for children under the age of five, because patients need to be able to concentrate on what the therapist is saying and to cooperate in the treatment. Atopic eczema often seems to be made worse by stress so that the irritation of the rash, which itself causes stress, creates a vicious circle. Hypnotherapy can break the vicious circle by teaching the child to relax and giving him suggestions that he will be less aware of the soreness and itching in his skin. Visualizations such as that mentioned in the section on psoriasis may be given and the child is made to feel that he has some control over his eczema. By helping the patient to relax, hypnosis may also be helpful in the treatment of other forms of eczema where attacks seem to be brought on by stress.

*Naturopathy*

A naturopath is likely to concentrate on finding out whether there is anything in the patient's diet that is making the eczema worse and will then advise on how any aggravating substances may be avoided.

*Nutrition*

Patients with eczema may have a calcium deficiency and an additional intake may be advised. Healthy skin is dependent on an adequate intake of vitamins A, E and C, and of zinc, so supplements of these (plus vitamin $B_6$ which is needed to help the zinc to work) may be recommended.

# Organizations

The National Eczema Society of Great Britain provides practical support. Most cities have a branch. Its headquarters are at Tavistock House East, Tavistock Square, London, WC1H 9SR (071-388 4097). A number of information packs are available from the society.

# Epilepsy

## Definition and Causes

The nervous system is made up of millions of tiny nerve cells, each of which has long arms or tendrils which allow it to communicate with the cells all around it. Electrical impulses travel from cell to cell, carrying messages which regulate all the body functions. The impulses that occur in the brain produce certain recognized patterns on an electroencephalogram (EEG, or brain wave trace). Their absence is one criterion that may be used by doctors to assess that a patient is dead.

Normally messages are carried correctly around the nervous system, enabling us to breathe, move, see, hear, digest and so on. But some people may have occasional discharges of abnormal electrical impulses in the brain, which send incorrect messages over a limited period of time – this is the condition of epilepsy.

Sometimes epilepsy may develop as the result of a head injury, but it may also be caused by a number of other conditions including a congenital abnormality in the brain, infection (such as meningitis), a brain tumour (benign or malignant) or addiction to alcohol or drugs. However, in the majority of cases there seems to be no obvious cause and the condition is said to be idiopathic. There are various types of epilepsy, each with different symptoms.

# Types of Epilepsy

## PETIT MAL

This occurs mainly in children, being slightly more common in girls than in boys. There is no convulsion but the patient's consciousness becomes impaired for a matter of seconds during which she stares straight ahead and fails to respond to stimuli. In many cases, this is accompanied by twitching of the eyelids and arms or by chewing and swallowing movements or fumbling with the fingers. Usually the patient stays upright and may even continue to walk or to ride a bicycle during the attack which comes on suddenly and disappears with equal suddenness. When the attack ends, some children are unaware that anything abnormal has happened and just continue to do whatever they were doing previously.

Petit mal rarely occurs before the age of four, with most cases starting between the ages of eight and twelve. The vast majority of patients have stopped having attacks by the time they are seventeen, although in a very few the condition may continue into adult life. Some go on to develop grand mal epilepsy.

The attacks may occur only occasionally or may be very frequent, with a patient having several hundred in a single day. In severe cases, the condition may seriously interfere with the child's schooling and special arrangements may have to be made. Usually an individual attack lasts between two and forty-five seconds but, on rare occasions, a patient may go into 'petit mal status' in which the attack is greatly prolonged.

## GRAND MAL

When epilepsy is mentioned, most people think automatically of grand mal convulsions, in which the patient falls to the floor and may thrash around. Grand mal epilepsy is a surprisingly common condition, affecting between four and eight people in every thousand. And it is estimated that as many as three people in every hundred have had a fit at some time in their lives. However, because in many cases the condition is well controlled by medication and because sufferers don't necessarily like to talk about their illness, most people are not aware of the extent of epilepsy in the population.

'Idiopathic' grand mal (where there is no apparent cause) usually starts in childhood, often between the ages of eight and twelve. However, about 75 per cent of those affected will have stopped having attacks by the time they are twenty. Cases that start when the patient is over the age of twenty usually have an underlying cause.

The fits often occur early in the morning or even when the patient is still asleep. Indeed, some people only ever have fits during the night. As in the case of petit mal, attacks may occur rarely or frequently; they may be brought on by late nights or the consumption of alcohol and may be more common in women around the time of menstruation.

For several hours before a fit, a patient may feel irritable or depressed or, conversely, unusually elated. The fit itself may begin with an aura in which the patient is aware of certain recognizable sensations, such as discomfort in the upper abdomen, twitches, numbness or tingling, flashing lights in front of the eyes or a bad taste or smell. The aura only lasts a few moments before the convulsion begins but may be long enough to enable the patient to get himself into a safe and comfortable position so that he will not hurt himself by falling to the floor.

Whether or not the patient has an aura, the first major sign that the fit is beginning is a sudden loss of consciousness. All the muscles go into a violent spasm. This is known as the tonic phase. The sudden contraction of the muscles of the chest forces air through the larynx (voice box) and may produce a characteristic cry. It is as he falls that the patient may bite his tongue, and blood and saliva may ooze from his mouth. His face becomes dusky, because the muscle spasm makes it impossible for him to breathe. After a few seconds, the spasm relaxes and is replaced by a series of violent jerking movements, which is known as the clonic phase. It is at this point that the patient may froth at the mouth, as air enters the lungs in a series of gasps, through the accumulated saliva. Some patients may wet themselves during this stage. After three or four minutes, the movements slow down and eventually stop. The patient is now completely relaxed, breathing deeply but still unconscious. After a few minutes he gradually regains consciousness but may remain confused and drowsy and may have a headache for several hours afterwards. Some patients go into an 'epileptic fugue', in which they wander off and do things of which they later have no recollection. Most patients sleep after an attack – for anything up to eighteen hours.

Individual patients and individual attacks vary, of course. Sometimes a clonic phase may last for half an hour. Some children may find they are paralysed after an attack – this usually affects only one side of the body and lasts between twelve and twenty-four hours before disappearing. Some 5–8 per cent of patients suffer at one time or another from status epilepticus, a condition in which one fit is followed by others, without regaining consciousness in between. This may be a life-threatening condition and needs urgent medical treatment.

PSYCHOMOTOR SEIZURES

This type of attack usually begins with a sudden alteration in mood and behaviour. An aura is common, in which the patient may experience upper abdominal discomfort, nausea, giddiness, hallucinations of various types (hearing, smelling, tasting or seeing things that aren't there) or the '_déjà vu_' phenomenon. The latter is something which many healthy people are aware of from time to time – the feeling that you have been in a particular place or situation before, but at the same time knowing that you haven't. The patient may feel that the world around him has become unreal and he may be aware of a feeling of fear, although he is unable to say what it is that frightens him.

The symptoms may vary according to where in the brain the abnormal discharges start. The patient usually becomes confused and may run round in circles, make chewing movements, smack or lick his lips and fiddle aimlessly with objects. Sometimes the limbs go into spasm or the head and eyes are turned sharply to one side. The patient may try to remove his clothes and, if restrained, may become violent. He may shuffle his feet, rub his hands or wet himself. The attack may end after a few minutes and be followed by confusion, or may progress into a grand mal convulsion. After the attack, the patient may be unable to remember anything about it.

## JACKSONIAN EPILEPSY

A Jacksonian attack is one that begins locally and then may become generalized. The first sign may be a change in the patient's behaviour but usually the attack itself begins with twitching of one hand, one foot or one side of the face. The movements are rhythmic and may occur in bursts. Gradually they spread to other muscles on the same side of the body. They can stop at any point or they may progress to involve the whole body in a generalized fit. Two thirds of all patients who suffer from Jacksonian epilepsy have generalized fits at some time during their lives. After the attack the muscles that were first involved may be weak or paralysed for several hours.

Some patients who suffer from Jacksonian epilepsy find that if they very firmly squeeze or press the muscles above those that are twitching, they can stop the attack from progressing.

## FEBRILE CONVULSIONS

Some five children in every hundred will have a fit during infancy or early childhood as the result of a high fever. A small proportion of these will turn out to be epileptic, the fever just precipitating the first attack, but in the majority of cases the fit is a result of the fever alone.

A child who has had one febrile fit is at risk of having another whenever his temperature starts to rise rapidly but most children grow out of their susceptibility by the age of three. Very rarely, a child may continue to have the occasional febrile fit until the age of seven or eight. The condition occurs more often in boys than in girls and the commonest cause is tonsillitis. Usually the fit, which takes the form of a generalized convulsion, is short, although two or three may follow each other in quick succession. After the fit there is a short period in which the child cannot be roused.

# Investigations

If epilepsy is suspected, an EEG, or electroencephalogram, is usually necessary. A number of wires are taped to the patient's head and these then record the brain's activity on a machine. Only the activity closest to the surface is picked up so, if the abnormal focus from which the fits are starting is deep in the brain, the EEG may appear normal. The test is best done soon after a fit.

Sometimes, when a generalized convulsion occurs in a previously healthy person, meningitis may be suspected. In such a case, a lumbar puncture will be done to confirm or exclude this diagnosis. Under local anaesthetic, a small needle is inserted between two of the vertebrae in the lower part of the back and a small quantity of the fluid that surrounds the spinal cord (the nervous tissue contained inside the backbone) is drawn off. If the patient is suffering from meningitis, the fluid may appear cloudy instead of clear and, when tested in the laboratory, will show evidence of infection.

In older patients, when it seems possible that the fits may be due to a physical abnormality in the brain, such as a cyst, a tumour or a blockage of a blood vessel, there are a number of investigations that may be used. These include plain X-ray of the skull, brain scan and arteriography. For the latter, a radio-opaque substance is injected into the bloodstream and allowed time to circulate; then X-rays of the head are taken on which the blood vessels of the brain can be seen clearly.

# Orthodox Treatment

PETIT MAL

In most cases, the attacks will be partly or wholly controlled by sodium valproate or ethosuximide, although in some patients the latter may cause drowsiness, dizziness, sensitivity to light and digestive problems.

An intravenous injection of diazepam may be needed to bring petit mal status to an end.

Medication has to be taken regularly until the patient has had four years without an attack or until he has reached his teens and a considerable amount of time has elapsed since the last attack.

## GRAND MAL

A number of drugs are available to treat grand mal and, in some cases, two or more may have to be used together in order to control the condition. All are capable of producing side effects, although some patients react more violently to one drug than another. This, as well as the effectiveness of individual drugs, is an important factor in the choice of long-term medication.

Phenytoin is safe and effective. Side effects are rare; they include skin problems, overgrowth of the gums, hairiness in women and anaemia. Used over a prolonged period, it may cause osteomalacia (softening of the bones). It is probably best avoided during pregnancy as there may be a risk to the unborn child.

Sodium valproate, too, should be avoided during pregnancy, since there is a possibility that it may cause foetal deformities. Its side effects include digestive problems, weight gain, hair loss, rashes and shaking.

Carbamazepine may cause skin problems, dizziness, fluid retention and, rarely, anaemia. But it has the advantage of being safe in pregnancy. Primidone, too, may cause dizziness and also drowsiness.

Phenobarbitone may cause drowsiness and loss of balance but usually only if too much is taken. Rashes may also occur. On the whole this is a very safe drug and is probably the safest to use during pregnancy.

Some female patients find that they have more attacks during pregnancy. So their medication may need to be changed not only to ensure that the baby is not at risk from the drugs but also to control the increased attacks. The contraceptive Pill, too, may increase the incidence of attacks and women suffering from epilepsy should use other methods of birth control.

All epileptic patients need regular follow-up by a hospital doctor for as long as the attacks continue. Once they have been free of attacks for some time, they are usually discharged back to the care of their GP.

## JACKSONIAN EPILEPSY

This is the hardest type of epilepsy to control completely and patients may need large doses of the drugs used to treat grand mal in order to prevent generalized fits.

## FEBRILE CONVULSIONS

Normally all that is required is prompt treatment by the parents if the child's temperature starts to rise rapidly. As soon as they become aware that the child is feverish, they should put him in a bath of tepid water and sponge him continuously until he appears to have cooled down. Older children may be given the sponge and allowed to play with it, which usually has the same effect.

If it seems likely that the fever is the result of a bacterial infection – for example tonsillitis or an ear infection – the child should be seen as soon as possible by the GP so that a course of antibiotics may be started.

In some cases, where a child has had a prolonged fit, the GP may think it advisable to prescribe phenobarbitone, to be taken on a regular basis until the child reaches the age of three.

# Complementary Treatment

*Acupuncture*
The points used in treatment will depend upon the individual symptoms. Febrile convulsions, for example, are seen as being due to an invasion of the body by wind which stirs up inner heat. The therapist will use specific points to expel wind, eliminate heat, relieve spasm and clear mental clouding.

*Bach Flower Remedies*
It has been observed by a doctor that giving a patient who is having an epileptic fit the compound Rescue Remedy will bring him round quite quickly. Indeed, this doctor has even found it possible to cut short status epilepticus by putting a few drops of this remedy into the patient's mouth. As a first-aid measure it is certainly worth trying, since it can have no harmful effects whatsoever.

*Herbalism*
Treatment may be given to reduce the severity and frequency of attacks. Scullcap is commonly used for this.

*Homoeopathy*
A wide range of remedies may be appropriate but belladonna may be particularly useful in the treatment of febrile convulsions, while cuprum may be given to a patient whose attack begins with twitching in the fingers and toes.

*Hypnotherapy*
Hypnosis may help to reduce the frequency of epileptic attacks. Occasionally, when a patient has warning that an attack is coming on, the use of self-hypnosis or of techniques learned while under hypnosis may help to abort the full attack.

*Nutrition*
Epileptic patients are often found to have a deficiency of manganese and a supplement of this mineral may be beneficial. The amino acid taurine may help to control attacks in some patients. It is taken initially in doses of 1 g daily but, because it accumulates rapidly in the body, this can soon be reduced to a maintenance dose of around 50 mg a day.

# Self-help

Attacks may be brought on by over-breathing or by watching flashing lights, so patients should avoid both of these.

As a first-aid measure for a patient in petit mal status, a paper bag placed over the mouth and nose may be helpful. This makes the child re-breathe the carbon dioxide that has been exhaled and this may help to bring the attack to an end.

It is a common belief that, during an attack of grand mal epilepsy, a patient is at risk of swallowing his tongue and that something should be pushed into his mouth to hold the tongue in place. However, there is, in fact, very little risk of the tongue being swallowed and if it is bitten this occurs right at the start of the attack and cannot be prevented. On the other hand, forcing something into a patient's mouth during a fit could seriously damage his teeth or his jaw and therefore should be avoided.

For some years a GP in Scotland has been conducting a campaign to publicize smother-proof pillows, since there is a small risk that a patient who has an epileptic fit during the night may be suffocated by his pillow. The smother-proof model is available from Melco Products Ltd, Tottington, Bury.

Anyone who has epilepsy is banned from driving a car but may re-apply for a driving licence once three years have elapsed since the last fit. But no one who has ever had a fit is allowed to drive a heavy-goods vehicle.

## Information

The drug company, Ciba Geigy, has published a booklet for children entitled *Learning about Epilepsy*. To obtain a copy, send a 9 × 6 inch stamped addressed envelope to Ciba Geigy Pharmaceuticals, Wimblehurst Rd, Horsham, West Sussex, RH I 2 4AB.

## Organizations

The British Epilepsy Association, Anstey House, 40 Hanover Square, Leeds, LS3 IBE (tel. 0532 439393), and the Epilepsy Association for Scotland, 48 Govan Rd, Glasgow, G5I IJL (tel. 041-427 4911), offer help, advice and information to sufferers.

The Chalfont Centre for Epilepsy, Chalfont St Peter, Gerrards Cross, Buckinghamshire, SL9 ORJ, offers medical assessment for people with epilepsy as an aid to rehabilitation. This is arranged by the patient's GP.

# Fibroids

## Incidence and Description

Fibroids are benign growths of muscle and fibrous tissue that occur in the uterus (womb). They affect about 20 per cent of women over the age of thirty although, in many cases, they produce no symptoms. When symptoms do arise, they are likely to do so between the ages of thirty-five and forty-five. Fibroids are commoner in black women than in white but, although they may cause infertility in between 25 and 35 per cent of white women, they do not have this effect in black women. Why this should be is not known. Nor is the cause of fibroids known. However, they are to some extent dependent on the woman's hormonal status, since they tend to enlarge during pregnancy and shrivel up after the menopause.

Fibroids may be single or multiple and vary enormously in size, although they grow only slowly. Usually they occur within the muscle of the uterus itself (interstitial or intramural fibroids). But they may arise on the outside of the uterus (subserous fibroids) or on the inside (submucous fibroids) and in these positions may become pedunculated (grow out on stalks). Rarely, they grow within the cervix (neck of the womb). Also rare is the so-called wandering fibroid. This is a large subserous fibroid which becomes attached to a band of tissue lying in the abdomen called the omentum. The omentum carries in it a number of blood vessels and, eventually, the fibroid may develop a blood supply from it. When this occurs, it may break off from its stalk so that it is now separated completely from the uterus.

## Symptoms

To a certain extent, the symptoms depend upon where in the uterus the fibroids are situated. Submucous fibroids have abnormally large blood vessels stretched over their surface and they increase the surface area of the inside of the uterus, so they often cause heavy periods (menorrhagia), although the periods themselves are not prolonged. Anaemia is a common result of this. These fibroids may also become infected, producing a discharge. Irregular vaginal bleeding may occur if they become ulcerated. A large pedunculated fibroid may descend through the cervix (neck of the uterus) and, in this position, may cause quite heavy bleeding. Pedunculated fibroids may cause colicky pain, as the uterine muscle tries to push them out. This may be particularly severe during a period (dysmenorrhoea). Large polyps may cause urinary symptoms of discomfort in the rectum (back passage) because of the pressure they exert on the surrounding organs. Patients may also suffer from infertility or recurrent abortion.

Intramural fibroids may first be noticed as a mass in the abdomen. Like submucous fibroids they may cause menorrhagia, pressure symptoms and infertility.

Women who have subserous fibroids frequently have no symptoms, although they may become aware of a mass in the abdomen. Occasionally they may develop severe abdominal pain due either to bleeding or to twisting of the stalk. Haemorrhage may occur either inside the fibroid itself or into the abdominal cavity. If the stalk of the fibroid twists (torsion), the blood supply to the fibroid is cut off and the pain persists until the fibroid dies.

Fibroids within the cervix are rare. They may be associated with urinary symptoms (pain on passing water, frequency or stress incontinence), bleeding, infection, pain on intercourse and infertility.

# Complications

As well as torsion of a pedunculated fibroid, there are several other complications that may occur. All of them are uncommon.

Pregnant women who have fibroids may develop severe pain in the second trimester of pregnancy (the middle three months) due to red degeneration, which is caused by the fibroid losing its blood supply so that it dies back. However, this only occurs with large fibroids.

Pressure on the bladder or ureters may cause acute retention of urine, repeated urinary tract infections or partial obstruction of urinary flow from the kidneys to bladder.

Malignant change occurs in about one in two hundred patients with large fibroids, which is why doctors always recommend that large fibroids be removed. Symptoms of malignant change include sudden rapid growth of the fibroid, pain and fever.

Fibroids may also interfere with pregnancy, producing recurrent abortion, premature labour and post-partum haemorrhage or infection. They may also prevent normal vaginal delivery and necessitate a Caesarean section.

# Investigations

Fibroids are first diagnosed by a vaginal examination. Their presence can then be confirmed by ultrasound investigation. Sometimes fibroids become calcified, especially in older patients, and, in this case, will show up on X-ray. If the patient has been having irregular vaginal bleeding, a scrape of the uterus (D & C) is necessary to rule out a diagnosis of cancer.

# Orthodox Treatment

Surgery is usually unnecessary if the patient has few or no symptoms and if the fibroids are small and either intramural or subserous. It is also avoided during pregnancy.

If the patient has been bleeding heavily, iron supplements may be necessary and, rarely, a blood transfusion. Infection is treated with antibiotics. It may be possible to control excessive bleeding in younger patients by prescribing progesterone or other drugs used for the treatment of menorrhagia.

When an operation is necessary, the simplest is a hysterectomy. However, for those women who dislike this idea or who wish to become pregnant in the future, it is possible to remove the individual fibroids (myomectomy), leaving the womb intact. Unfortunately, myomectomy carries the risk of post-operative bleeding and infection, and fibroids recur in between 5 and 20 per cent of cases.

## Recent Advances

A Dutch trial has found that fibroids can be shrunk by a monthly injection of an LHRH analogue (the hormone-like substance described in the section on the treatment of prostate disease). Six patients have had the treatment in Holland, and another twelve were treated with a similar preparation in Canada, where the results were the same. Mild hot flushes seemed to be the main side effect. However, treatment would have to be continued until the patient reached the menopause in order to prevent the fibroid re-establishing itself, and so is unlikely to be used for women other than those for whom an operation is not advisable.

## Complementary Treatment

_Herbalism_
Some herbs may help to prevent fibroids from becoming any larger and may relieve the patient's symptoms. Helonias root improves the function of the ovaries and helps to maintain menstrual regularity. Agnus castus also has a hormone-like effect, acting on the pituitary gland in the brain, whose hormones control other glands in the body, including the ovaries. Life root relieves spasm in the uterus as do blue cohosh, motherwort and black cohosh.

_Homoeopathy_
The remedy chosen for an individual patient will depend on her symptoms and may include any of those mentioned in the section on menstrual problems.

# Organizations

The Hysterectomy Support Group, 11 Henryson Rd, Brockley, London, SE4 1HL (tel. 081-690 5987), offers support and coun-selling to women who are about to have, or have had, a hysterectomy. For information about local support groups, phone 071-251 6332 on Monday, Wednesday, Thursday or Friday between 11 a.m. and 5 p.m.

# Gallbladder
# Disease

## The Function of the Gallbladder

Because fat cannot be dissolved in water, a special system has evolved for its digestion and its absorption through the intestinal wall. Bile is an essential factor in this, since it contains substances that allow fats to be emulsified. It also stimulates the secretion of an enzyme concerned with the breakdown of fats. Bile is secreted by the liver and stored in the gallbladder until needed. When fat is eaten, this stimulates the gallbladder to contract and bile flows down the cystic duct, into the common bile duct and through the ampulla of Vater into the intestine.

As well as acting as a storage vessel, the gallbladder concentrates the bile within it by removing water through its wall. Thus if the gallbladder is removed, although bile still flows into the intestine from the liver, fat digestion may be less efficient because the bile is not concentrated.

## Gallstones (Cholelithiasis)

The commonst disorder of the biliary tract (gallbladder and bile ducts) is gallstones. This occurs very frequently in developed countries and may be associated with eating a diet that is high

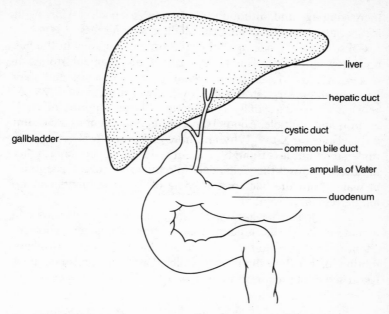

*The relationship between the liver, gallbladder and duodenum*

in fat and refined carbohydrates and low in fibre. Probably 10–20 per cent of the population over the age of forty have gallstones but only in a minority do symptoms occur. If gallstones are found by chance on an X-ray taken for some other reason it is standard practice to leave them alone if they are causing no symptoms, since the risk of developing problems is slightly less than the risk from a major operation. However, if a patient with symptomless gallstones is having an abdominal operation for another reason, the gallbladder may be removed at the same time.

Medical students learn that the typical patient with gallstones is 'fair, fat, female, fertile and forty'. However, this is rather a simplification. Certainly obese patients have a greater risk of developing gallstones, as do women, especially those who have had a number of children. Taking the contraceptive Pill also increases the risk. But the condition becomes commoner with increasing age and, although it is rare in Asians and Africans, it is especially common among the Mediterranean races.

Gallstones are made up of the substances contained in the bile and may be described as cholesterol stones, pigment stones or mixed. About 20 per cent contain pure cholesterol and may occur as single large stones. The majority of stones (about 75 per cent) are mixed (usually containing a large amount of cholesterol) and multiple. About 10 per cent contain enough calcium to be visible on X-ray. Why and how gallstones form is not fully understood but it is thought that, in some cases, an abnormality in function causes the gallbladder to remove an excessive amount of water from the bile so that some of its constituents can no longer remain in solution.

The problems that gallstones can give rise to are various and include cholecystitis (inflammation of the gallbladder), choledocholithiasis (stones in the common bile duct), cholangitis (inflammation of the bile ducts and gallbladder) and gallstone ileus (obstruction of the intestines by a gallstone).

## Chronic Cholecystitis (Biliary Colic)

Both these names are somewhat of a misnomer, since this is not a chronic inflammatory condition and the pain it produces is not colicky. (True colic comes and goes in waves but the pain of biliary colic is constant during the attack.)

Of those patients who have symptoms from their gallstones, the majority will suffer from 'chronic cholecystitis'. The attacks are caused by a stone becoming stuck either in the junction of the gallbladder and the bile duct or in the duct itself. The muscle in the wall of both gallbladder and duct contracts in an effort to move the stone and this produces intense pain which is usually felt under the ribs on the right-hand side of the abdomen. However, the pain may also be felt under the V of the ribs or may extend right across the abdomen and spread round to the back, below the right shoulderblade. The patient may vomit and is usually restless. After several hours, the stone either falls back into the gallbladder or, by virtue of the muscle contractions, is passed down the bile duct and into the intestine.

Some patients suffer from a constant dull ache in the upper abdomen and many complain of discomfort and flatulence after eating a fatty meal.

ORTHODOX TREATMENT

Patients who are otherwise healthy should have a cholecystectomy (removal of the gallbladder) to prevent further recurrences. If an operation is inadvisable because the patient is frail, elderly or has severe heart or lung disease, it may be possible to control the symptoms with painkillers and anti-emetics (drugs to stop vomiting) but, ultimately, surgery may still be necessary if the pain becomes intolerable or if complications, such as jaundice, occur. A low fat diet and weight reduction will also help these patients and those who are waiting for surgery.

In some patients who are not fit for surgery, it may be possible to dissolve the stones by giving them chenodeoxycholic acid or ursodeoxycholic acid. These preparations are taken by mouth and excreted in the bile. However, they will only work if the gallbladder is seen on investigation to be functioning (see below) and if the gallstones are very small and contain very little calcium (making them invisible – or radiolucent – on a plain X-ray of the abdomen). This treatment is not suitable for women of childbearing age nor for those with any form of liver disease. It has the disadvantage that, although 80 per cent of stones may be dissolved after six months' or a year's treatment, they frequently re-form after the medication has stopped.

# Acute Cholecystitis

Twenty per cent of those who develop gallbladder symptoms suffer from this condition, which most frequently affects women between the ages of twenty and forty. Like 'chronic cholecystitis' it is caused by a stone becoming jammed either in the junction of the gallbladder and duct or in the duct itself, and many patients have previously suffered from biliary colic, indigestion or flatulence. The pain of acute cholecystitis stems from inflammation which, at first, is probably caused by the chemicals in the bile. However, a bacterial infection then supervenes in 50 per cent or more of cases.

The pain comes on suddenly and is severe and constant. It is felt across the right and central parts of the upper abdomen and under the right shoulder-blade. The patient usually vomits and is quite ill and feverish. If the common bile duct becomes swollen, slight jaundice may occur as bile from the liver is prevented from passing into the intestine and enters the bloodstream instead.

ORTHODOX TREATMENT

At least 90 per cent of cases settle on a regime of bed rest, painkillers and antibiotics. Rarely, complications may occur which include abscess formation, peritonitis and septicaemia.

The patient is admitted to hospital and is given fluids intravenously. If she is vomiting, a tube is passed through the nose into the stomach in order to keep it empty.

If complications occur, emergency surgery is necessary. In most cases, however, the symptoms are allowed to settle down and an operation is performed to remove the gallbladder at a later date. Nowadays many surgeons like to do this two or three days after the patient's admission to hospital. Some, however, prefer the traditional gap of two or three months between the acute attack and surgery. Waiting for a few months has the advantage that obese patients have the chance to lose some weight, reducing the risks of operation, and that the surgeon can be certain that all the inflammation has settled. However, 10 per cent of patients get another attack while waiting for their operation.

# Choledocholithiasis (Stones in the Common Bile Duct)

Some 10 per cent of patients who have gallbladder symptoms have stones in the common bile duct. Some of these stones actually form in the duct itself while others originate in the gallbladder and then pass into the duct where they gradually enlarge. This condition occurs more frequently in older patients.

Various complications may arise as the result of stones becoming lodged in the common bile duct. They may prevent bile from getting through, causing jaundice as the bile escapes into the bloodstream. They may result in an infection in the gallbladder (suppurative cholangitis) in which the patient has a high fever and becomes extremely ill. Occasionally, acute pancreatitis (inflammation of the pancreas) may occur. Rarely, the back pressure that builds up in the duct may affect the liver and cause liver failure (biliary cirrhosis).

Because some of these complications may be life-threatening, it is usual to remove ductal stones when they are diagnosed, even if they are not producing any symptoms. When symptoms occur, they are usually recurrent, lasting for a few hours or days at a time, and consisting of pain, jaundice and fever. The pain, which is felt in the right upper abdomen and under the V of the ribs, is usually severe and the patient may vomit. While the patient is jaundiced, the stools are pale and the urine dark because the pigments from the bile that normally colour the stools can no longer get through to the bowel and are being excreted in the urine.

## ORTHODOX TREATMENT

Usually the acute episode is allowed to settle before surgery is performed, although a very ill patient with jaundice may need an emergency operation. Painkillers are prescribed and, if necessary, antibiotics. Once the symptoms have subsided, the patient is taken to theatre, the common bile duct is opened and all the stones are removed. Because it is easy to miss stones, a cholangiogram (see below) is performed during the operation to see whether the duct has indeed been cleared. During the operation a T tube is inserted into the duct. This is a piece of plastic tubing in the shape of a T. The crossbar is inserted into the duct and stitched in snugly using catgut, which will then slowly dissolve. The long vertical part of the T is brought out to the surface and is anchored to the skin with a stitch. Bile drains from the tube and is collected in a plastic bag. About nine or ten days after the operation, a substance that will show up on X-ray is injected down the tube and into the bile ducts and an X-ray is taken. If there is no evidence of any stones or blockage in the duct, the skin stitch is removed and the T tube comes out easily. Within about a day the tiny hole left in the bile duct has closed up and bile is flowing normally again. If, however, the X-ray shows that there are still stones in the duct, it is usually possible to remove them through the T tube, either physically or by injecting the solvent, mono-octanoin. Another operation is only rarely necessary.

Elderly or frail patients who are at increased risk from a major operation may be treated by endoscopic sphincterotomy rather than by surgery. This technique, which has a 90 per cent success rate, consists of inserting a flexible telescope through the mouth down into the small intestine. The muscular band at the mouth of the common bile duct is cut into and large stones can be removed in this way.

# Cholangitis

This is a bacterial infection involving the gallbladder and bile ducts and it may be mild or severe. It often occurs as a result of an obstruction in the ducts – from a gallstone, congenital narrowing, scarring from a previous operation, or malignant growth. The patient has severe pain in the gallbladder area, fever, shivering fits and, often, jaundice. The right upper section of the abdomen is very tender.

Complications include the development of a liver abscess and liver failure. If, despite treatment, the symptoms continue, septicaemia may occur. This condition is known as acute suppurative cholangitis.

ORTHODOX TREATMENT
Acute suppurative cholangitis needs emergency treatment. The patient is admitted to hospital and is given intravenous fluids and large doses of antibiotics. As soon as she is in a fit condition, an operation is performed at which the obstruction to bile flow is relieved and bile is drained out. The simplest and quickest procedure possible is used, in order to minimize the risk to the patient. (Various methods are available to the surgeon.) Once

the patient has fully recovered, another operation may be necessary to ensure that further episodes do not occur.

The treatment of milder forms of cholangitis consists of antibiotics and, if necessary, intravenous fluids; the operation to relieve the obstruction can be delayed until the patient has recovered from the acute attack.

Patients who have recurrent attacks of mild cholangitis but who are not suitable for surgery may be helped by long-term courses of antibiotics.

Because cholangitis may be precipitated by operative procedures, any patient who is to have surgery on the biliary tract or investigative procedures such as ERCP or PTC (see below) will be given a course of antibiotics as a preventive measure.

# Gallstone Ileus

This is an uncommon condition which usually occurs in older women. The gallstone responsible is an inch or more across. Having taken some years to achieve this size, it ulcerates through the wall of the gallbladder into the duodenum. It passes down the small intestine and then becomes lodged lower down where the intestine becomes narrow. The patient develops a colicky pain, as the muscles of the intestinal wall contract in an attempt to dislodge the stone, and vomits profusely. Often the symptoms settle and then recur, because the obstruction of the intestine is not complete. The vomit contains food at first, then bile and, finally, material from the lower part of the bowel which consists of the waste left over after food has been digested.

An operation to remove the stone is essential.

# Cancer of the Biliary Tract

Cancer of the gallbladder is rare. Cancer of the bile ducts is rarer. Gallbladder cancer usually occurs in elderly women and the first symptom is jaundice or pain in the gallbladder area. The outlook is not good since the tumour has usually spread by the time symptoms develop.

Cancer of the bile ducts usually occurs in men over fifty and more frequently in people who suffer from ulcerative colitis, although the reason for this is not known. Symptoms include jaundice, pain in the gallbladder region and weight loss. As with cancer of the gallbladder, the outlook is poor but radiotherapy is sometimes helpful and, if the tumour is entirely confined within the liver, a liver transplant may be possible.

## Investigations for Disease of the Biliary Tract

There are a number of investigations that are in use to diagnose gallbladder and bile duct disease and to differentiate the various conditions from each other.

Three types of blood test are used. The first is a full blood count. A raised number of white cells in this suggests that the patient has an infection (although not necessarily in the biliary tract). Thus the count will be raised in acute cholecystitis and cholangitis but normal in chronic cholycystitis or if there is a stone in the bile duct.

Blood may also be taken for liver function tests. These measure certain enzymes and other substances produced by the liver. Various abnormalities suggest different biliary tract problems.

If a patient is thought to be suffering from acute cholecystitis or cholangitis, blood may be cultured in order to detect whether there are any bacteria in it.

There are also three types of X-ray in use. The first is the plain abdominal X-ray which will demonstrate the 10 per cent of gallstones that are radio-opaque because they have a large amount of calcium in them. A cholecystogram is a test which has been in use for many years. The patient is given a radio-opaque dye which she takes by mouth the night before the X-ray. This is absorbed from the intestine and excreted by the liver into the bile. An X-ray will show the gallbladder full of the dye and, if there are stones present, these will appear as dark holes. However, if the gallbladder is not functioning, the dye will not be concentrated by it and nothing more will be seen than was apparent on a plain X-ray. Other reasons for the gallbladder not being shown are the loss of the dye from vomiting or diarrhoea before it can be absorbed from the intestine.

The third type of X-ray is intravenous cholangiography. In this, the radio-opaque dye is injected into a vein. It is excreted in a concentrated form by the liver and often it is possible to see the bile ducts as well as the gallbladder. It is particularly useful when the biliary ducts need investigation after the patient has had the gallbladder removed.

More recent techniques include ultrasonography, biliary scintigraphy, endoscopic retrograde cholangiopancreatography and percutaneous transhepatic cholangiography. The first of these consists of using a small instrument which sends an ultrasound beam through the body tissues and analyses the beam which they reflect back. It is an extremely safe and easy procedure and, since it is as accurate as a cholecystogram and can provide more information, it is tending to replace the older investigation in many centres. In acute cholecystitis it often demonstrates gallstones and an inflamed, distended gallbladder. It also shows up the bile ducts and the liver. It is particularly useful in patients in whom cholecystography is useless (those with a non-functioning gallbladder and those who are jaundiced) and in patients in whom it is inadvisable (such as pregnant women who should avoid all unnecessary X-rays).

Biliary scintigraphy involves the use of a radioactive chemical which is injected into the bloodstream and is then excreted into the bile. A scan shows the bile ducts and gallbladder.

Endoscopic retrograde cholangiopancreatography (ERCP) is used to examine the bile ducts and the pancreatic ducts and is especially useful in patients who are jaundiced. A flexible telescope (endoscope) is passed through the patient's mouth into the small intestine and a radio-opaque dye is injected through the ampulla of Vater. This travels up and flows into the biliary and pancreatic ducts. X-rays are then taken which allow diagnosis of abnormalities within the ducts.

Percutaneous transhepatic cholangiography (PTC) consists of an injection given, under local anaesthetic, through the skin into the liver, using a very fine flexible needle. A radio-opaque dye is injected and this outlines the bile ducts within the liver and the larger ducts which arise from them. This investigation can be especially helpful in locating the position and determining the cause of an obstruction in the biliary tract and it is used particularly for jaundiced patients who have been shown, on ultrasound, to have abnormally dilated bile ducts within the liver.

## Recent Advances

A technique known as extra-corporeal shock-wave lithotripsy (ESWL) which has for some time been used in the treatment of kidney stones has recently been used for gallstones. A shock wave is transmitted through water to the gallstone region and this causes the stones to shatter. The gravel that remains passes easily down the bile duct into the intestine. A German trial in which 200 patients were treated found that over 90 per cent remained free of stones a year later. Since then, a new machine had been developed. When this is used together with ultrasound to locate the stones, the treatment takes less than an hour, an anaesthetic is usually unnecessary and the patient need only stay in hospital for two days. It is thought likely that this form of treatment will be suitable for about 25 per cent of all patients.

Attempts to dissolve stones using chenodeoxycholic acid and ursodeoxycholic acid, mentioned above, have not been very successful due to the high rate of recurrence after treatment is stopped. However, at the Mayo Clinic in Rochester, Minnesota, another substance, methyl tertbutylether (MTBE), was injected into the gallbladder. After several treatments, the stones were found to dissolve rapidly. This technique was used in a modified form by doctors in Glasgow, who inserted a long fine tube into the ampulla of Vater, using an endoscope with its upper end protruding from the patient's nose. MTBE was then injected down the tube. The subjects were ten elderly patients whose stones were too large to be removed endoscopically. In eight, the bile duct was found to be completely free of stones after an average of eight hours' treatment. The other two patients were operated on and were found to have stones low in cholesterol which, it seems, are less likely to respond well to MTBE.

# Complementary Treatment

*Acupuncture*
Jaundice is said to be due in some circumstances to damp heat in the Gallbladder channel and specific points will be used to eliminate this and to remove the obstruction to the flow of Chi which has resulted.

*Aromatherapy*
Several oils may be recommended for patients with gallstones, such as bergamot, eucalyptus, chamomile and hyssop.

*Herbalism*
Certain herbs known as cholagogues stimulate the flow of bile, helping to prevent stagnation within the gallbladder. Dandelion leaves, for example, stimulate the liver and help to reduce cholesterol levels. Echinacea may be prescribed for an infection in the biliary tract.

*Homoeopathy*
A large number of remedies may be suitable for the treatment of biliary colic, including berberis, dioscorea and chelidonium, and may help to prevent further attacks.

*Nutrition*
Lecithin, which is a natural emulsifier, can be taken as a supplement to help to keep cholesterol in solution in the bile and prevent the formation of stones. Globe artichokes stimulate the flow of bile and may prevent stagnation in the gallbladder.

# Glandular Fever

## Incidence and Symptoms

Glandular fever, otherwise known as infectious mononucleosis, is a very common condition. It can attack people of any age but usually tends to affect adolescents and young adults. It seems likely that in younger children it takes the form of a slight flu-like illness, because there are many people who can be shown to be immune to glandular fever but who have no recollection of ever having had the disease. It is caused by a virus, known as the Epstein Barr (or EB) virus but is not particularly infectious. However, mini-epidemics do occur, usually in boarding-schools, military barracks or other institutions where young people live in close proximity to each other. The virus is thought to be transmitted in the saliva and therefore can be passed on by kissing – in fact, glandular fever is sometimes referred to as 'the kissing disease'.

The onset of the illness is usually gradual, with fever, headache and a general feeling of being unwell. After a few days, the lymph glands swell up, especially those in the neck, armpits and groins. However, they are not usually tender and, unless the swelling is severe, may not be noticed. Between 50 and 80 per cent of patients develop a sore throat and in some cases this may be very severe, with badly inflamed and ulcerated tonsils. The fever rarely goes above 40°C (104°F) but may last up to three weeks.

In 95 per cent of cases, the liver is affected and this can be demonstrated by blood tests. However, only 5 per cent of patients develop jaundice (although occasionally this may be the first sign of illness) and liver failure is rare. The liver (which is situated under the ribs on the right) is often enlarged, as is the spleen (which is under the ribs on the left). Very rarely, the spleen may rupture – a potentially fatal condition in which the patient develops severe abdominal pain and rapidly becomes pale and sweaty with a thready pulse due to internal bleeding. Urgent hospital treatment is required.

Between 10 and 40 per cent of patients develop a generalized red rash. In most cases, the lining of the nose and throat becomes slightly swollen and, very rarely, this may be severe enough to cause problems with breathing. Other rare complications include meningitis and paralysis, which usually resolve of their own accord, and disorders of the immune system.

However, an almost universal symptom of glandular fever is fatigue. Although full recovery is normal, the patient may continue to suffer from fatigue for a long time after the other symptoms have disappeared.

## Investigations

Glandular fever is diagnosed by a blood test, known as a Paul-Bunnell test. Abnormal white cells (mononuclear cells, which give the disease its alternative name) can be seen when the blood is examined under a microscope.

## Orthodox Treatment

Treatment consists of bed rest and gradual rehabilitation as the symptoms recede. However, in some cases, steroids may be used. Prednisolone given for twelve days in decreasing doses is known to speed recovery and its use seems justifiable in patients who have an important event coming up – for example, those who are about to take final examinations or to get married. Hydrocortisone is used to reduce severe swelling of the lining of the nose and throat and steroids are also given to patients who develop some of the rarer complications such as paralysis.

Patients with glandular fever should not take part in contact sports until they are completely recovered, because of the risk to the spleen. A ruptured spleen requires emergency treatment consisting of blood transfusions and surgery to stop the intra-abdominal bleeding.

People whose immune systems are functioning poorly (for example, those taking anti-cancer drugs) may be given the antiviral agent, acyclovir, for seven to ten days to help them to fight the infection.

Sometimes prolonged symptoms of fatigue may be helped by a two-to-three-month course of antidepressants.

## Complementary Treatment

_Aromatherapy_
Lavender, eucalyptus, peppermint or bergamot may be recommended.

_Herbalism_
Herbs may be given to strengthen the nervous system (such as St John's wort or vervain), to help to fight the infection (such as echinacea or marigold), to reduce the fever (such as elderflower or yarrow) and to cleanse the lymphatic system (such as wild indigo, poke root or marigold).

_Homoeopathy_
Carcinosin is usually the remedy of choice for glandular fever. However, in some cases, other remedies may be appropriate – for example, phytolacca if the glands remain swollen and sore after the fever has subsided and the patient complains of headaches and generalized pains. For cases where symptoms have been present for a long time, bacillinum, kali iod., calc. iod. or baryta carb. may be prescribed.

# Hair
# Loss

## The Mechanism of Hair Growth

The average person has about 100,000 scalp hairs and loses between twenty and a hundred of these each day. Hair growth is not continuous – a hair will only grow to a certain length before dropping out and being replaced by another. The length of hair varies according to its site and according to the individual. Thus the eyebrows and body hair are shorter than the scalp hair and, whereas some people can grow their hair until they can sit on it, with others it will never grow much beyond shoulder-length.

Each hair follicle, from which the hair itself grows, goes through a cycle that starts with great cellular activity (the catagen phase). This is followed by the anagen or growing phase in which the hair develops and lengthens, and, finally, the telogen phase during which the hair is shed and the follicle rests before once again entering the catagen phase. In a normal person about 85 per cent of the scalp hairs are in anagen at any one time.

Hair loss can be divided into two main groups – diffuse and patchy. Patchy hair loss can then be broken down into primary hair loss, in which the problem lies in the hair or its production, and secondary hair loss, in which hair cannot be produced because the follicles have been damaged.

# Male Pattern Baldness

CAUSE AND SYMPTOMS

This is the commonest form of primary diffuse hair loss, affecting many men in middle age, although it may begin as early as the teens. It is an inherited condition but only occurs in the presence of male hormones, so that a eunuch would not go bald. (Perhaps this underlies the popular idea that bald men are sexy!)

Once the hair loss has begun, it is usually progressive, but the length of time over which it occurs is very variable. Some men become quite bald over a period of two or three years, while others gradually lose some hair but never become completely bald. Hair is lost at the front of the scalp and on the temples and also on the crown. However, even in the most severe cases, a ring of hair always remains at the base of the skull and the sides.

ORTHODOX TREATMENT

Until recently, orthodox medicine had little to offer the balding man although, for some, hair transplants have proved effective. Hair plugs are taken from the area at the base of the skull which, it seems, are unaffected by the male hormones, and are inserted into the bald areas, where they continue to grow.

However, a new drug has been produced which can induce regrowth of hair in bald areas. Known as Regaine, its active ingredient is minoxidil which is used, in tablet form, to treat high blood pressure. One side effect of these tablets is increased hairiness in some patients and it was the observation of this that led to the research which resulted in the production of Regaine. Unfortunately the preparation does not work for everyone. It is most likely to be effective in men who have recently started to go bald and it is unlikely to help those who have been balding for more than ten years or whose bald patch is more than 10 cm (4 in) across. It comes as a fluid which, to begin with, must be applied twice a day to the bald patch for at least four to six months. If it has not worked within this time, it is unlikely to do so. Once it has started to work, it must continue to be used, as stopping treatment will allow the baldness to take over again. Several trials of minoxidil have shown that over 50 per cent of patients have significant regrowth of hair within a year of starting treatment, and many of the other patients notice a slowing down or stopping of the balding process. Side effects include irritation and redness of the bald area and, because some of the drug gets absorbed through the scalp into the blood stream, increased hair growth in other areas such as the beard or the ear. Minoxidil is available only on private prescription and is quite expensive.

## Female Baldness

Some middle-aged and elderly women tend to lose their hair but the loss is usually just from the crown and rarely proceeds to total baldness of the area. It may occur in young women, in which case it is often associated with an excess of male hormones and can be treated with hormone therapy.

Sometimes baldness can result from underlying diseases, the commonest being thyroid disorders and iron-deficiency anaemia. Tension on the hair caused by styles involving tight plaiting, or by wearing rollers for prolonged periods, may produce bald patches, and both perming and bleaching may damage the hair.

## Telogen Effluvium

Sometimes a large number of hair follicles suddenly go into the resting phase (or telogen) so that the hair is shed. The reason for this is unknown but the condition is most commonly precipitated by a severe illness or by childbirth. Hair loss usually begins three or four months after the event and may be quite severe. Nail growth may also be affected. However, the hair cycle returns to normal within a few months and the hair starts to grow again. Other conditions which may be associated with telogen effluvium are thyroid disease, iron deficiency and rapid weight loss from dieting.

# Drug-induced Alopecia

Some drugs may cause hair loss. Commonest among these are the cytotoxic drugs used in the treatment of cancer. Others include anticoagulants, thyroid drugs, allopurinol (used in the treatment of gout), the contraceptive Pill and the retinoids used in the treatment of skin conditions such as acne and psoriasis. Hair growth usually begins again when the patient stops taking these drugs.

_PRIMARY PATCHY HAIR LOSS_

# Alopecia Areata

This is a fairly common condition, affecting both sexes and producing small or large patches of hair loss. It usually affects children and young adults, only 25 per cent of patients being over the age of forty. One quarter of those affected have a close relative who has also suffered from the condition. Many patients have had atopic conditions (eczema, asthma or hay fever), or these diseases may run in the family. Alopecia is sometimes seen in patients suffering from auto-immune diseases (in which the body is attacked by its own immune system), such as thyrotoxicosis, Addison's disease and pernicious anaemia, and this has led to the theory that a disorder of the immune system may be involved in this type of hair loss.

Women are affected as often as men. Usually there is a fairly sudden onset, with the discovery of a round or oval bald patch, frequently on the head but occasionally in the beard area or elsewhere on the body. The hair loss may be complete or there may be so-called 'exclamation mark' hairs visible. These short hairs, usually seen at the edges of the patch, derive their name from their appearance, since they taper towards their base. If they are pulled with tweezers, they come out very easily. In children, it is more common to see black dots on the bald surface, indicating the position of the abnormal hair follicles. The skin itself is normal, although sometimes it may be a little pinker than usual. Sometimes the nails become pitted and deformed and, in the most severe cases, may be lost completely.

Rarely, all the scalp hair is lost – this is known as alopecia totalis and is commonest in children who have had atopic conditions. Even more rarely, loss of all the body hair may occur as well – alopecia universalis. In one study of alopecia areata, it was found that 54 per cent of children and 24 per cent of adults who had the disease progressed to alopecia totalis and, of these, 21 per cent of children and 30 per cent of adults did not get their hair back again.

In most cases, however, the hair begins to regrow – often within two to three months and usually within a year. At first the new hair is fine and downy and often white but it becomes stronger and pigmented with time. In some cases, as the hair regrows other bald patches appear. The more extensive the hair loss, the less likely is a complete recovery. However, sometimes hair may start to grow again after many years of baldness.

ORTHODOX TREATMENT
Steroids given by mouth will induce regrowth of hair in many cases but patients often relapse once the treatment is stopped. In addition, it is inadvisable to give children steroids unless it is unavoidable. Injection of steroids into the scalp (by a special technique which uses pressure to force the fluids in and is therefore painless) is often helpful. Some cases respond to PUVA (see section on psoriasis) and others to minoxidil (see above).

# Trichotillomania

Some patients (usually children) develop bald patches because they get into the habit of rubbing a particular area of the scalp or pulling a section of hair. The hairs can be seen to be broken off close to the surface. Most children grow out of the habit but if it is associated with other anxieties or problems, patients may need psychiatric help.

SECONDARY HAIR LOSS

# Destructive or Scarring Alopecia

This may result from burns, severe infections of the scalp or X-ray therapy to the scalp. Some skin disorders such as lichen planus, scleroderma and discoid lupus erythematosus may also cause localized baldness. Scarring may be seen but is not always apparent. When a bald patch is small and due to a non-recurring cause, such as a burn, plastic surgery may be possible.

# Complementary Treatment

*Aromatherapy*
Oils of lavender, sage or thyme may be recommended.

*Herbalism*
Because alopecia areata often seems to be brought on by stress, herbs with relaxant properties, such as chamomile, balm and vervain, may be helpful.

*Homoeopathy*
Phos. ac. or staphysagria may be helpful if hair loss follows emotional problems, and cinchona if it appears after an illness.

*Hypnotherapy*
Because alopecia areata may sometimes be precipitated by an emotional upset, hypnosis may speed recovery by relieving anxiety and teaching the patient how to cope with stress.

# Herpes Simplex

There are two types of herpes simplex virus, known as HSV 1 and HSV 2. Both are very common. HSV 1 is mainly responsible for causing cold sores while HSV 2 produces genital herpes. However, approximately 5 per cent of cases of genital herpes are due to the HSV 1 virus, the infection probably having been transmitted during oral sex.

## Cold Sores

Eighty per cent of the population have antibodies to HSV 1 which means that, at some time, they must have been infected with the virus. However, only a minority – about eight million people in the UK – have recurrent symptoms.

The first attack, or primary infection, usually occurs in childhood. Mothers who have HSV 1 antibodies pass them through the placenta to their infants, who are thus protected for the first year or so of their lives. But after this, the immunity dwindles and primary infection is commonest between the ages of one and five.

In a large number of cases, no symptoms at all occur at the time of the primary infection. However, some children react quite severely to the virus. The mouth and throat become painful and the child is feverish, unwell and unwilling to eat. The gums swell and may bleed. Shallow white ulcers develop on the tongue, gums and the lining of the mouth and throat, and saliva may dribble from the mouth if the child finds it painful to swallow. The lymph glands in the neck may become swollen and tender. In mild cases, the worst is over within three to five days but in more severe cases the infection may take up to two weeks to subside. If the child is unable to drink because of the pain from the ulcers, hospital admission may be necessary so that fluid can be given by an intravenous drip.

Occasionally one of the fingers may be the site of primary infection in the form of a herpetic whitlow. The area becomes swollen and painful and then blistered over a period of seven to ten days, finally subsiding over the next month.

Once the herpes virus has got inside the body it can lie dormant in the tissues, ready to cause trouble if the patient's resistance drops, through stress, injury or illness. Fortunately, the recurrences are never as severe as the primary infection can be. Attacks may also be brought on by cold, exposure to strong sunlight or menstruation. A group of small blisters appears, usually on the lips or round the mouth; after a few days, they burst and then scab over. Healing normally takes ten to fourteen days.

## Genital Herpes

This is a very common infection which is usually sexually transmitted. In 1985 there were over 20,000 new cases in the UK. As in the case of cold sores, the primary infection is usually the most severe although, in women, there may be no symptoms if all the blisters develop high up in the vagina.

In genital herpes, either in the primary infection or the recurrence, blisters may occur in the vagina, on the cervix and on the vulva in women, on the shaft of the penis in men, around the anus or even on the buttocks and thighs. In male homosexuals they commonly involve the anus and back passage. The patient may be aware of a burning, tingling or itching sensation in the affected skin for a few hours before the blisters appear. These then break down to form shallow, very painful ulcers. Female patients may have a watery vaginal discharge. The lymph glands in the groins may become enlarged and tender, and, if there is an ulcer close to the urethral opening, passing water may be very painful. Indeed, this may be so severe as to cause complete urinary retention, which needs urgent medical treatment.

An individual attack lasts between three and five days, and patients may have many attacks during the course of a year, although the average is three to four. The infection may continue to recur over a number of years before eventually dying out.

## Complications of Herpes Infections

The commonest complication, especially of cold sores, is bacterial infection. If this occurs repeatedly, there is a risk that the affected skin will become scarred.

Patients who suffer from eczema (even if it is quiescent at the time) may react very severely to a herpes infection, developing eczema herpeticum or Kaposi's varicelliform eruption, in which there is a widespread rash and fever. In severe cases, the blisters cover a large amount of the body surface and, if untreated, almost 10 per cent of patients will die. This type of infection may also occur in people who are suffering from burns. It is therefore vital that anyone with an active cold sore should avoid all contact with patients who have eczema or burns.

One of the most worrying complications of cold sores is the development of ulcers on the surface of the eye, since not only are these painful but they can cause scarring which may lead to blindness.

If a patient's resistance to infection is very low, he may develop a generalized herpes infection which, in severe cases, can cause death from hepatitis or encephalitis. This is most likely to occur in patients whose immunity has been lowered by intensive cancer therapy or by AIDS, or in newborn babies whose mothers are suffering from a genital herpes infection at the time of delivery. In the case of a baby, the first symptoms of fever, vomiting, diarrhoea, breathing problems, jaundice and convulsions usually appear on the fifth day of life. Often the infection is fatal. It is standard procedure, therefore, to do a Caesarean section for any mother who is suffering from herpes when her pregnancy comes to term, rather than allow a vaginal delivery.

## Investigations

These are usually unnecessary since the diagnosis is obvious in most cases. However, a swab taken from a blister can be cultured to show the virus.

## Orthodox Treatment

Drying agents such as surgical spirit encourage the ulcers to crust over and help to diminish the pain. Povidone-iodine also works in this way as well as having a mild anti-viral action and its use may help to prevent bacterial infection from occurring.

In recent years, specific anti-viral agents have been developed, including idoxuridine and acyclovir (ACV). Both of these, in ointment form, have been used in the treatment of herpes eye infections, while ACV, given as tablets or intravenously, has been found to reduce considerably the mortality from generalized herpes. Intravenous ACV may also be necessary for patients whose genital herpes has caused retention of urine. Applied locally, ACV can be useful in the treatment of both cold sores and genital herpes but needs to be used as soon as symptoms begin and before the blisters appear. Patients who suffer from frequent severe recurrences of genital herpes can be treated with ACV taken orally over a period of several months.

## Recent Advances

In 1985 it was announced that research had shown that it was possible to produce a vaccine which could reduce the frequency and severity of recurrent attacks of herpes. However, at the time of writing, this has yet to be developed.

# Complementary Treatment

*Aromatherapy*
Lavender, lemon and geranium are among the oils that may help to dry up a cold sore.

*Herbalism*
Echinacea may be used to promote the body's defences against viral infection. Golden seal, St John's wort, myrrh or calendula tinctures may be applied topically to act as an antiseptic and to promote healing. St John's wort is also a painkiller.

*Homoeopathy*
Any number of remedies may help to prevent recurrences of cold sores or genital herpes but the prescription depends very much on the individual patient.

*Nutrition*
The herpes virus needs the amino acid arginine in order to thrive; lysine, however, will prevent it from flourishing. A diet that is low in arginine and high in lysine is therefore likely to be recommended during an attack, plus a supplement of lysine. Arginine is found in peanuts, cashew nuts, pecan nuts, almonds, chocolate, edible seeds, peas, non-toasted cereals, gelatin, carob, coconut, wholewheat and white flour, soya beans, wheatgerm, garlic and ginseng. Fish, chicken, beef, lamb, milk, cheese, beans, brewer's yeast and mung bean sprouts are high in lysine and low in arginine.

# Self-help

Because it seems as though there may be a link between genital herpes infection and cancer of the cervix, all women who have recurrent attacks should have a cervical smear every year.

Female patients with cold sores should take care when applying or removing make-up to avoid spreading the virus. All patients should, when washing, dry their eyes before drying the infected area and should also avoid kissing or sharing cups, cutlery, towels or flannels during the course of the infection.

Fresh lemon juice applied to a cold sore as soon as the itching begins may promote rapid healing.

## Organizations

The Herpes Association, 41 North Road, Islington, London N7 9DP (tel. 071-609 9061), provides information and advice for people suffering from herpes.

# High Blood Pressure

## (Hypertension)

---

## Definition

In medical parlance, high blood pressure is known as hypertension, tension in this respect meaning pressure. Blood pressure is measured using an instrument known as a sphygmomanometer ('sphyg' for short) of which there are now various types available. The traditional sphyg has a column of mercury which travels up a graduated glass tube to show the pressure that is being exerted on the patient's arm by an inflatable cuff. Blood pressure is therefore measured in millimetres of mercury (abbreviated to mm Hg). Two readings are taken as the pressure in the cuff is slowly released. The first is where the doctor, listening with a stethoscope over an artery at the patient's elbow, starts to hear the sound of a pulse and the second is where that sound becomes muffled or disappears. The first reading is known as the systolic pressure and corresponds to the pressure in the arteries when the heart contracts, pumping blood through them. The second reading is the diastolic pressure, which corresponds to the pressure in the arteries when the heart relaxes allowing it to fill up with more blood.

Normal blood pressure is usually said to be 120/80 but, in fact, there is a range of values around this which could all be taken as normal. For example, 110/70 or 125/85 are normal for many people. Because of this range, it is difficult to say exactly where high blood pressure begins. The World Health Organization defines hypertension as a level of 165/95 or more, recorded in a sitting patient. Below 140/90 is defined as normal and the range between 140/90 and 165/95 is regarded as 'borderline'.

Usually, when trying to diagnose hypertension in a patient, a doctor will take a series of readings, since there are many factors which can affect the level of the blood pressure. For example, anxiety or excitement can cause it to rise but it will drop when the patient is very relaxed or asleep.

## Essential and Secondary Hypertension

In the vast majority of cases, no underlying illness can be found to account for the patient's hypertension, which is therefore said to be 'essential'. It has been suggested that the condition of the blood vessels and their response to a number of hormonal and nervous stimuli may be partly responsible but it seems likely that, in any one case, a combination of many factors is involved. In many cases, hypertension and atheroma (hardening of the arteries) seem to go hand in hand. Each seems to make the other worse and it is hard to say whether one condition initially caused the other (a chicken-and-egg situation) or whether a third factor is responsible for causing both.

Essential hypertension usually begins during the thirties or forties and, very often, there is a family history of the condition. It is particularly common in black people, in whom it may be quite severe. However, in some 5 per cent of patients, some definite abnormality can be found which has resulted in 'secondary' hypertension. This may occur at any age.

Twenty per cent of all cases of secondary hypertension are due to kidney disease. Because it is vital that blood flows steadily through the kidneys to have its waste products and excess water removed, the kidneys have a special mechanism for controlling their own blood flow. If the blood pressure drops, a substance known as renin is released, which acts on a protein in the blood (angiotensin I) to produce angiotensin II. This latter substance not only acts directly on the blood vessels, constricting them and thus raising the blood pressure, but also stimulates the secretion of the hormone aldosterone, whose effect is to raise the blood pressure. Thus the flow of blood through the kidneys returns to normal and, when it has done so, no more renin is secreted. It is thought that kidney disease causes hypertension by interfering with this mechanism and causing a steady excretion of renin.

The commonest form of kidney disease to produce hypertension is chronic pyelonephritis (described in the section on urinary tract infections). When only one kidney is affected, its removal may bring the blood pressure back to normal. Another condition which can be treated surgically is renal artery stenosis. In this, the artery which supplies blood to the kidney is constricted, so that the blood flow is reduced.

A similar condition affecting the aorta (the main artery leading from the heart) is known as coarctation and, like renal artery stenosis, it is commoner in males than in females and can be corrected surgically. Coarctation is rare and only causes hypertension in the upper part of the body, making it relatively easy to diagnose. It is usually apparent before the patient reaches the age of thirty.

Other causes of secondary hypertension (all of which are rare) include conditions in which the adrenal glands produce an excess of hormones that have the effect of raising the blood pressure. In Cushing's syndrome excessive quantities of steroids are secreted. In the very rare Conn's syndrome the hormone produced is aldosterone. And the tumour known as a phaeochromocytoma (or 'phaeo' for short), which may occasionally be found outside the adrenals, produces large amounts of adrenaline and noradrenaline.

In Cushing's syndrome, the patient may become obese, although the legs remain thin, and his face becomes moon-shaped and flushed. Woman may notice that they are becoming hairy. Patients suffering from Conn's syndrome may complain of weakness, headache, cramps and tingling, and may pass large amounts of urine. The symptoms of a patient with a phaeochromocytoma are often intermittent, as is the hypertension, and attacks may be precipitated by a number of things, such as emotional upsets or exertion. The symptoms include severe headache,

211

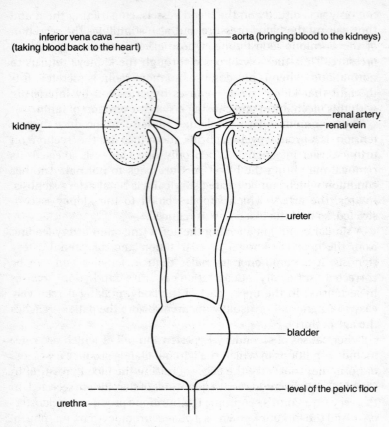

inferior vena cava
(taking blood back to the heart)

aorta (bringing blood to the kidneys)

kidney

renal artery
renal vein

ureter

bladder

level of the pelvic floor

urethra

_The urinary tract_

nausea, vomiting, abdominal pain, sweating and a rapid heart rate. Fortunately, removal of the tumour will cure the condition.

## Investigations

Because hypertension can be secondary to other conditions, it may be necessary to do a number of investigations before making a definite diagnosis of essential hypertension. This is especially the case if the patient is relatively young.

*Examination*
The doctor may feel the pulses in the patient's groins – if they are less full than they should be, this may be a sign of coarctation of the aorta. An abdominal examination will enable him to feel whether the patient's kidneys are abnormally large. He may also listen to the abdomen with a stethoscope, since a murmur can be heard in 50 per cent of the patients who have renal artery stenosis.

*Urine*
The urine may be examined for protein and blood since these may be found in kidney disease or in advanced cases of hypertension. It may also be tested for sugar, which is sometimes found in the urine of patients who have Cushing's syndrome or a phaeochromocytoma. If protein is detected, a collection of the total urine passed over twenty-four hours may be required for an assessment of kidney function.

*Blood*
Blood may be taken to test for urea (a waste product whose level rises in kidney failure) and for potassium (which may be low in Conn's syndrome, Cushing's syndrome and renal artery stenosis). It may also be taken when the patient is fasting to test for cholesterol and fats, since high levels of these may be associated with hypertension and an increased risk of heart attack.

*Ophthalmoscopy*
The doctor may examine the back of the patient's eyes with an ophthalmoscope, since this is the one place in the body that a clear view can be obtained of the blood vessels. Early signs of hypertension include spasm of the arteries, which appear narrowed. As the condition advances, the vessel walls become thickened and opaque, which gives them, at first, a coppery appearance and, later, a silvery look. Little patches of blood may be seen where the vessels have leaked. In the severe form of high blood pressure known as malignant hypertension (see below), the optic disc which is visible as a light-coloured circle at the back of the eye becomes swollen and its edges become blurred.

Small haemorrhages and fluffy-looking white patches, or exudates, formed by protein leaking from the vessels may also be visible.

*Aortography*
This is done only if renal artery stenosis is suspected. A needle is inserted into the aorta (usually through the femoral artery in the groin) and a dye is pumped in which will show up on X-ray. The renal artery branches off from the aorta and will be clearly outlined by the dye.

*X-rays*
A chest X-ray may be done, since it will show up any enlargement of the heart that has resulted from long-standing hypertension. (Such enlargement will also be shown by an electrocardiogram or ECG.) Occasionally an X-ray of the kidneys may be performed.

*Tests for Cushing's, Conn's and Phaeochromocytoma*
Various specialized tests are available to diagnose these conditions, most of which involve collection of the urine over twenty-four hours, plus blood tests.

# Symptoms of Hypertension

In the early stages, patients may have few symptoms. Indeed, it is not at all uncommon for hypertension to be discovered during the course of a routine medical examination, the patient having been quite unaware that his blood pressure was raised.

Among the symptoms that may occur are headaches, which are often at the back of the head and present on waking and which tend to wear off during the course of the day. Nosebleeds are not uncommon. Patients may also complain of noises in the head, dizziness, irritability, visual problems or palpitations.

As the hypertension progresses, further symptoms may arise as a result of the damage that it causes to various parts of the body.

# Dangers of Hypertension

High blood pressure is always treated, even if the patient has no symptoms, because of the damage that it can do. Borderline hypertension is usually treated if the patient has symptoms.

Surveys have shown that patients with hypertension have an increased risk of stroke, heart failure, coronary heart disease and kidney disease. Treatment has been shown to reduce the mortality from strokes and kidney failure and, although there is less evidence that it protects patients from heart attacks, the newest medications have not been in use for long enough to be assessed in this respect.

### Left Ventricular Failure (LVF)

Hypertension puts strain on the left side of the heart, which receives blood from the lungs and pumps it out to the rest of the body. As a result, the left side of the heart enlarges (left ventricular hypertrophy) and, ultimately, may be unable to cope with the work, in which case its function deteriorates (left ventricular failure). Patients who have LVF may experience shortness of breath due to the pooling of blood in the lungs. This is commonest when they lie down and they may wake feeling breathless during the night.

### Coronary Heart Disease

One of the commonest sites at which atheroma (hardening of the arteries) occurs is within the coronary arteries that supply the muscle of the heart with blood. The rate at which atheroma is formed is speeded up in patients with hypertension and may cause angina or a heart attack.

### Cerebrovascular Disease

The arteries supplying the brain may also get furred up. High blood pressure may result in weaknesses appearing in the walls of these arteries, which can then haemorrhage, causing a stroke or even death.

*Kidney Damage*
The kidneys may be damaged by high blood pressure, even when kidney disease has had nothing to do with causing the condition. In severe cases, kidney failure may occur.

*Malignant Hypertension*
In some 2 per cent of cases, the blood pressure rises very high and can cause widespread damage, resulting in death within about a year if it is untreated. Fortunately, the introduction of modern drugs now means that the life expectancy for these patients is almost normal once they are on treatment.

Malignant hypertension is commoner in men than in women and usually occurs between the ages of forty and sixty. The small blood vessels in the kidneys, eyes and brain are severely damaged, resulting in renal failure, deteriorating eyesight and mental confusion. Left ventricular failure also occurs. If untreated, the patient may have fits, lapse into coma and die from renal failure or from a stroke.

# Orthodox Treatment

## SECONDARY HYPERTENSION
Treatment will depend upon the underlying cause. Often, as in the case of coarctation of the aorta and renal artery stenosis, it is surgical. Surgery also has a part to play in the treatment of Cushing's and Conn's syndromes and phaeochromocytoma, when the tissue responsible for the excessive hormonal secretion may be removed, after which any residual hypertension is treated with drugs. Kidney disease which is causing hypertension may require the kidneys to be removed and either dialysis or a transplant performed.

## ESSENTIAL HYPERTENSION
The GP may suggest some or all of the measures given under 'Self-help' below. They are all worth trying, since, it is sometimes possible to reduce the blood pressure to normal levels without the use of drugs.

*Thiazide Diuretics*

These are often the first drugs to be given to a patient with hypertension. Their main action is to make the kidneys excrete more water, thus reducing the volume of blood circulating round the body, but they probably also cause a relaxation in the blood vessels, both of these actions resulting in a drop in the blood pressure.

Although they may take up to eight weeks before their full benefit is felt, the thiazide diuretics have many advantages. They have minimal side effects and rarely need to be stopped because of these. They can be used in combination with other blood-pressure drugs and will enhance their effect. In addition, they are useful in the treatment of black patients, who often don't respond to some of the other drugs, such as beta blockers.

The main disadvantage of thiazide diuretics is that they cause the body to lose potassium. Although this may not be a problem in the short term, it may ultimately produce symptoms such as weakness and muscle cramps. Patients who are on the heart drug digoxin are particularly likely to develop abnormal heart rhythms if they become short of potassium, and so will always be given a potassium supplement if they are put on thiazide diuretics. Some doctors like to give all patients on thiazides a potassium supplement and combined preparations are available.

Thiazide diuretics may cause a build-up of uric acid in the blood and so are unsuitable for patients who suffer from gout. They may also precipitate gout in those who have not previously suffered from it. Rashes may occur and, occasionally, dizziness and tiredness during the first few weeks of treatment.

Drugs in common use include bendrofluazide, chlorothiazide and cyclopenthiazide.

*Loop Diuretics*

These work in a different way from the thiazide diuretics and are not commonly used in the treatment of hypertension. However, they are useful for patients who are suffering from kidney disease. They, too, may cause the potassium level to fall and the uric acid level to rise, and they may cause disturbances in the levels of fats, calcium and other minerals in the blood. They include

217

frusemide and bumetanide, which are also available combined with a potassium supplement.

## Potassium-sparing Diuretics

These diuretics, which include amiloride and triamterene, have the advantage that they do not cause a drop in potassium levels in the blood. They are also less likely than the other diuretics to cause a rise in uric acid, although this may still occur. They are unsuitable for patients with kidney failure and may cause sexual side effects such as impotence. Weakness, cramps, swelling of the breasts in men and disturbance of the menstrual cycle in women may also occur.

## Beta Blockers

These are probably the commonest drugs to be used in the treatment of hypertension. Although they may sometimes produce unpleasant side effects, they have been available for a considerable time and are therefore tried and tested.

The way in which beta blockers act to reduce blood pressure is not absolutely clear. It is known, however, that they prevent the hormones adrenaline and noradrenaline from acting on so-called beta receptors in the brain, heart and lungs, and in the muscle layers in the walls of the blood vessels. Stimulation of the beta receptors in the brain causes a rise in blood pressure, of those in the heart (known as beta-1 receptors) an increased rate and force of heartbeat, and of those in the blood vessels and lungs (known as beta-2 receptors) relaxation of the vessels and of the bronchioles of the lungs. Beta blockade produces the opposite effect. The earliest beta blockers prevented all beta stimulation and therefore were unsuitable for use in asthmatic patients, since they could cause constriction of the bronchioles and precipitate an asthmatic attack. These non-selective blockers, which can also cause cold hands, fatigue and unpleasant dreams, include propranolol and oxprenolol, which are still used for suitable patients. However, propranolol seems to work less well in smokers.

Selective beta blockers block only the beta-1 receptors and include metoprolol and atenolol. They are more suitable for asthmatics and can be used for insulin-dependent diabetics, whereas the non-selective blockers may mask hypoglycaemic attacks and are therefore not suitable.

Side effects of the beta blockers include a slow heart rate, fatigue – especially on exercise – dizziness and sexual problems such as impotence.

## Vasodilators

Vasodilators – drugs that cause dilation of the blood vessels – are normally used in combination with a diuretic or a beta blocker or both.

### HYDRALAZINE

Although vasodilators are useful drugs, they have a considerable range of side effects which may, however, be reduced if they are used in combination with other types of anti-hypertensive therapy. Hydralazine may cause headache, a rapid heart rate, palpitations, tremor, nausea, dizziness, weakness, tiredness and flushing of the skin. However, it is safe in pregnancy. A derivative of hydralazine is minoxidil.

### PRAZOSIN

This is less likely to cause palpitations than hydralazine but patients may faint after the first dose due to a sudden drop in the blood pressure. Advice is usually given, therefore, to take the very first dose on going to bed at night. It is customary to start with a small dose and gradually increase it during the following weeks.

### ALPHA BLOCKERS

Prazosin is thought to prevent constriction of the blood vessels by blocking stimulation of the so-called alpha receptors in their walls. Another drug, labetalol, is both an alpha and beta blocker. At the time of writing a preparation called dozazosin has been developed but not yet licensed for use. It seems to give effective control of the blood pressure in both black and white patients and has the advantage of lowering the blood cholesterol while raising the levels of HDL (high density lipoprotein), which appears to have a protective effect against atheroma. It seems to be safe for use in patients with diabetes, asthma or gout, and, unlike beta blockers, does not cause impotence. There may be side effects, however, and these include tiredness, dizziness, fluid retention, blurring of vision, headache and constipation.

*Calcium Antagonists*

These drugs, which include nifedipine and verapamil, have only recently come into general use but are becoming increasingly popular. Originally they were thought to act by controlling levels of calcium in the body fluids but the mechanism has been shown to be a great deal more complicated than this.

They can be used in patients who have diabetes or angina, and indeed they seem to have a preventive effect against the development of atheroma. They also seem to relieve spasm in the coronary arteries that supply the heart muscle and are therefore useful in the treatment of patients with angina. Unfortunately, they produce an effective lowering of blood pressure in only about 50–60 per cent of patients, although others may respond if one of the drugs is combined with a beta blocker or an ACE inhibitor (see below). The main side effects include headache, palpitations, nausea, swelling of the ankles and flushing, but these are less likely to occur with slow-release preparations. A recent discovery is that the calcium antagonists may also cause swelling of the breasts in men, although this will subside once the drug is stopped.

*ACE Inhibitors*

These, too, are recently developed drugs. ACE stands for angiotensin-converting enzyme, an enzyme which plays a vital role in the conversion in the blood of angiotensin I into angiotensin II. The action of the drugs is to prevent this reaction from taking place. Angiotensin II has a powerful constricting effect on the blood vessels and its production is stimulated by the excretion of renin from the kidneys (see above).

The ACE inhibitors, which include captopril and enalapril, are effective in about 90 per cent of patients but may need to be used together with a loop diuretic or a calcium antagonist.

*Older Drugs*

Before the beta blockers came on the market, the drugs in use for the treatment of hypertension worked in a fairly crude way on blood-pressure-controlling receptors in the brain. As a result, they had many side effects and, since the development of newer therapies, they have tended to be used less and less. However, two – methyldopa and clonidine – are still used in certain situations and, like other older drugs, continue to be used for patients who have been taking them for years and are happy on them.

Methyldopa is the drug of choice in pregnancy, since it is known to be perfectly safe. Indeed, if a woman who is hypertensive is planning to get pregnant, her GP may decide to change her medication so that she is already established on methyldopa by the time she conceives. There will therefore be no risk to the baby. It may be combined with hydralazine, which is also safe in pregnancy.

Methyldopa and clonidine are useful drugs for patients with renal problems because they do not reduce the flow of blood to the kidneys. In the United States, clonidine is now available as a transdermal patch – a sticking plaster which contains the drug and slowly releases it into the skin over a period of time.

Side effects of methyldopa and clonidine include drowsiness, dizziness and a dry mouth. Methyldopa may cause headaches and clonidine may cause constipation. An additional problem with clonidine is that it must not be stopped suddenly after a prolonged period of therapy, since this may result in the blood pressure rising rapidly. It is important, therefore, that patients who take clonidine never run out of their tablets.

# Complementary Treatment

*Acupuncture*

Hypertension is said to be due to hyperactivity of the yang (or masculine, positive) aspect of Chi or to an accumulation of phlegm and damp. Treatment consists either of reducing yang and stimulating yin (the balancing, feminine, negative aspect) or of expelling phlegm and damp. There are also some specific points whose use will bring down the blood pressure.

*Aromatherapy*
Clary sage, lavender, melissa, lemon and ylang ylang are some of the oils that may be prescribed.

*Herbalism*
Mistletoe, hawthorn, lime blossom and garlic are among the remedies used by herbalists in the treatment of hypertension. Mistletoe dilates the blood vessels, slows and steadies the heart rate, and is a diuretic. Hawthorn dilates the coronary blood vessels and slows and stabilizes the contraction of the heart. Lime blossom is particularly useful for patients who are anxious or tense since, as well as dilating the blood vessels and being a diuretic, it has a relaxant effect. Garlic dilates the blood vessels and also reduces the amount of cholesterol in the bloodstream.

*Homoeopathy*
The choice of remedy is vast since there is no set pattern of symptoms for patients with hypertension. However, glonoine may be effective for patients who suffer from pounding head-aches, palpitations and a feeling of fullness in the chest, while those complaining of weakness, dizziness and a fear that they will collapse may respond well to gelsemium.

*Hypnotherapy*
By teaching the patient to relax and to cope with stress, hyp-notherapy can be useful in the treatment of hypertension.

*Manipulation*
This may help in so far as it can relieve physical tension and muscle spasm.

*Nutrition*
Vitamins C, B complex and E will help to keep cholesterol levels down and regulate blood clotting; vitamin C also keeps the arteries healthy.

# Self-help

There are a number of steps that the hypertensive patient can take which should help to control his blood pressure. Indeed, in some cases of mild hypertension such self-help measures may be all that is necessary and the use of drugs may therefore be avoided.

Blood pressure tends to be higher in overweight, sedentary people and in those who smoke. The patient should therefore try to keep relatively slim, give up smoking and take regular gentle exercise. Recent studies have shown that reducing alcohol intake is beneficial for hypertensive patients. The role of salt in the development of hypertension is still being debated by specialists. However, studies have shown that in communities where the salt intake is low throughout life, high blood pressure tends not to occur. Some studies have shown benefits in reducing the amount of salt in the diet but the effects seem to be a highly individual thing – possibly genetically determined. It is worth reducing one's salt intake, therefore, to see whether it is helpful in one's own case. A low fat diet is also beneficial, but a study done in the United States has shown that a certain amount of olive oil in the diet can help to reduce the blood pressure. Fresh fruit and vegetables contain potassium and this, too, seems to have a lowering effect on the blood pressure.

Naturopaths may recommend excluding sugar, coffee and red meat from the diet.

Certain drugs may contribute to a rise in blood pressure. It is usually recommended that women whose blood pressure rises while they are on the contraceptive Pill should come off it. If necessary, they may take the progestogen-only Pill, since it is the oestrogen component which is responsible for the rise. Anti-inflammatory drugs (NSAIDs) which are taken by arthritic patients may also affect the blood pressure, but substituting a simple painkiller such as paracetamol may bring it down again.

Anything which will help to reduce stress and promote relaxation, such as yoga or meditation, will also be beneficial.

# Impotence

## Definition

Impotence is defined as the inability to achieve or sustain an erection adequate for satisfactory intercourse. It is extremely common, affecting about one man in every ten at some time or another.

## Causes

Both erection and ejaculation are reflex involuntary actions, governed by nerves running from the spine to the genitalia. However, they are also controlled to some extent by psychological stimuli and are dependent on an adequate output of male hormones (androgens). But because they are reflex actions, they cannot be made to happen voluntarily – a man cannot decide to have an erection in the same way that he can decide to raise his arm or open his mouth.

It is thought that just over half of all cases of impotence are psychogenic – that is, they are due to psychological problems. Temporary impotence is common during any illness or if the patient is anxious, depressed or under stress. Very often, one episode of impotence occurs when the man is tired or has had

224

too much to drink and, as a result, he begins to worry about his sexual performance. This makes it more difficult for him to have an erection next time he tries, and a vicious circle arises in which his impotence causes anxiety and his anxiety causes impotence.

Of those cases that are due to a physical cause, 27 per cent are caused by diabetes, and 32 per cent by injury. Long-term or permanent impotence may be due to disease of the blood vessels, hormonal abnormalities, diseases involving the nervous system (particularly diabetes), alcohol or drug abuse, certain prescribed medicines, damage to the spine or pelvic area, unavoidable damage during a prostatectomy or operations on the bladder or rectum, or problems affecting the penis itself.

The penis contains two spongy compartments which, when a man becomes sexually excited, fill up with blood, causing it to become stiff. If the blood vessels which run into the penis are badly affected by atheroma (hardening of the arteries), blood cannot flow as readily and this may be a cause of impotence. When atheroma is widespread, resulting in inadequate amounts of blood being delivered to the legs and causing pain on walking and poor healing, the condition is referred to as peripheral vascular disease. Fifty per cent of men who suffer from this will be affected by impotence.

To achieve an erection a properly functioning nervous system is necessary, since this controls the initial dilation of the blood vessels supplying the penis and the relaxation of the muscles in the spongy compartments which allows blood to flow in. It is probably also responsible for closing down the outflow of blood from the penis, thus helping to keep it erect. Diseases that interfere with this will cause impotence. Diabetes is the commonest of these (see section on diabetic neuropathy). Other causes include multiple sclerosis and damage to the lower end of the spinal cord, from which the nerves run to the penis.

Patients who have low circulating levels of male hormones will suffer from impotence but, because the hormonal lack will also reduce their libido (sex drive), they rarely complain about their impotence. Medication with oestrogen, in the treatment of cancer of the prostate for example, will have the same effect.

Both illegal and prescribed drugs may cause impotence. Those that most commonly do so are cannabis, opiates (such as morphine and heroin), barbiturates, drugs that lower the blood pressure (particularly bethanidine, guanethidine, methyldopa and beta blockers), diuretics and the tricyclic antidepressants. Alcohol frequently has the same effect.

Peyronie's disease is a problem affecting the penis in which fibrous plaques develop, so that it is no longer soft and mobile. When an erection occurs, the penis can't stretch correctly and becomes deformed. This may be associated with pain. The cause is unknown but some cases seem to resolve after a few years.

## Diagnosis

It is very important that impotence due to a psychological cause should be differentiated from that due to a physical cause. Sometimes this will be apparent from the history. A patient who still has early morning erections and who can masturbate satisfactorily has psychogenic impotence. This type usually has a sudden onset whereas physical impotence, in which an erection becomes impossible under any circumstances, is more likely to come on gradually.

Impotence may also be classified as primary or secondary. A man with primary impotence has never been able to have intercourse whereas secondary impotence comes on later in life, after a previously satisfactory sex life. The type of onset, however, gives no clue as to the cause.

## Investigations

If it is suspected that a man has physical impotence, there are various investigations that may be used to determine the cause. Initially, the doctor will examine the penis and testes, looking for signs of any abnormality, and will take the patient's blood pressure. He will also check the pulses in the legs and feet, since absence of these will suggest that there is a problem with the blood vessels. The urine will be tested for sugar in case impotence is the first sign of diabetes. Checking the reflexes in the legs and testing the genital area for sensation to touch and vibration will indicate whether or not the problem is one involving the nervous system.

If a hormonal problem is suspected, blood will be taken to test for hormone levels. If the patient is referred to a hospital consultant further investigations may be undertaken, including the use of a special stethoscope to measure the blood pressure in the penis. The ability to have an erection while asleep can also be determined. Normally, some degree of erection will occur during periods of rapid eye movement (which correlate with episodes of dreaming). This is known as nocturnal penile tumescence or NPT. Patients with psychogenic impotence will continue to have normal NPT, while in those whose impotence is due to a physical cause it will be reduced or absent. NPT is usually measured by a small device called a mercury strain gauge, consisting of a piece of mercury-filled tubing put round the penis and attached to a measuring instrument.

The injection of papaverine into the penis will always cause an erection unless the blood supply is seriously impaired or blood is leaking out of the penis as fast as it is flowing in. Patients who fail to have an erection after such an injection may then be investigated by more sophisticated tests to determine the exact problem that affects their blood vessels. These include the injection into the bloodstream of a substance that shows up on X-ray. Screening then shows whether the failure of the erection is due to blood leaking out of the penis.

## Orthodox Treatment

If impotence is due to psychological causes these have to be treated. In simple cases, where impotence has occurred as a result of the man's anxieties about his own performance, reassurance may be all that is necessary. In other cases, psycho-sexual counselling may be very helpful in restoring the patient's sexual function to normal. However, where there is a long-standing problem or the cause is a very deep-rooted one, it may be a considerable time before the patient responds to therapy.

Various substances can be injected into the penis to produce an erection, the most popular of these being papaverine. As mentioned above, this will not help patients whose impotence is due to disease of the blood vessels, but all others will respond, including those with psychogenic impotence. It is sometimes prescribed for patients whose problem is psychological, since it can be remarkably effective in restoring their self-confidence. Usually they only need to use it a few times but have the assurance of knowing that they can resort to it again if it is ever necessary. Patients with physical problems, however, need to continue with the injections long term. Once they have been taught how to inject themselves, most patients find it very simple. It is important that the correct dose is determined from the start, since an overdose can produce a prolonged erection (priapism) which, after a number of hours, can become very painful. There is then the risk of the blood clotting and gangrene occurring. Fortunately, only 4 per cent of those using the injection develop a prolonged erection and this can be treated by an injection of metaraminol and heparin, which will counteract the papaverine and get the blood flowing again.

In young men whose impotence is due to problems with the blood vessels leading to the penis, surgery is now available which attempts to restore the blood flow. This is a very specialized technique and has about a 50 per cent success rate. For those patients whose blood flow is poor because of atheroma in the larger blood vessels supplying the lower part of the body, an operation on these vessels may restore potency as well as improving the blood supply to the legs. Surgery may also be able to prevent blood leaking from the penis during an erection.

When a patient is unsuited to any of these forms of treatment, a penile implant may be the answer. These devices are of two basic types – those that are semi-rigid and those that can be made rigid by pumping fluid into them. One type has a fluid-filled reservoir implanted into the patient's abdomen and a pump into the scrotum. Squeezing the pump causes an erection and, at the end of intercourse, pressing a valve releases the fluid back to the reservoir. The simplest, semi-rigid, implant makes the penis permanently erect, but can be bent into position. The implant does not interfere with ejaculation or with the patient's fertility.

Although the insertion of an implant is a simple and quick operation, waiting-lists on the NHS are long. A private hospital which has recently opened in the Bristol area claims to be the first to specialize in the treatment of impotence. Patients have to be referred by their own general practitioner and treatment may cost several thousand pounds.

## Recent Advances

Research in Canada has shown that a new drug, called yohimbine, may be helpful in the treatment of both psychogenic and physical impotence. At the time of writing, it is still in the experimental stage.

A device known as ErecAid has been produced which, for some patients, may be a practical alternative to a penile implant. It consists of a type of condom which is placed over the penis and it uses suction to bring on an erection. The erection is then maintained by placing a constriction band around the penis. The device is being used in the United States and a study of its use by ten diabetic patients at Leeds General Infirmary showed that most of them found it easy to use and effective. ErecAid is available through general practitioners from Cory Bros., Hospital Contract Co. Ltd, 4 Dollis Park, London, N3 1HG (tel. 081-349 1081), and cost £199 in 1989.

## Complementary Treatment

_Acupuncture_
Impotence is said to be due to a lack of the yang (positive, male) aspect of the Chi of the kidney or to damage to the Chi of the heart, spleen and kidney, which may result from emotional problems. Points are chosen which will strengthen the yang of the kidney or the Chi of heart, spleen and kidney.

_Aromatherapy_
Various oils may be recommended, including cinnamon, clove, mint and pine.

## Herbalism

Certain herbs have a hormone-like effect on the male reproductive system and may be used in the treatment of impotence. They include damiana and saw palmetto. Ginseng, too,
may help to improve the hormone balance. Other herbs with a
relaxant effect may be helpful for patients with psychogenic impotence.

## Homoeopathy

Impotence in the elderly or impotence which has occurred as
the result of an illness may respond well to sabal serrulata. If
it follows injury, arnica may be helpful. In the early stages
agnus castus may restore the patient's sexual function to
normal but for chronic cases lycopodium may be prescribed.
If impotence is associated with anxiety, arg. nit. may be
appropriate.

## Hypnotherapy

Hypnosis can be very valuable for treating any complaint which
is triggered off or made worse by anxiety and so may be appropriate for the patient with psychogenic impotence. Not only
can techniques be used to teach the patient to relax and to
relieve him of his anxiety about his sexual performance, but
analytical techniques may, in certain cases, be used to try to find
out the underlying reasons for his problems.

## Nutrition

Impotence may be associated with low levels of zinc, so supplements of this mineral may be recommended, together with
vitamin $B_6$, which works with it in the body.

# Organizations

Although a general practitioner may refer patients for psycho-
sexual counselling, it is also available through some family
planning clinics. Information about other clinics offering psycho-
sexual counselling is available from the Association of Sexual
and Marital Therapists, PO Box 62, Sheffield, SIO 3TS.

Information about all aspects of impotence is available from the National Impotence Information Centre, Freepost, Staines House, 158–162, High St, Staines, TW18 1BR.

# Incontinence

## Incidence

Incontinence of urine is a very common problem, mainly involving women. It is estimated to affect about 5 per cent of young women who have never been pregnant, 10 per cent of all young to middle-aged women and 20–40 per cent of older women. But in a recent survey, over 50 per cent of those women suffering from incontinence said they were too embarrassed to discuss the problem with their GPs. Many thought it would clear up by itself and nearly a third waited over five years before seeking help. This is a sad state of affairs, since, if left, the condition will not improve and may get worse, whereas treatment offers an excellent chance of cure.

## How the Bladder Works

(See the diagram of the urinary tract on p. 212.) The bladder receives urine from the kidneys in frequent small spurts. Two rings of muscle, or sphincters, at the base of the bladder prevent leakage into the urethra, the tube which leads to the outside. One of these rings, the internal sphincter, is under the control of the autonomic nervous system which regulates automatic reactions over which we cannot exert will-power, such as breathing and digestion. The second ring, the external sphincter, is under voluntary control and it is this that we consciously relax when we wish to pass water. During urination, the muscle in the bladder wall (the detrusor muscle) contracts and helps to push the urine out. For this system to function normally, the entire bladder and the upper part of the urethra have to maintain their position above the muscle layer that makes up the 'pelvic floor'; if the pressure becomes raised in the abdomen (for example, by coughing, sneezing, laughing, straining or other exercise), it will affect the urethra as well as the bladder. However, if the bladder drops, any rise in pressure will affect the bladder alone and will force urine through the sphincters and down the urethra. Women are more likely to suffer from incontinence than men because the muscles of the pelvic floor and the urethral sphincters can be damaged during childbirth.

## Causes of Incontinence

Stress incontinence is a condition in which any rise in intra-abdominal pressure (from coughing, laughing and so on) causes a slight loss of urine. This happens when the urethral sphincters are not functioning correctly and is usually due to damage to the sphincters themselves or to the ligaments that hold the bladder in position, or both. In mild cases, vigorous activity or a bad fit of coughing may be necessary for incontinence to occur but in severe cases a slight cough or even a change of posture may result in urinary loss. Patients are usually women over 40 who have had one or more children. The condition may, however, appear for the first time during pregnancy, although it usually clears up after the baby is born.

Urge incontinence is the condition in which the patient suddenly feels the need to pass water and may be unable to get to the toilet in time. This is due to abnormal contractions in the detrusor muscle of the bladder which increase the pressure within the bladder above that which can be controlled by the urethral sphincters. It may occur as a result of urinary infection, diabetes or a disease of the nervous system but, in many cases, the cause is unclear. Very occasionally, it may be produced by a slipped disc which is pressing on the nerves that supply the bladder.

Some patients suffer from a combination of stress incontinence and urge incontinence. In such cases, the urge incontinence usually disappears once the stress incontinence has been treated.

Incontinence may also be due to retention in the bladder of abnormally large amounts of urine. As more urine flows into the bladder from the kidneys, the pressure overcomes the urethral sphincters and overflow occurs in which some urine is passed but the bladder is not completely emptied. Usually this condition results either from an inability of the bladder to contract and expel its contained urine or from an increased resistance, which prevents normal emptying. If the pressure within the bladder becomes abnormally high, there may be back-pressure on the kidneys which can be damaged as a result. Retention with overflow may be due to damage affecting the nerves that supply the bladder, for example injury to the spinal cord, multiple sclerosis or extensive surgery in the pelvic area, so that the patient can no longer sense when the bladder is full. Increased resistance, preventing normal emptying, may be due to an enlarged prostate gland in men or a large fibroid or ovarian tumour (benign or malignant) in women.

Rarely, patients may have an abnormal exit (fistula) between the ureter, bladder or urethra and the skin surface or the vagina, which means that they are permanently wet. This may be due to a congenital abnormality or may result from injury or surgery.

## Investigations

An initial assessment can be made by the GP and sometimes this is all that is necessary for a diagnosis to be made. He will test the nervous system by looking in the patient's eyes and checking her reflexes and the strength of her muscles, and will examine the abdomen to see whether the kidneys are unduly large or whether any abnormal mass can be felt. An examination of the back passage will allow the doctor to assess the size of the prostate gland in a male patient and will also tell him whether there is any faecal impaction – a condition of chronic constipation in which rock-hard faeces (stools), accumulate in the back passage. This can cause transient incontinence in patients of either sex, particularly in the elderly. In a woman, an internal examination through the vagina will allow the doctor to detect any degree of prolapse, which may be associated with stress incontinence. The patient may be asked to cough and, if this causes a leak the doctor may proceed to do Bonney's test in which he places two fingers high up in the vagina, so that they are supporting the bladder neck. The patient is then asked to cough again. If, under these circumstances, there is no leak, it suggests that an operation which lifts the bladder neck back up above the pelvic floor will cure the condition.

For patients in whom the diagnosis is not so clear, further tests may need to be undertaken by a specialist. Uroflowmetry necessitates the patient attending the clinic with a full bladder and then passing water, in privacy, into a special machine which records the rate of flow. Somewhat less sophisticated is the pad test in which the patient drinks a large amount of fluid and then, wearing a special pad which will absorb the urine, performs various physical exercises over a period of thirty to sixty minutes. This may be useful if the patient is uncertain about the degree of activity that causes her to be incontinent.

If it seems that a neurological disorder may be the cause of the patient's problems, measurements can be taken of the activity of the muscles of the pelvic floor, using a special instrument.

A slightly uncomfortable but very useful test is cystometry, which actually measures the pressure within the bladder and can differentiate between excessive resistance at the bladder neck and an under-active or over-active detrusor muscle. A fine tube (catheter) is passed into the bladder and another into the back passage, through which the intra-abdominal pressure is measured. A known amount of fluid is put into the bladder and the level at which the patient feels a desire to pass water is noted. In a normal bladder, the desire is first felt when it contains about 150 ml and becomes strong at around 400 ml.

The pressure within the bladder is measured and, when the pressure in the back passage is subtracted, this gives an estimate of the pressure being exerted by the detrusor muscle. Finally, the patient is asked to pass water into a special machine which measures the rate of flow. The whole test takes about thirty minutes. Sometimes the fluid instilled into the bladder is one which can be seen on X-ray and a film can be taken of the whole sequence. This is known as videocystourethrography, or VCU.

## Orthodox Treatment

The treatment of incontinence depends on the cause. If there is any evidence of infection, this will be treated with antibiotics. If the patient has a fistula, this can be treated surgically.

For patients who are suffering from stress incontinence, particularly younger women, exercises which increase the strength of the pelvic floor may be useful. After the menopause, weakness in these muscles may be due to a lack of oestrogen, so hormone replacement therapy may be effective.

A comparatively new method of treatment which seems to be proving successful is the use of a series of vaginal cones. These are made from plastic, are 5 cm long and contain different metal weights. One is inserted into the vagina with its pointed end downwards. It tends to fall out, so the patient has to use her muscles to keep it in place. When she becomes skilled at retaining the cone, she replaces it with another which is heavier. By the time she can keep the heaviest cone in place, her pelvic muscles will be working well.

In the post-menopausal patient, incontinence may result from thinning of the tissues of the urethra. The use of an oestrogen cream, applied to the vagina, can sometimes be remarkably effective in such cases, as mentioned in the section on the menopause.

For those in whom these methods fail, there are several types of operation available which raise the bladder up into the abdomen, either by passing a sling (about 1 cm wide) under the bladder neck or by attaching the vagina walls to tissues higher up in the pelvis, so that the urethra is lifted. About 80 per cent of patients are cured by operation, good results being less likely in those who are obese. However, even after an initial failure, a second operation may be successful. Following an operation, patients must be very careful to avoid heavy lifting or straining as these may undo the good results.

Urge incontinence may be helped by drug treatment in about 60 per cent of cases. The drugs used have an effect on the nervous system, reducing the excessive activity of the detrusor muscle. They include propantheline, terodiline and imipramine (which is also used in the treatment of bed-wetting in children). Unfortunately, many patients complain of side effects, which include a dry mouth, blurred vision and constipation. Occasionally, an injection into the bladder wall of local anaesthetic or phenol solution may reduce its irritability.

For a patient who has no apparent neurological cause for her urge incontinence, bladder retraining may be helpful. For seven days, she keeps a diary in which she records how much she drinks, how often she passes water and how much urine she produces. Then she tries to increase the length of time she can go without urinating and, over several weeks, works at developing better control of her bladder. Another method is biofeedback, in which the patient has up to eight one-hour treatment sessions during which a catheter is inserted into her bladder and, as fluid is instilled into it, she is taught how to use various techniques to reduce her feeling of needing to pass water. Both these methods can be very successful but may have a high relapse rate if patients do not continue to practise the techniques.

The treatment of retention with overflow is the treatment of the primary cause. When no specific treatment (such as prostatectomy) is appropriate, surgical enlargement of the urethra may be helpful. Various drugs may be used, including prazosin, bethanechol and carbachol, and antibiotics if necessary. Some patients may have to practise intermittent self-catheterization in which they insert a tube into the bladder in order to empty it completely.

If all else fails, or if the patient is unsuitable for or refuses surgical treatment, there are two alternative methods of treatment. In mild cases, incontinence pads or appliances may be appropriate. The most modern versions are well designed so that discomfort and smell are reduced to a minimum. For more severe cases, the patient may need a permanent catheter which is linked to a collecting bag taped to the upper leg.

Recently an artificial urinary sphincter has been developed which has proved revolutionary in the treatment of some patients who had seemed condemned to a life of catheters. It consists of an inflatable cuff which goes round the bladder neck and which is connected by a fluid-filled tube first to a pump near the skin surface and then to a reservoir of fluid in the pelvis. The patient can activate the pump which deflates the cuff and the bladder then empties slowly over a couple of minutes. After this, the cuff automatically reflates. Unfortunately the device is very expensive and the surgeon needs special training in order to be able to insert it, so it is not widely available. Complications include a breakdown of the mechanism, so that the bladder cannot be emptied, and irritation of the surrounding tissues by the cuff. However, in over 80 per cent of cases, the device has proved successful.

## Recent Advances

In Norway, doctors have found that electrical stimulation of the pelvic floor by a device inserted into the back passage for several hours a day over a period of nine months produced a significant improvement in over 60 per cent of the 121 women taking part. All had been incontinent for a considerable number of years and 40 per cent had regained complete continence by the end of the course.

## Complementary Treatment

_Acupuncture_
Incontinence is said to be caused by a deficiency of Chi in the kidney and spleen. Treatment consists of using specific points to strengthen Chi in these organs and their related channels.

*Aromatherapy*
Oils of cypress or pine may be recommended.

*Herbalism*
Various herbs may be used in the treatment of incontinence,
including agrimony, horsetail, marshmallow root and yarrow.

*Homoeopathy*
Gelsemium may be helpful in the treatment of men whose
incontinence is associated with an enlarged prostate. For stress
incontinence or a slow stream with dribbling, causticum may be
effective. Baryta carb. and cantharis may be appropriate for
elderly patients.

## Self-help

Because the intra-abdominal pressure may be raised by constipation or obesity, these should be avoided. A high fibre diet containing plenty of fresh fruit and vegetables is helpful. Patients with
incontinence tend to reduce the amount they drink but this may
be counterproductive, since it may result in constipation or
urinary infection. They should therefore drink plenty, although
reduced amounts at night may be sensible. Another reason for
drinking plenty is that dilute fresh urine has very little smell.
Therefore patients using pads who change them regularly and
who do not allow their urine to become concentrated need have
little fear of having a detectable odour.

Advice is available from a number of sources. Coloplast is a
company which manufactures incontinence pads and appliances.
It has a confidential advice service which is manned by trained
nurses and which offers help on all aspects of incontinence. To
contact the service, dial 100 and ask the operator for Freephone
Coloplast. The company also produces some helpful leaflets.

Another pharmaceutical firm has published a series of booklets
including one on self-catheterization. These are available from
Simcare, Peter Rd, Lancing, W Sussex, BN15 8TJ (tel. 0903
761122).

Age Concern has produced a series of leaflets on incontinence aimed at elderly patients. They are available free, with a stamped addressed envelope, from Age Concern England, Bernard Sunley House, 60 Pitcairn Road, Mitcham, Surrey, CR4 3LL (tel. 081-640 5431).

Advice on laundry services and home-help services for the incontinent is available from local social services departments (addresses in the phone book).

# Infertility

## Incidence

Most people, when they get married, expect to be able to have a family. For those who find that they cannot, the discovery can be very traumatic. Nowadays, infertility is not an uncommon occurrence – it affects some 10–15 per cent of all couples. The increased incidence may be due to a number of causes, not least of which is the fact that many women are delaying their first pregnancy until their late twenties or early thirties and many of them have used contraception such as the Pill or the IUCD (coil) for several years beforehand. It is thought that the Pill may interfere with the hormone balance in susceptible women – indeed, in a few, it may cause long-term loss of periods (amenorrhoea) – and the IUCD may act as a focus of infection, resulting in pelvic inflammation and blocked tubes. Even if she has not used these methods, an older woman may find it harder to get pregnant, since fertility declines after the age of thirty-five and after forty-five pregnancy is rare.

However, if one looks at 100 women who have just started trying to get pregnant, 25 will be successful during the first month, another 38 in the following five months, a further 12 in the next three months and, by the end of a year, between 80 and 90 of the group will have become pregnant. The more

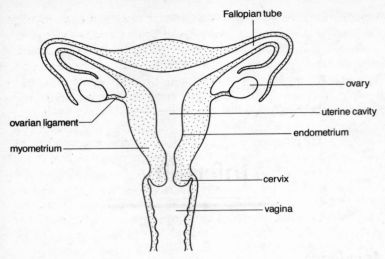

*The female reproductive system*

frequently a couple has intercourse, the greater the likelihood of pregnancy, with 83 per cent of those having intercourse more than three times a week being successful within six months. However, during the same period, only 16 per cent of those who have intercourse less than once a week will get pregnant.

## Causes of Infertility

In those couples who do not conceive, there may be one or more reasons for their failure. The man may have too low a sperm count; the woman may not be ovulating or the egg, when produced, may not be able to travel down the Fallopian tube to the womb. The womb itself may be abnormal – for example, there may be fibroids present, which can interfere with the implantation of a fertilized egg. Or the sperm may be unable to swim into the womb because of hostile secretions in the vagina. In some 10 per cent of cases, the cause of infertility is never established.

Ovulation – the maturation of an egg and its release from the ovary into the Fallopian tube – is dependent upon normal hormone levels, each stage of the egg's development being under hormonal control. Because the sex hormones are themselves controlled by other hormones produced by the pituitary gland in the brain, anything that disrupts the working of this gland may interfere with the reproductive cycle. It may also interfere with the activity of the adrenal glands and the thyroid, which, like the ovaries, are under pituitary control.

Some 5 per cent of cases of infertility that occur in young women are caused by a condition known as the Stein–Leventhal (or polycystic ovary) syndrome in which large numbers of cysts develop on the ovaries, preventing ovulation. Patients may also have problems with their periods (which can be scanty or infrequent), may become hairy or overweight, and may develop acne.

Blockage of the tubes, so that an egg cannot travel through to the womb, is usually due to a previous infection.

Two conditions which may sometimes cause infertility– fibroids and endometriosis – are dealt with in separate sections (endometriosis will be found in the section on menstrual problems).

In one third of all cases of infertility, it is the male partner who has the problems. Damage to the testes, from mumps or an injury, for example, may result in a low sperm count. Raising the temperature of the testes may have the same effect, which is why a man with a varicocoele (a varicose vein in the scrotum) may be infertile, the heat from the increased blood flow acting to inhibit the maturation of sperm. Male hormones, like female hormones, are under the control of the pituitary gland so, here again, an imbalance may result in reduced fertility. A low sperm count may also be caused by more generalized conditions such as kidney disease or diabetes.

The tube (vas) which carries the sperm from the testes to the penis may, like the Fallopian tubes, become blocked as a result of infection or trauma so that, although healthy sperm are produced, they don't get through into the ejaculate.

## Investigations

Before any investigations are performed, the doctor will need to take a full history from the couple involved to try to see whether

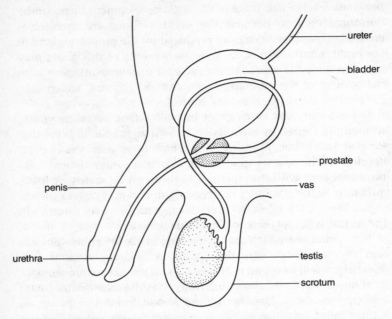

*The male reproductive system, prostate and bladder*

this gives any clues as to what may be causing the problem. Rarely, there may be some obvious abnormality. For example, if the woman has never had a period this suggests that her reproductive system could be underdeveloped or even absent. This may result from a defect in her chromosomes, which can be determined from a blood test.

However, in most cases, the first test to be done is a sperm count. The male partner has to produce a specimen of sperm, by masturbation, which has then to be delivered very rapidly to the local hospital laboratory. Because it is essential that the specimen is kept warm and is looked at within two hours of ejaculation, most hospitals provide facilities for the specimen to be produced on the premises.

If the sperm count is normal, the woman will then be investigated. This usually begins with a full examination, a cervical

244

smear and swabs taken from the vagina and neck of the womb to ensure that there is no infection present. Repeated blood tests may be taken at different stages of the monthly cycle, to see whether her hormones are rising and falling correctly, and she may be asked to take her temperature on waking every morning, since ovulation is often preceded by a rise in temperature.

If it seems that she is not ovulating, other tests may be done to find out why. One reason may be an excessive secretion of the hormone prolactin by the pituitary. This hormone is normally secreted during pregnancy to suppress ovulation and, if excessive amounts are produced when a woman is not pregnant, it will have the same effect and may also interfere with the menstrual cycle. It is a condition that may be brought on by stress (a minor form is the so-called 'boarding-school amenorrhoea', in which young girls stop having periods temporarily after leaving home for the first time) and it may also be due to an enlarged pituitary gland, certain drugs, thyroid deficiency and kidney disease. If a prolactin excess is suspected, blood may be taken for thyroid function tests and the skull may be X-rayed to see whether there is any evidence of enlargement of the pituitary gland.

Ultrasound may be used to investigate the ovaries, to detect cysts or to follow the development of an egg before its release. In order to discover whether or not the tubes are blocked, a hystero-salpingograph or a laparoscopy ('lap.') and dye may be done. In the hysterosalpingograph, a dye is injected into the womb, and X-rays are then taken to follow its flow through the tubes. If there is an obstruction, the exact site will be seen. The advantage of this test is that no anaesthetic is necessary, unlike the lap. and dye, in which a dye is injected into the womb and a small telescope inserted into the abdomen just next to the umbilicus. The gynaecologist can then watch to see whether the dye emerges from the ends of the tubes. Although this method has the added advantage that the ovaries can be inspected for abnor-malities, it does not allow the exact site of a blockage in the tubes to be demonstrated.

If both ovulation and sperm production appear to be normal and there is no evidence of tubal obstruction, a post-coital test may be done to see whether there is some incompatibility between the sperm and the mucus in the neck of the womb. For this, it is necessary for the couple to have intercourse not more than six hours before the woman attends for examination. The test is usually done at mid-cycle, when the cervical mucus should, under hormonal influence, be in such a condition that sperm can pass through easily. A specimen of the cervical mucus is taken and examined under the microscope. The sperm should be seen in considerable numbers, swimming vigorously.

In cases where the man is found to have a low sperm count, the woman will usually be investigated too, to ensure that her reproductive system is functioning normally, but additional tests are carried out on the man. Follicle-stimulating hormone (FSH) is produced by the pituitary gland and its secretion is controlled, via a feedback mechanism, by hormones from the testes. If a man with a low sperm count has high levels of FSH in his blood, it suggests that his testes have been damaged; however, if the levels are normal, this may indicate that there is a blockage in the vas, preventing sperm from being ejaculated. In such a case, a biopsy of the testes may be taken under anaesthetic in order to determine whether or not they are functioning normally.

## Orthodox Treatment

A variety of drugs have been developed to stimulate ovulation in the non-ovulating woman. One of these is clomiphene citrate which is given for five days at the beginning of each cycle. Side effects include hot flushes, palpitations, blurring of vision, abdominal discomfort and depression, which may be quite severe. There is also a risk that, if a woman gets pregnant using clomiphene, she will have more than one baby – 15–20 per cent of cases result in a multiple birth. Another drug, tamoxifen, seems to have fewer side effects, but many gynaecologists prefer not to give either of these drugs for longer than a few months.

Gonadotrophins – hormones that stimulate the ovaries into action – may be given by injection. They are usually given daily for five days or so to bring about the rise in the level of oestrogen necessary for the egg to mature, and then a final injection of a different hormone is given to trigger ovulation. This form of treatment may be continued for up to six months, if necessary, and some 60 per cent of patients get pregnant this way. Again, multiple pregnancy occurs in about 20 per cent of cases.

If an excessive secretion of prolactin from the pituitary is suppressing ovulation, it can be controlled with bromocriptine. Side effects of this drug include dizziness, depression, nausea, vomiting and headache, although these tend to diminish as treatment progresses. If a tumour of the pituitary is responsible for the excessive secretion, bromocriptine may be able to shrink it. However, in some cases, surgery may be necessary.

Patients with the Stein–Leventhal syndrome may respond to treatment with clomiphene but the most successful treatment seems to be to remove a section from each ovary. This restores normal function in up to 80 per cent of cases.

Any infection that is discovered in the course of the investigations will, of course, be treated, but treatment of blocked Fallopian tubes is seldom satisfactory.

If the male partner's fertility has been reduced by the increased heat generated by a varicocoele, an operation may be performed to tie the vein off, so that the testes can return to their correct temperature.

Nowadays, the idea of the 'test-tube baby' is widely accepted and treatment is available, to a limited extent, on the NHS. However, waiting-lists, naturally, are very long. IVF (in vitro fertilization) is used for women whose tubes are blocked, who have been unable to conceive over a long period of time for no apparent reason or whose cervical mucus remains hostile to sperm. It is also used in some cases of male subfertility. The mature egg is removed from the ovary, fertilized and allowed to grow a little before being replaced into the womb where, with luck, it will implant. The egg can be removed either at laparoscopy, the surgeon using the same telescope as in the lap. and dye, or by needle, which he inserts through the vagina, using ultrasound to guide him. Ovulation is usually stimulated by clomiphene and gonadotrophins but recently specialists have found that a newer hormone-like drug, buserelin, is more effective. In one trial, it produced a 50 per cent pregnancy rate, compared with a 25 per cent rate when using clomiphene.

Another form of treatment is GIFT, in which the egg is mixed with the sperm and immediately transferred back into the Fallopian tube so that fertilization occurs there. This technique may be used in cases of unexplained infertility or sperm problems.

AIH (artificial insemination by husband) is used where the only problem preventing pregnancy is a mechanical one – impotence or an inability to ejaculate on the part of the man. AID (artificial insemination by donor) may be used where the male partner is severely subfertile or where a hereditary disorder makes the likelihood of an affected child very probable. The medical history of a potential sperm donor is investigated thoroughly before he is accepted and no one in poor health, with a family history of inherited disorders or with an increased risk of catching AIDS is allowed to become a donor. Once accepted, donors have regular HIV antibody (AIDS) tests, their sperm only being used after each test is shown to be negative. The donor's semen is deposited in the neck of the womb around the time of ovulation. Sixty per cent of women treated become pregnant within the first three months but this form of treatment can be very stressful psychologically.

## Complementary Treatment

_Acupuncture_
The reproductive system is said to be under the control of the kidney and points may be used to stimulate the kidney and the flow of energy through its meridian.

_Aromatherapy_
Geranium, melissa, jasmine and rose may be prescribed.

_Herbalism_
A mixture of herbs may be indicated to promote normal function in the reproductive organs and ensure a proper hormone balance. Among those used are helonias (or false unicorn) root, blue cohosh and agnus castus, which work on the ovaries, pituitary and womb, and, for men, damiana and saw palmetto, which stimulate the function of the testes. Other herbs, such as black

cohosh and liquorice root are useful for both male and female patients.

## Homoeopathy

Conium may be given if infertility is associated with scanty periods, sepia when it is accompanied by a loss of sex drive, apathy and irritability, or aurum when the patient is depressed. Other remedies may also be used depending upon the patient's symptoms.

## Hypnotherapy

A woman who is unable to conceive easily may become very anxious as a result. Unfortunately, this anxiety may, itself, make matters worse by affecting the patient's hormone balance. Hypnotherapy may help to reduce her anxiety levels, by teaching her how to relax.

## Nutrition

Zinc is vital for fertility in both sexes and, since many people are mildly deficient, a supplement of 15 g a day, or more, may be recommended. In addition, vitamin C supplements may help to increase a low sperm count and to promote fertility. Octacosanol and essential fatty acids, which are found in cold pressed vegetable oils, are also important to the normal functioning of the reproductive system. A tablespoon each day of cold pressed vegetable oil, in the form of a salad dressing, is an adequate supplement.

The amino acid arginine may be helpful in cases where sperm motility is reduced. (Not only do sperm have to be plentiful, they also have to be mobile in order to enter the womb and fertilize an egg.) Up to 8 g a day may be prescribed but arginine should not be taken by anyone with a history of schizophrenia.

## Radionics

Some radionics practitioners have a very good record for treating infertility.

## Self-help

Recent studies have shown that men tend to be less fertile if they smoke and that women's fertility can be reduced by a high caffeine intake (from coffee, tea and fizzy drinks). Stopping smoking and cutting down on caffeine is probably advisable for any couple wishing to start a family.

Women whose periods are irregular may find it very hard to know when they are at their most fertile. They, and other women who are having difficulty conceiving, may find an ovulation prediction test helpful. This simple test can be bought at the chemist without a prescription but, unfortunately, is quite expensive. However, it is capable of predicting ovulation thirty-six hours in advance, by measuring a hormone whose level rises just before an egg is released. Brand names include First Response and Clearplan.

## Organizations

The British Pregnancy Advisory Service, Austy Manor, Wootton Wawen, Solihull, West Midlands, B95 6BX (tel. 05642 3225), is a non-profit-making charity which offers services including infertility investigation and treatment, artificial insemination and sterilization reversal.

The National Association for the Childless, Birmingham Settlement, 318 Summer Lane, Birmingham, B19 3RL (tel. 021-359 4887), is a self-help support group which offers advice and information to infertile couples.

# Insomnia

## Incidence and Definition

Insomnia is a very common problem, affecting almost all adults at some time in their lives but women twice as frequently as men. The average adult sleeps between six and eight hours a night but sleeping patterns change as we get older and most elderly people sleep less than this. It is understandable, therefore, that it is among the elderly that most complaints of insomnia are to be found.

Insomnia can be described as transient (when it is due to some unusual experience which interferes with sleep – for example, sleeping in a strange bed), short term (when it is often due to worry or stress) and long term (when it may be due to a variety of factors such as depression, alcohol abuse, drug dependency, pain or habit). A recently recognized form of insomnia is known as sleep apnoea, in which the patient (frequently an obese man) wakes repeatedly during the night as a result of his airway being temporarily cut off by the fat around his neck.

Insomniacs complain that it takes them a long time to get to sleep, that once they are asleep they wake often and that they don't feel refreshed in the morning. Patients with sleep apnoea also complain of nodding off frequently during the day.

# Orthodox Treatment

Doctors are far less willing than they used to be to prescribe sleeping pills, or hypnotics. Barbiturates fell out of favour because they were dangerous in overdose and were addictive. The newer drugs, benzodiazepines, have also been shown to cause dependence, although they are somewhat safer in overdose. However, it is estimated that patients can become tolerant to them (need a larger dose for the same effect) after only a few days' continuous use and it is usually recommended that they are taken for no longer than a few weeks. The patient who is coming off benzodiazepines needs to do so slowly, since stopping suddenly may cause insomnia that is worse than it was before treatment. Some specialists recommend that patients who need benzodiazepines for insomnia take them only every other night or every third night. In this way they can be sure that they will get two or three good nights' sleep a week but will reduce their risk of becoming dependent on the drug. Benzodiazepines may also produce hangover effects although this is less likely with the newer, short-acting preparations.

The longer-acting benzodiazepines include nitrazepam, flurazepam and flunitrazepam. The shorter-acting preparations include loprazolam, lormetazepam, temazepam and triazolam. The latter group may be less suitable for patients who wake early in the morning and are unable to get back to sleep.

Other hypnotics include chloral hydrate (a tried and trusted medication but less pleasant to take than the benzodiazepines) and its derivatives dichloralphenazone and triclofos sodium. A drug with no hangover effects, which is therefore especially suitable for elderly patients, is chlormethiazole. Children should not be given hypnotics but, if absolutely necessary, an antihistamine with a sedative effect such as promethazine or trimeprazine may be used for a short period.

For patients whose insomnia stems from depression, treatment with an antidepressant drug may bring rapid relief. The tricyclic antidepressants such as imipramine and trimipramine have a particularly sedative effect.

Sleeping pills should not be taken by patients with sleep

apnoea, since they can make the problem worse. Patients are advised to lose weight, avoid alcohol after 6 p.m. and stop smoking. In severe cases, a special device can be provided by a chest physician which consists of a mask placed over the patient's nose and a pump which forces air through and keeps the airway open.

# Complementary Treatment

*Acupuncture*
Classical Chinese theory says that insomnia may result from a number of different causes. These include a deficiency of energy in the spleen resulting from anxiety, a lack of yin (the negative, feminine aspect of Chi) in the kidney resulting in fire in the heart, mental depression causing fire in the liver, and retention of phlegm and heat due to indigestion. Other causes are a weakness of the heart and stomach, an imbalance between the liver and gallbladder and a disturbance of the Chi of the spleen and stomach. Whichever organ is affected, the aim of treatment is to restore a normal flow of Chi through it. Fire and phlegm are eliminated where necessary. Where Chi, or its yin aspect, are lacking, these are stimulated. The spirit is said to reside in the heart and points along the Heart channel are used, in appropriate cases, to calm the spirit.

*Aromatherapy*
Oils of chamomile, lavender, neroli, rose, basil and marjoram are among those which have a relaxant effect and which may be helpful in the treatment of insomnia.

*Bach Flower Remedies*
Patients who are suffering from mental and physical exhaustion may be helped by olive. However, when exhaustion has resulted from over-effort by a highly strung person who finds it hard to relax, vervain may be appropriate. White chestnut may be beneficial if the patient's mind is unable to relax and thoughts continue to go round and round endlessly.

*Herbalism*
Many herbs have a relaxant or sedative effect. These include chamomile, balm, St John's wort, lime blossom, passiflora and hops. Vervain and scullcap are useful when insomnia results from nervous tension. On the whole, herbal remedies are non-addictive but valerian, which is a powerful relaxant, may be habit-forming and so is reserved for severe cases and, usually, used for only a short period.

*Homoeopathy*
If insomnia is associated with restlessness and anxiety, aconite may be helpful. If it results from overwork and lack of exercise or from indigestion or excessive alcohol, nux vomica may be appropriate. Sulphur may be prescribed for the patient whose insomnia is worse in the early hours and who is awakened by the slightest noise. If insomnia is associated with nightmares when the patient does fall asleep, belladonna may help. Coffea cruda may be beneficial for the patient who is unable to sleep because her mind is going round and round. For children, chamomilla is often the remedy of choice. For the patient who is unable to sleep until after midnight and then wakes at about 3 a.m., often getting up to have a snack or a drink, pulsatilla may be helpful. A number of other remedies may also prove useful in the treatment of patients suffering from insomnia.

*Hypnotherapy*
Hypnosis can be remarkably effective in the treatment of insomnia. There are three ways in which it may be used. Firstly, it can teach the patient to relax so that she is less likely to be kept awake by anxieties or muscular tension. Secondly, she can be taught how to hypnotize herself and can be given the suggestion that if she does this when she is in bed, she will very quickly fall asleep. In fact, if a patient is left quietly in a hypnotic trance for any length of time, it is quite natural for her to fall asleep, so the suggestion just reinforces this. Thirdly, if there are deep-seated reasons for the patient's insomnia, these can be investigated under hypnosis and she can be helped to resolve them.

*Nutrition*

Calcium, magnesium and vitamin B$_6$ have a tranquillizing effect. Calcium and magnesium are combined in tablet form as dolomite and are also found in seeds, nuts and vegetables. Vitamin B$_6$ must always be taken with zinc, since the two work together in the body. The amino acid tryptophan is a very effective treatment for insomnia, is non-addictive and has no known side effects in the short term. However, its long-term use is not recommended. It takes about an hour to work and is effective for up to four hours. It must not be taken by pregnant women or by those hoping to become pregnant nor by patients who are taking MAOI antidepressants.

# Self-help

Insomnia may start as a transient phenomena and become long term simply because the patient begins to worry about it. It is important, therefore, to remember that a few nights' sleeplessness does no harm and that most people sleep longer than they think they do.

Patients should go to bed only when they are sleepy – going to bed at a set time will almost inevitably result in lying awake on some nights. The bedroom should be warm and quiet. Alcohol and caffeine should be avoided in the hours before bedtime. Some quiet relaxation in the form of a hot milky drink, some music or a good book is helpful. Very often when children can't sleep it is because they have gone to bed in an overstimulated state, having been watching an exciting programme on television or playing an exciting game right up to bedtime.

People who wake in the night should, once they are sure that they will not drop off again right away, get out of bed and do something – read, listen to the radio, write letters or make a hot drink – until they feel tired again.

# Irritable Bowel Syndrome

### (Spastic Colitis)

## Definition and Symptoms

The irritable bowel syndrome (IBS) is a very common condition which can cause recurrent bowel disturbances and attacks of abdominal pain over a long period of time. The cause is unknown but some authorities suggest that it may result from an initial attack of food poisoning or dysentery which makes the bowel hypersensitive, while others think that some of the cases are due to an allergy to a certain foodstuff or to a deficiency of fibre in the diet. Recently it has been suggested that the disorder may lie in the nerves that supply the bowel. The section of bowel affected is the colon (which is why this condition used to be called spastic colitis or spastic colon). Normally, in order to pass its contents along, the muscles in the wall of the colon gently contract and relax, an action known as peristalsis. However, in patients with IBS the colon contracts more than is usual and is also unduly tender.

Although in about 20 per cent of cases painless diarrhoea is the only symptom, most patients with IBS complain of abdominal pain. Classically, this is in the lower left side of the abdomen and is usually relieved by passing a stool or wind. However, the pain may appear on the right lower side of the abdomen, mimicking appendicitis, or on the right side under the ribs, mimicking

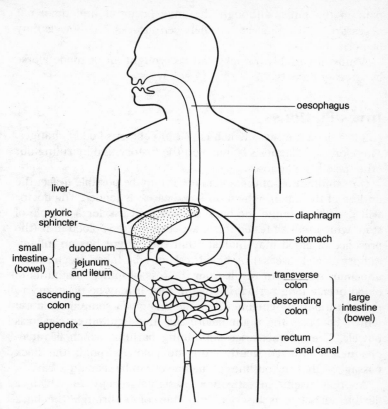

*The digestive system*

gallbladder disease. It may occasionally take the form of indigestion and may be associated with nausea. It can be dull or colicky (coming in spasms) and can sometimes be quite severe. It may be brought on or be made worse by eating and, during an attack, fatty or gas-forming foods (such as vegetables) may make it considerably worse.

The patient may also have constipation or diarrhoea, or both alternately. Sometimes there is mucus in the stools, which may be small, like pellets, or long and thin. After passing a stool, the patient may still feel that he needs to go. Occasionally, there is pain in the anus, although this may occur at any time, not necessarily during defecation. Between attacks, the bowels may be normal.

Almost invariably, attacks can be brought on or made worse by stress or anxiety.

## Investigations

IBS is a benign disease which causes no obvious bodily changes. Therefore the diagnosis is made on the history and by ruling out other possible diagnoses.

On examination of the abdomen, it may be possible to feel the outline of the colon, which, in some cases, is tender. The doctor will usually examine the back passage and ask for a sample of stool which will be tested to see whether there is blood in it (the presence of blood may indicate that the patient has an inflammatory bowel disease). A blood test may be taken to check for anaemia, which can result from the loss of minute amounts of blood over a long period. Following this, it may be necessary to perform a barium enema. The patient is given some medication which he takes the night before the investigation to clear his bowels. Then a substance containing barium, which is radio-opaque, is pumped gently into the colon through the back passage so that the outlines of the bowel can be seen on X-ray.

Another useful investigation is sigmoidoscopy in which a flexible telescope is inserted into the colon through the back passage and the walls of the bowel are inspected. A tiny piece of tissue (biopsy) may be taken in order to exclude an inflammatory disorder. This is a relatively painless procedure and, as well as ruling out more serious diseases, it may help to confirm the diagnosis of IBS. In order to help the sigmoidoscope pass up the bowel, air may be pumped in and this sometimes produces the identical pain that the patient with IBS feels during an attack.

# Orthodox Treatment

Various types of treatment are recommended. It is important for the patient to try to avoid stress and, occasionally, psychotherapy may be appropriate for a particularly anxious person. Between attacks a balanced high fibre diet should be eaten and patients should only avoid specific foodstuffs if repeated incidents have proved that they cannot eat them without bringing on an attack.

Antispasmodic drugs, such as mebeverine or propantheline, can be helpful. A 'stool-bulking agent' which makes the stools larger and firmer is useful in reducing diarrhoea and also has a role to play in constipation since, by making the stools softer, it allows them to be passed more easily. Such agents, which include ispaghula husk, methylcellulose and sterculia, come in the form of granules or drinks.

One study of patients with IBS showed that, after a time, 30 per cent stopped having attacks, 60 per cent had recurrent mild symptoms with which they could cope and in 10 per cent the condition continued to cause problems.

# Recent Advances

In 1986 doctors in Italy tried the anti-allergic drug disodium cromoglycate (which is used in the treatment of asthma) on twenty-eight patients suffering from IBS. These patients seemed to have allergies to certain foods and their symptoms had improved when they cut these foods out of their diets. Twenty of them responded well to treatment with this drug. However, it is unlikely to become a universal treatment for IBS since it is probably only in a small proportion of patients that the symptoms are due to allergy.

In 1988 doctors at the University Hospital in Manchester, acting on the theory that calcium has a lot to do with the contraction of the muscle in the bowel, gave some patients with IBS an injection of nicardipine. This is a calcium antagonist, used in the treatment of high blood pressure. Another group of patients was given an injection of saline and the contractions in each patient's bowel were measured after he had taken a 100 calorie liquid meal. In the patients who had been given the saline, there was increased contraction over a period of several hours whereas there was no increase in those who had been given nicardipine. The drug seemed to have little in the way of side effects but more work needs to be done before it is offered generally to treat IBS.

## Complementary Treatment

*Herbalism*
Meadowsweet, marshmallow root, bayberry, slippery elm and comfrey can all be used to reduce irritability in the wall of the intestine. Linseed may be prescribed for constipation.

*Homoeopathy*
Ignatia may be prescribed for patients who have spasms of abdominal pain and diarrhoea after emotional upsets. For those who suffer from pain which is relieved by passing offensive-smelling wind and whose stools are bulky and may contain mucus, graphites may be appropriate. A patient who suffers from sudden cramp-like pains which are relieved by bending over but made worse by eating or drinking may respond to colocynthis.

*Hypnotherapy*
Because attacks of IBS are often brought on by anxiety or stress, hypnosis can be an effective treatment. Patients are taught how to relax and how to cope with stressful situations and suggestions are given while they are under hypnosis that their bowel symptoms will no longer trouble them.

## Further Reading

*How to Improve Your Digestion and Absorption* by Christopher Scarfe (published by ION Press).

# Ischaemic
# Heart Disease

(Angina and Heart Attacks)

## Definition, Mechanism and Incidence

The word 'ischaemic' means having an inadequate blood supply
and is used to describe those heart conditions which are caused
by blockages of the coronary arteries. These arteries carry blood
containing oxygen to the muscle of the heart; having released its
oxygen, the blood absorbs and removes the waste products
which are formed as a result of the heart's work. If the blood
supply is inadequate, the muscle receives insufficient oxygen to
be able to work efficiently, while waste products accumulate
which further interfere with the heart's function and which
cause pain by stimulating nerve endings within the muscle.

By far the commonest cause of ischaemic heart disease is
atheroma, or hardening of the arteries. Atheroma (whose name
derives from the Greek word for porridge) is a fatty substance
which is laid down in plaques along the inside of arteries. Not
only does it narrow the artery but there is the risk that thrombi
(clots) may form on it, shutting off the blood flow altogether. No
one is quite sure what initiates the formation of atheroma but
there are a number of risk factors which make its development
more likely. These include smoking, obesity, an unbalanced diet,
high blood pressure, a high level of cholesterol in the blood,
physical inactivity and diabetes. There is also some evidence that

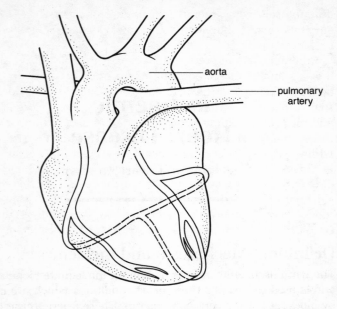

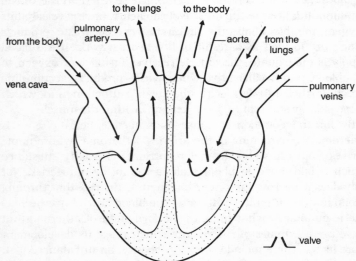

*The blood flow through the heart*

drinking soft water, more than six cups of coffee a day or large amounts of milk may increase a person's chances of developing severe atheroma.

Atheroma is found to a certain extent in everybody. Although it is rare in childhood, post-mortem examinations of young men between the ages of twenty and thirty often show evidence of some atheroma. A 'high-risk' man (that is, one whose life-style and medical condition include several risk factors) has a one in three chance of developing angina or having a heart attack within ten years. Recent surveys have shown that Asians living in Britain have a higher risk of developing ischaemic heart disease than other ethnic groups but the reason for this has not yet been discovered. There is also a small group of people who have hyperlipoproteinaemia running in the family. This is a condition in which there is an excess (hyper-) of fats (lipoproteins) in the blood (-aemia) and these tend to cause the deposition of atheroma at an early age.

Ischaemic heart disease has a great deal to do with life-style – it is the leading cause of death in all affluent countries and yet was hardly known before the turn of the century. In the United Kingdom it kills over 138,000 people each year and over half of the men who die from it are under sixty-five. Women seem to be protected by their hormones until the menopause and in the forty to fifty age group ischaemic heart disease is six times more common in men. After the menopause, however, the proportion of women with the disease steadily increases and eventually catches up.

## Angina Pectoris

### SYMPTOMS

The literal translation of the Latin term agina pectoris is 'a strangling sensation in the chest'. Patients usually complain of a constricting or crushing pain which may be felt right around the chest but is worst across the front or beneath the breast bone. It may travel up into the shoulders, the neck and the jaw, and is commonly associated with a heavy sensation, tingling or pain down one or both arms. If only one arm is affected it is usually the left. Rarely, pain may also be felt in the teeth or in the abdomen. Occasionally there may be pain in the arms and not in the chest.

There are several types of angina of which 'classical' or 'exertional' angina is by far the commonest. This, as its name implies, is brought on by exertion. It is particularly likely to occur if the patient is walking uphill or against the wind or has just eaten a meal or if the weather is cold. Some patients can walk long distances on the flat and only develop pain if they try to walk up a slope. Anger, excitement or mental stress can also bring on an attack which may last up to twenty minutes. However, if the pain has occurred during exercise, it will usually disappear within five minutes if the patient sits down to rest. Some people find that the pain disappears if they carry on walking, but this may be dangerous and the onset of an attack should always be a signal to rest.

Other types of angina include angina decubitus (which may be associated with exertional angina), in which pain comes on when the patient lies flat and is eased by sitting up, and the rare Prinzmetal's angina, in which the pain occurs at rest, especially during the night or early morning, being caused by spasm in a coronary artery.

Unstable angina is a term used to describe a condition which is steadily worsening, being provoked more easily and responding less readily to treatment than before. Vigorous treatment is needed for such patients in order to avoid the onset of a heart attack.

INVESTIGATIONS

Many conditions can cause chest pain and it is very important that an accurate diagnosis is made. It is not unknown for a patient suffering from angina to think that his pain is due to indigestion. Usually the patient's description of the pain, together with the details of when it occurs and how long it lasts, will indicate to the GP that he is dealing with a case of angina. However, in the majority of cases, there is nothing abnormal to find on examination, although some patients may have a raised blood pressure. Most cases of angina are confirmed by an ECG (electrocardiogram). Wires are attached to the patient's ankles, wrists and chest, and a record of the electrical impulses received from them, which reflect the impulses occurring in the heart, is traced out on a strip of paper. Very often, the ECG is normal and it is not until the patient is asked to perform some gentle exercise that changes are seen on it which suggest that the heart muscle is ischaemic.

In cases where there are few changes even on exercise but where the history strongly suggests a diagnosis of angina, further investigations may be performed. Ultrasound can be used to assess how well the heart muscle contracts. Radionuclide ventriculography consists of injecting a mildly radioactive substance into the bloodstream and scanning it as it travels through the heart, a technique which allows the heart's function to be measured accurately. In nuclear imaging another mildly radioactive substance, thallium 201, is injected and this is absorbed into the healthy heart muscle, leaving a blank 'cold spot' on the scan in any area which is ischaemic. The thallium is usually given during exercise and a scan is taken soon afterwards and then again after another three to four hours, when the disappearance of the cold spot confirms that the ischaemia was brought on by exercise and relieved by rest.

If the diagnosis is still uncertain or if the patient is suffering from severe attacks and surgical treatment is being contemplated, coronary angiography may be performed. In this, a substance which is radio-opaque (shows up white on X-rays) is introduced into the coronary arteries and X-rays are taken to try to demonstrate the position of the blockages.

ORTHODOX TREATMENT
The general condition of a patient with angina is very important. He will therefore be advised to stop smoking and, if he is overweight, to go on a diet. Regular gentle exercise is encouraged since it may help to open up the smaller vessels that bring blood to the heart muscle, but vigorous exercise and over-excitement should be avoided.

An acute attack of angina is normally treated with glyceryl trinitrate (sometimes referred to as GNT). This comes in the form of little tablets which are dissolved under the tongue. Once the pain has been relieved, the tablet is spat out, to try to avoid the main side effect of nitrates – a pounding headache. Unfortunately, once a bottle of tablets has been opened they deteriorate within a few weeks and in recent years sprays have been developed which have the same effect when applied to the tongue, but which can be kept much longer.

Nitrate preparations are also used in the long-term treatment of angina and patients are advised to take them before embarking on something that might provoke an attack, rather than waiting for symptoms to appear. Long-acting preparations include isosorbide dinitrate or isosorbide mononitrate, buccal pellets which are allowed to dissolve between the upper lip and the gum, and ointments or patches which are applied to the skin and from which nitrate is slowly released. They all have the effect of relaxing the blood vessels and therefore reducing the work that the heart has to do by decreasing the resistance it has to overcome.

In an acute attack of angina, 75 per cent of patients get immediate relief from taking a tablet of glyceryl trinitrate, while another 15 per cent have a slightly delayed response. Fortunately, glyceryl trinitrate is not addictive and its effect does not diminish even if taken repeatedly over a long period. However, it has recently been ascertained that, for nitrate preparations to work maximally, the patient should have a 'nitrate-free' period of about eight hours a day. This means that patches should be removed at bedtime and that the last dose of the isosorbide preparations should be taken in the early evening. Elantan LA, a long-acting preparation which is taken once a day, keeps the nitrate circulating in the blood for about sixteen hours only and therefore gives the patient eight hours free of the drug.

A nitrate preparation is usually the first that a patient with angina receives. For patients whose pain is not controlled adequately by this, beta blockers or calcium antagonists are added. (These drugs are more fully described in the section on high blood pressure.) Some doctors like to prescribe beta blockers routinely with nitrates.

The effect of beta blockers, of which propranolol is probably the most widely used, is to reduce the heart rate, the blood

266

pressure and the force with which the heart contracts, and, as a result, to reduce the amount of work that the heart has to perform and its need for oxygen. Calcium antagonists, such as nifedipine, verapamil and diltiazem, also reduce the heart's force of contraction and its need for oxygen, at the same time relaxing the coronary arteries, thus allowing more oxygen to be brought to the heart.

Unfortunately, all these drugs have side effects. The nitrates can cause headaches, facial flushing, dizziness, nausea and light-headedness. Beta blockers can cause tiredness, muscle weakness, impotence, sleep disturbance and cold hands and feet. (This last effect is less likely with labetalol, which has some alpha blocking action – see the section on hypertension.) Calcium antagonists may cause headache, dizziness, flushing and palpitations, all of which may be reduced by using a slow-release preparation. Nifedipine may cause ankle swelling and diarrhoea; verapamil may cause constipation.

For patients with high levels of cholesterol in the bloodstream, medication such as clofibrate may be needed in order to lower it.

When the attacks of angina continue to be frequent and severe, surgical treatment may be suggested. The simplest form is coronary angioplasty. In this a very thin catheter (tube) with a balloon on its end is inserted into an artery and fed through into the partially blocked coronary vessel by the doctor, who uses an X-ray screen to guide him. Once in place, the balloon is inflated with a substance which shows up on the X-ray. It is deflated and inflated a number of times and the pressure it exerts on the atheromatous plaques cracks and demolishes them, clearing the obstruction. This is an especially useful treatment for patients in whom atheroma is limited to one or two patches. It is successful in 60–80 per cent of cases but patients need to have follow-up arteriography after six to twelve months because, in 20–30 per cent of those helped, the condition will recur. Angioplasty has the great advantage that patients can return to work within a few days, whereas those who have bypass surgery usually have to convalesce for several months.

Two types of bypass surgery are performed. In one, a vein is removed from the leg and sewn into place between the aorta (the large vessel that carries blood from the heart to the arteries) and the section of the coronary artery that lies beyond the obstruction. In the other, the internal mammary artery, which runs down the inside of the chest wall, is loosened and fed into the far end of the blocked artery. There is a slight risk associated with the operation, which has a 1–2 per cent mortality rate but, since surgery is usually offered only to patients who are in danger of having a heart attack, this is usually considered to be an acceptable risk. Results are very good, with about 90 per cent of patients being free of symptoms in the year following the operation. This falls to 75 per cent after five years, since some of the grafts gradually become blocked. However, a bypass operation offers a patient not only an improved quality of life but also an increased life expectancy.

## COMPLEMENTARY TREATMENT
### Acupuncture
Chest pain is divided into two types by acupuncturists – the shi type in which there is an excess of energy (Chi) and the xu type in which Chi is deficient. In both types the channels of the heart are obstructed. Treatment consists of using points that will restore the flow of Chi to normal, overcoming the obstructions.

### Aromatherapy
Aniseed may be recommended.

### Herbalism
There are a number of herbs that have an effect on the heart and blood vessels. Hawthorn dilates the arteries, including those supplying the heart muscle, and slows the heart rate. Yarrow, too, can dilate arteries. Garlic not only dilates arteries but also helps to reduce cholesterol levels in the blood and acts to prevent abnormal blood clotting.

### Homoeopathy
The remedy prescribed will depend not only on the patient's symptoms but on his general personality. For example, nux vomica may be suitable for someone who is outwardly calm but

bottles up anger, whereas arsenicum may be appropriate for an over-anxious perfectionist who finds it hard to express emotions or fears. Aconite may be of value during the acute angina attack when there is severe pain that is made worse by activity.

*Nutrition*
Eicosapentaenoic acid (EPA) is an extract obtained from fatty fish which has remarkable effects upon the cardiovascular system. The reason why heart attacks are rare among Eskimos seems to be that they eat large amounts of raw fatty fish. EPA prevents abnormal blood clotting, stops arteries going into spasm and reduces the level of cholesterol in the blood. EPA is available in capsule form and is nowadays prescribed by doctors as well as by nutrition therapists.

# Heart Attack (Myocardial Infarct or Infarction)

MECHANISM AND SYMPTOMS
This is the commonest cause of death in the UK and other developed countries, and is nearly always due to the sudden deposition of blood clots on an atheromatous plaque inside a coronary artery. This is usually the end result of an obstruction which has caused the blood to run more and more sluggishly through the artery until it comes to a standstill. The section of heart muscle that is supplied by the artery dies and, if the patient survives, is replaced by scar tissue. However, if the area of muscle is a very large one, the heart may cease to function and the patient dies suddenly at the time of the infarction.

The symptoms are similar to those of angina but are more severe, continue when the patient is at rest and may last for a day or more. However, a few patients (usually among the elderly) may have no symptoms at all or may develop breathlessness or an abnormal heart rhythm without any pain occurring. Half the patients who have heart attacks have had increasingly severe angina during the previous weeks but, for the others, the attack is the first indication that they are suffering from ischaemic heart disease. As well as the pain, the patient may feel sick and faint, and may vomit, sweat and become short of breath.

## INVESTIGATIONS

Usually it is fairly clear from the condition of the patient that he has suffered a heart attack and this can normally be confirmed by an ECG. He is likely to be transported to hospital solely on the basis of his symptoms and all investigations will be done once he has arrived there.

When heart muscle dies, it releases chemicals known as cardiac enzymes into the bloodstream. These enzymes, which include lactic dehydrogenase (LDH), aspartate aminotransferase (AST) and creatine phosphokinase (CPK), can be measured by a blood test to confirm the results of the ECG. This test is particularly useful in the 5 per cent of cases where the ECG remains normal for a few days after the attack.

A scan may be helpful in distinguishing a heart attack from a bad attack of angina. The thallium nuclear-imaging technique mentioned above will continue to show a 'cold spot' after several hours if an infarct has occurred. A pyrophosphate scan uses the chemical pyrophosphate labelled with a mildly radioactive substance which is taken up by recently dead heart muscle. It is injected into a vein between one and five days after the attack and, a few hours later, a 'hot spot' will be seen on the scan at the site of the infarct.

## PROGNOSIS

Once over the first two or three hours following the attack, the patient has a very good chance of survival. However, complications may occur, the most important of which are abnormalities of heart rhythm. Some abnormality is almost universal in the first few hours, but only in a small percentage of cases does it seriously interfere with the heart's function.

## ORTHODOX TREATMENT

The immediate treatment for a patient who has suffered a heart attack is bed rest, preferably in a coronary care unit. However, for those who do not summon medical help until twenty-four hours or more have elapsed since the start of the attack, or for those patients who are over seventy and seem to have no complications, bed rest at home may be an acceptable alternative, since, in such cases, the stress of the move to hospital may cancel out the advantages of hospital care.

Strong painkillers such as morphine or diamorphine are given, together with a drug to stop the vomiting which they may induce. The patient is put to bed for 36–48 hours and his heart is constantly monitored on a screen to which he is attached by wires secured to his chest.

The main purpose of the monitor is to detect any abnormalities of rhythm (arrhythmias) as soon as they occur so that they can be treated. In most cases, treatment consists of lignocaine (a drug which is also used in other circumstances as a local anaesthetic) given intravenously through a drip. However, some patients with arrhythmias need the digitalis derivative digoxin and those with abnormally slow heart rates require intravenous atropine. Two per cent of patients develop ventricular fibrillation (VF) in which the heart starts to contract in a totally uncoordinated way and therefore fails to pump out blood normally. This is an emergency, with the patient ceasing to breathe and becoming unconscious. However, prompt electric shock treatment to the chest followed by cardiac massage will bring most patients round. Another 6 per cent of patients will develop heart block, in which the chambers of the heart which receive blood from the lungs no longer pump in time with the chambers that pump blood out to the body. This results in greatly decreased efficiency and in some cases it may be necessary to implant a pacemaker to ensure that normal function is restored. For some patients, this may only be a temporary measure since the block corrects itself in time.

Heart failure may occur, in which the damaged heart is unable to cope with the demands put on it and fluid accumulates in the lungs (where it causes shortness of breath) and in the ankles( where it causes swelling). In these cases, diuretics (as described in the section on high blood pressure) need to be given, together with digoxin.

Recently a lot of work has been done on the use of a group of drugs known colloquially as 'clot busters'. The main drug in this group is streptokinase, a protein derived from bacteria which, given soon after a heart attack, dissolves the clots that have formed within the coronary artery and thus restores the blood flow and limits the damage to the heart muscle. Given intravenously it is effective in up to 60 per cent of cases and seems to reduce the death rate in the first weeks after the attack by up to 25 per cent. If aspirin is given in addition, the death rate is reduced by over one third. However, the drugs have to be given in the first few hours after the start of the attack and, at the time of writing, streptokinase is not universally available, although specialists seem to think that it soon will be. Meanwhile, scientists have developed other similar substances such as urokinase, eminase and tPA. The latter two seem to be even more effective than streptokinase but, as yet, are being used on an experimental basis only.

Since arteries unblocked by streptokinase are likely to block up again, it may still be necessary for patients who are treated in this way to have a bypass operation. Long-term therapy may be given in the form of aspirin or beta blockers, both of which seem to reduce the incidence of a second attack and of sudden death.

## COMPLICATIONS

Modern coronary care is now so good that the great majority of patients make an uncomplicated recovery and are able to return to work within six weeks of the attack. However, some may continue to be troubled by arrhythmias and this may necessitate long-term medication or the fitting of a pacemaker. Patients who had no chest pain previous to their attack may find that they now suffer from angina.

An uncommon complication is the shoulder–hand syndrome in which the left shoulder becomes stiff and painful and the left hand may swell. Physiotherapy is often helpful but the condition can take several months to subside.

Patients who earned their living from driving may have problems following a heart attack, since an HGV licence will be revoked. Driving of any sort is forbidden for two months after an attack and the patient is duty-bound to inform the DVLC of his condition. Patients must also stop driving if they find that doing so brings on angina, if they have had bypass surgery but continue to have angina or if their medication makes them feel drowsy.

# Recent Advances

In 1986 surgeons in France used the first coronary stent – a coiled stainless steel spring which, inserted into the coronary artery after angioplasty, holds the walls apart and prevents the artery from blocking up again. By early 1988 it had been used to treat seventy-six patients, mainly in Lausanne, and surgeons at the National Heart Hospital in London had started to use it on an experimental basis.

In October 1987 a patient at the Musgrove Park Hospital in Taunton was given an epidural stimulator – the first to be used in this country. This new device, designed to treat patients whose angina does not respond either to drugs or to surgery, consists of a box which is implanted, under local anaesthetic, into the patient's chest wall, and which is linked by a wire to an electrode implanted in the spine. Stimulation of the nerves associated with sensation in the chest blocks their recognition of pain and relieves the pain of angina. The device is either used continuously or switched on and off by means of a magnet run over the skin.

In July 1988 surgeons working at the Freeman Hospital in Newcastle reported that they had carried out over a hundred operations during the past ten years in which they had cured dangerous arrhythmias by removing the tiny piece of heart muscle which was stimulating the abnormal beat. So far only 80 per cent of patients had survived the operation but they were expecting this figure to rise to 95 per cent within five years. Meanwhile, doctors at the Brompton Hospital in London had treated thirty patients with arrhythmias by shocking the abnormal piece of heart muscle with an electric charge.

New drugs, too, are being developed, including beta blockers, which seem to have fewer side effects than those at present available.

# Organizations

The Chest, Heart and Stroke Association, which is based at Tavistock House North, Tavistock Square, London wc1h 9je (tel. 071-387 3012), publishes a booklet called *Living with Angina* which gives guidance on the factors that cause attacks and advises on how, with care, a patient can live a full and active life. The Association also has offices at 65 North Castle St, Edinburgh, EH2 3LT (tel. 031-225 6963), and at 21 Dublin Rd, Belfast, BT2 7FT (tel. 02323 20184), and, at the time of writing, has plans to set up a nationwide network of support groups for people who have suffered heart attacks.

The Coronary Prevention Group, 60 Great Ormond St, London, WC1N 3HR (tel. 071-833 3687), offers information and advice on how to avoid ischaemic heart disease.

Cardiac Lifeline is an organization which came into being in June 1988, claiming to be the first to offer a twenty-four-hour service in which patients can have their ECGs analysed whenever they are concerned about their heart condition. (There were already other organizations offering a more limited service.) For a fee of several hundred pounds, the patient (who has to be referred by his doctor) is supplied with a portable ECG recorder that can transmit the signals down the telephone wire. If he is worried about his symptoms he attaches himself to the recorder and rings the organization. His ECG is immediately assessed by doctors who can advise him on what action to take. Cardiac Lifeline is based at 18 Marylebone Mews, London, W1N 7LF.

# Menopause

## Definition

The term 'menopause' is used loosely to describe the end of a woman's reproductive life and all its associated changes. Strictly speaking, though, the menopause is just the ceasing of the periods. The medical term applied to the period of time over which the body changes and the reproductive organs become non-functional is the climacteric.

The ovaries, which secrete the hormones that regulate the menstrual cycle, have a limited life span and, usually during the forties, their function begins to decline. Most women have their last period somewhere around the age of forty-nine or fifty, although the menopause may occur in younger or older women (up to the age of about fifty-five). If it occurs before the age of forty it is described as premature and this may often run in families. However, the commonest cause of a premature menopause is surgical removal of the ovaries or their treatment with radiotherapy.

The menopause is considered to have occurred when a woman has not had a period for over six months. Although in some women the periods may just suddenly stop, in many cases the cycle will change in the years leading up to the menopause. The periods may become increasingly scanty or infrequent, or both.

Very occasionally there may be no bleeding for several months, followed by an exceptionally heavy period (see section on menstrual problems). Heavy bleeding around the time of the menopause or bleeding occurring more than a year after the last period always requires investigation (usually a D & C or 'scrape'), since, occasionally, it may herald the onset of a malignant condition.

## Symptoms and Changes Occurring at the Menopause

Fifty per cent of women are said to have few symptoms at the menopause except, perhaps, for the occasional hot flush. Of the remaining 50 per cent, one half have symptoms with which they can cope while the others have symptoms that interfere with their lives and can become disabling. Smokers are more likely to have problems than other women.

The symptoms that may occur are numerous and include giddiness, palpitations, pain in the chest, dizziness, shortness of breath, headaches, extreme fatigue, loss of appetite and digestive upsets. The skin tends to become more fragile and wrinkled and the hair becomes thinner on both the head and body. Hot flushes are the commonest symptom and are experienced by about 85 per cent of all women. Lasting for a few seconds or minutes at a time, the woman is aware of a sensation of heat in her chest, neck and face. Her skin may flush and she may sweat. Twenty-five per cent of women have their sleep disrupted by hot flushes and night sweats. Often the flushes are made worse by a hot atmosphere and may be brought on by anxiety or by eating hot food or drinking a hot drink. Thus they may seriously interfere with a woman's life, making it difficult for her to go shopping in a crowded store, or to eat or even have a cup of tea in company. For 80 per cent of those affected, the flushes persist for at least a year, while 25 per cent have to suffer them for over five years.

Other symptoms are associated with changes in the reproductive and urinary tracts, caused by the lack of oestrogen in the bloodstream. The muscles supporting the womb (the 'pelvic floor') become slack, as do the ligaments that hold the womb in place, so that prolapse is more likely to occur (see separate section). The wall of the vagina becomes thinner and drier and the vagina itself may contract, becoming shorter and narrower. As a result the vagina may become sore (atrophic vaginitis) and discomfort on intercourse may occur. The increasing fragility of the skin around the entrance to the vagina (the vulva) may result in a persistent itch (pruritis vulvae). The lining of the urinary tract may be affected in a similar way, causing discomfort on passing water; the woman may have to pass water frequently and may also have to get up during the night to empty her bladder. Stress incontinence (the passage of small amounts of urine when laughing, coughing or sneezing) and urge incontinence (the inability to hold water once the need to urinate has become apparent) may occur, partly because of weakness in the muscles of the pelvic floor (see section on incontinence).

Psychological problems, such as depression, anxiety, irritability, panic attacks and sleep disturbances, may develop around the time of the menopause. (Insomnia may partly stem from the hot flushes and the need to get up to pass water.) Such problems are more likely to affect women who have previously suffered from psychological problems or from premenstrual tension.

A major cause of ill health after the menopause is osteoporosis (see separate section).

# Orthodox Treatment

*Hormone Replacement Therapy (HRT)*
There has been a revolution in the treatment of menopausal symptoms in recent years with the introduction of hormone replacement therapy. However, many specialists are concerned that there are a large number of women who could benefit from this treatment, but who are not yet receiving it.

The hormones used are those which are produced by the ovaries during the reproductive years – oestrogen and progestogens. Oestrogen stops the hot flushes and the night sweats, reduces vaginal dryness and discomfort, controls the urinary symptoms and prevents the bone loss that causes osteoporosis. Progestogens also control hot flushes and have some effect on preventing bone loss, although they are not as powerful as oestrogen. However, progestogens are less likely to cause side effects than oestrogen.

Usually oestrogen is used together with a progestogen because, on its own, it is thought to cause an increased risk of cancer of the womb. However, it is quite safe for a woman who has had a hysterectomy to take oestrogen alone.

Not all women are suitable for hormone replacement therapy. Surprisingly, an inability to take the contraceptive Pill because of side effects is not necessarily a contra-indication to HRT. However, women who have had cancer of the breast, ovaries or womb, or have suffered from liver disease, high blood pressure, various tumours or otosclerosis (deafness due to fusion of the tiny bones in the ear) should not have hormone replacement. Some women who have had thrombosis, fibroids, diabetes, gall-bladder disease, varicose veins, non-malignant breast problems or high levels of blood cholesterol may also be unsuitable.

Once on HRT, the patient may stay on it for many years, since this will give her continued protection against osteoporosis. However, the effect of oestrogen and progestogen on the lining of the womb is the same as if the hormones were being produced naturally and most women on HRT continue to have monthly bleeds, which some find unacceptable.

There are various combinations of oestrogen and progestogen, most of which are given for twenty-one days, with a break of seven days between courses. Women with no womb, who can safely be treated with oestrogen alone, may take this daily. Recently a transdermal patch has been introduced – a sticking plaster which, when applied below the waist, will release a constant flow of oestrogen into the skin and thus into the bloodstream. This has the advantage of producing fewer side effects than oestrogen taken by mouth, since much smaller doses can be used as the hormone is absorbed directly into the bloodstream. However, some 3–5 per cent of women are unable to use the patch because it causes skin irritation. At the time of writing, there is not yet a combined oestrogen/progestogen transdermal patch but one is being developed.

Injections and implants into the skin are other methods that are used to give oestrogen but the implant has the disadvantage that the treatment cannot be stopped quickly should side effects develop. If a woman who still has her womb is treated in this way, she will need to take a progestogen by mouth in addition.

Side effects of hormone replacement therapy include vaginal discharge, breast tenderness, pain at the time of the monthly bleed, weight gain, fluid retention and premenstrual syndrome.

*Vaginal Oestrogen Cream*
This may be very helpful in treating vaginal dryness and irritation, especially when these occur in patients who are unable to take HRT. It may also have an effect on the urinary system. At a Scandinavian geriatric centre, it was found that the application of a small amount of oestrogen to the vagina controlled incontinence to such an extent that the unit's expenditure on incontinence appliances and pads was reduced by 90 per cent.

However, if the cream is used over a prolonged period, a certain amount may be absorbed into the bloodstream, so its use must be carefully monitored in those patients for whom HRT is considered unsuitable. Another problem that may occur is the absorption of oestrogen by the patient's husband, which may lead to swelling of his breasts. To avoid this, intercourse should not take place until several hours have elapsed after the insertion of the cream.

*Non-Hormonal Treatment*
Clonidine hydrochloride, a drug used in the treatment of high blood pressure, may be helpful in controlling hot flushes when used in low doses.

# Complementary Treatment
*Acupuncture*
As in all forms of acupuncture therapy, the aim of treatment is to balance the energy flow whose disruption is causing symptoms. Treatment of menopausal patients will depend upon the '

particular symptoms that the individual is experiencing. There are some points that are specific for the treatment of hot flushes.

## Aromatherapy
Geranium, chamomile, cypress and sage are among the essential oils used.

## Bach Flower Remedies
Impatiens, olive and walnut are the three Bach flower remedies that are likely to be most useful at the time of the menopause. Impatiens is indicated for irritability and tension, olive for severe fatigue and walnut for people who are going through a major change in their lives.

## Herbalism
Herbs such as false unicorn (helonias) root and agnus castus have an effect on the hormonal system and may be used in the treatment of menopausal symptoms. Others, such as hawthorn tops and sage are effective in controlling hot flushes.

## Homoeopathy
Pulsatilla may provide relief in a woman who is weepy and in need of reassurance, who suffers from hot flushes and whose symptoms are worse for heat and tight clothes and better for gentle exercise and fresh air. Sepia, too, is useful for patients who are weepy and have hot flushes, but those who respond to this remedy are more likely to be anxious, complain of low dragging backache and be worse for cold and better for vigorous exercise. If hot flushes that are worse for heat and tight clothes are also worse first thing in the morning, and if other symptoms include headache, sweating, dizziness and tightness in the chest, lachesis may be useful. Several other remedies, too, may be helpful in the treatment of hot flushes. These include glonoinum, belladonna, sanguinaria, amyl nit., strontia carb., aconite and veratrum viride.

## Self-help

Vitamin E can help to relieve hot flushes when taken in doses of 400 i.u. a day. However, people who are suffering from high blood pressure should not start off with this dose as there is a risk that it may push their pressure still higher. They should begin with a dose of 100 i.u. a day and increase it by a further 100 i.u. each month until they are taking the full 400 i.u.

## Organizations

Women's Health Concern, PO Box 1629, London, w8 6au (tel. 071-602 6669), offers counselling and advice to women suffering from gynaecological and obstetric problems. It also publishes a number of books, including one on the menopause.

# Menstrual Problems

## Terminology

The two commonest menstrual problems are excessively heavy periods and painful periods, the latter being the commonest of all gynaecological disorders.

Heavy bleeding during periods which occur regularly is known as menorrhagia, while irregular heavy periods are referred to as metrorrhagia. Dysmenorrhoea is the term used for painful periods.

In order to understand how some of these problems occur, it is necessary to understand the basic physiology of the reproductive cycle in women. A diagram of the female reproductive organs will be found on p. 242.

## Physiology of the Reproductive Cycle

Each month a cell in one of the ovaries develops to form an ovum – an egg, capable of being fertilized and developing into a baby. As this cell develops, the cells surrounding it (the follicular cells) start to secrete oestrogen. Some of this oestrogen is retained in the fluid around the developing ovum and some is taken up by the blood and circulated around the body. Halfway through the cycle (day 14 of a twenty-eight-day cycle), the follicle surrounding the ovum bursts and the ovum is released. It passes down the Fallopian tube and into the womb (uterus) where the lining (endometrium) has become thick under the influence of the secreted oestrogen. If the ovum is fertilized, it will implant into this thickened endometrium.

Meanwhile, the part of the ovary that contained the ovum is being replaced by other cells known as the corpus luteum. These cells secrete progesterone and oestrogen which, again, enter the circulation. If the egg is fertilized and implants into the endometrium, the developing placenta begins to secrete a hormone which stimulates the corpus luteum to continue its production of progesterone so that the pregnancy is maintained. If, however, the egg is not fertilized, this does not occur and, towards the twenty-fourth day of the cycle, the corpus luteum begins to shrink, producing less progesterone. As a result, the thickened lining of the uterus begins to break down and is shed as the monthly period.

# Dysmenorrhoea

Over 50 per cent of all menstruating women have some discomfort during their period but for 10 per cent the pain is so severe that they become incapacitated for between one and three days each month. Dysmenorrhoea is divided into two types – primary and secondary.

*Primary Dysmenorrhoea*
This condition, which may run in families, usually begins within two or three years of the first period and accounts for 75 per cent of all cases of dysmenorrhoea. It is unusual for it to occur in the first few periods since these are commonly anovulatory cycles (that is, cycles in which the ovaries do not produce an egg) and primary dysmenorrhoea is associated only with ovulatory cycles (those in which an egg is produced). Usually the pain starts as the bleeding begins, although it may come on the day before the onset of the period. It is felt mainly in the lower part of the abdomen but may also travel through to the back and down the front of the thighs. It may last only a few hours or may

continue for two or three days. Other symptoms, such as nausea, vomiting, diarrhoea, loss of appetite, headache, dizziness, tiredness and nervousness may occur in addition to the pain. Usually, after a number of years, primary dysmenorrhoea improves, often helped by the birth of the first child.

There have been many theories as to what causes dysmenorrhoea, including one which said that the pain was 'all in the mind'. However, in recent years research has shown that its probable cause is an excess of the hormone-like substances, prostaglandins, in the uterus and the bloodstream. Prostaglandins, which were discovered during the 1970s, play a vital role in the control of many essential body functions but an imbalance of them (as of any hormone) will produce unwanted effects. It is thought that progesterone, which is produced during the second half of the monthly cycle, stimulates the production of prostaglandins, which are released as the lining of the uterus breaks down and is shed as the monthly period. Women who suffer from primary dysmenorrhoea seem to have high levels of prostaglandins in the muscle of the uterus, making it abnormally contractile and liable to go into spasm, while prostaglandins that escape into the bloodstream are likely to be responsible for the other symptoms that occur.

Primary dysmenorrhoea is more common in women who smoke and who either drink heavily or have done so in the past. The highest incidence is among those aged between fifteen and twenty-four and among women who have had fewer than two children. It also seems commoner among migraine sufferers. The fact that such patients often seem particularly prone to migraine attacks around period time may be due to the increase in circulating prostaglandins.

It has been suggested that anaemia, dieting, diabetes, chronic illness, overwork and emotional problems may be associated with a lowering of the pain threshold and that, therefore, dysmenorrhoea may be more likely to occur in patients suffering from these conditions.

### Secondary Dysmenorrhoea

This begins later in life than primary dysmenorrhoea and is due to some other condition affecting the uterus, such as endometriosis, adenomyosis, pelvic venous congestion, pelvic inflammatory disease or fibroids. Pelvic inflammatory disease (previously known as salpingitis) is a condition in which an infection travels upwards through the uterus and into the tubes, which may become blocked as a result. As the disease becomes chronic, all the reproductive organs may become inflamed and, later, scarred. Endometriosis, adenomyosis and pelvic venous congestion are described later in this section, while fibroids are dealt with in a separate section.

The pain of secondary dysmenorrhoea may start a few days before the period begins, gradually increasing in severity; it may continue all through the period and, sometimes, persist after it has finished.

# Menorrhagia

Between 5 and 10 per cent of menstruating women suffer from menorrhagia, which is defined as periods that occur more frequently than every twenty-one days, or last longer than seven days, or in which the loss is so heavy that the patient can't cope even if she uses the most absorbent pads. Cigarette smokers are five times more likely to be affected than other women.

Specialists have noticed that there is an increased incidence of anxiety and depression among women suffering from menorrhagia. However, although the condition itself may be partly responsible for this, it is possible that emotional and psychological problems may cause menorrhagia, since they can interfere with the normal functioning of the hormone-producing glands. Other causes may include abnormally high levels of circulating oestrogen which are not balanced by progesterone (see metropathia haemorrhagica, below), an increase in prostaglandins production (in which case, the patient will also suffer from dysmenorrhoea), pelvic inflammatory disease affecting the ovaries, fibroids, pelvic venous congestion, endometriosis or polycystic ovaries (a condition in which the ovaries develop cysts which interfere with their function). Sometimes women complain of increasingly heavy periods following a sterilization operation. The exact cause of this is uncertain, but it has been suggested that in some cases it is because the woman has come off the contraceptive Pill on which her periods were lighter and is now experiencing 'normal' periods. Very occasionally, what seems to be a rather late and very heavy period is, in fact, a very early miscarriage.

## Endometriosis

The endometrium is the lining of the uterus – that section which, each month, grows thick in response to hormonal stimulus and, if a fertilized egg is not implanted in it, breaks down and is shed as the monthly period. In the condition known as endometriosis, endometrial tissue is found elsewhere in the body, and not just within the uterus. Usually this occurs in the pelvic cavity, around the reproductive organs, the commonest site being on the ovaries. But endometrial tissue is also found in the bowel in up to 35 per cent of cases, in the urinary tract in between 10 and 20 per cent and, rarely, in other parts of the body such as the lungs, where, it is assumed, it must have been carried in the bloodstream. Quite why and how endometrial tissue is encouraged to grow in abnormal sites is unknown, although the latest theory suggests that affected women may have a deficiency in the immune system which, normally, would eradicate such cells.

Like pelvic inflammatory disease, endometriosis tends to cause neighbouring structures to stick to each other, resulting, ultimately, in scar tissue involving all the reproductive organs, so that they are locked into abnormal positions.

Endometriosis usually makes its first appearance between the ages of twenty-five and thirty, although it is not unknown in the teens nor in post-menopausal women. Some 30–40 per cent of affected women are infertile as a result of the disease. In many cases this is probably because it inhibits the normal mobility of the Fallopian tubes, through which the mature egg travels to the uterus, and therefore hinders the egg's passage. However, if it affects the ovaries, it may also prevent ovulation. In addition, the deep internal tenderness associated with endometriosis may lead to less frequent intercourse. Miscarriage, too, is more common.

The main symptoms of endometriosis are dysmenorrhoea and

pain on intercourse. Menorrhagia may occur but is rarely the first symptom. The endometrial patches, although growing in abnormal positions, still respond to the sex hormones in the same way as the endometrium in the uterus. Therefore, they thicken during the weeks leading up to a period and break down and bleed when the period begins. On the ovary, cysts tend to form, called chocolate cysts because of their colour. These may become very large before finally bursting and releasing their contents into the pelvic cavity. Both the monthly bleeding from the endometrial patches and the bursting of a cyst cause pain, and in the latter case may be severe enough to warrant hospital admission.

To begin with, the pain or discomfort is usually confined to one side of the abdomen but, in time, is likely to spread and become more severe. It usually starts before the period and may continue for some days after bleeding has begun. The deep pain which is felt during intercourse, and sometimes for several hours afterwards, is usually present throughout the month, although it tends to be worse just before the period. Patients may be aware of an increased need to pass water during a period, often associated with some discomfort, and, rarely, may notice blood in the water. They may experience pain when passing stools and may have either diarrhoea or constipation just prior to a period. If the bowel is affected by endometriosis, there may be blood in the stools.

## Adenomyosis

This is a fairly common condition which may cause both dysmenorrhoea and menorrhagia. Like endometriosis, it is caused by endometrium growing in the wrong place, in this case within the muscle (myometrium) of the uterus. As a result the uterus becomes enlarged and, occasionally, polyps may develop. Anything which grows into the uterine cavity, such as a polyp or a fibroid, may cause dysmenorrhoea, since the uterine muscle contracts in an attempt to expel the mass with the menstrual flow.

Adenomyosis tends to affect women in their thirties and forties who have had at least one pregnancy. They suffer from increasingly severe dysmenorrhoea together with pain on intercourse and, occasionally, irregular bleeding.

## Metropathia Haemorrhagica

Although commonest around the time of the menopause, this condition may also affect teenagers. It results from a failure of the follicle containing the mature ovum to burst, so that the ovum is not released and the follicular cells continue to secrete oestrogen into the circulation. As a result the endometrium becomes thicker and thicker until, eventually, it can no longer be controlled by the oestrogen and begins to break down. The symptoms are therefore those of heavy bleeding occurring considerably later than the time at which the period was expected.

## Pelvic Venous Congestion

This is a condition which has only been recognized in recent years and is thought by some specialists to account for the many cases in which women suffer from dysmenorrhoea, pain on intercourse, lower abdominal pain and, sometimes, heavy periods without there being any apparent cause. Doctors at a leading London hospital who have taken a special interest in pelvic venous congestion have estimated that whereas 15 per cent of women who suffer from the typical symptoms of secondary dysmenorrhoea can be shown to have a cause such as endometriosis, some 72 per cent can be shown to have dilated pelvic veins through which the blood moves only very sluggishly.

Patients complain of a dull, aching pain which is worse on exercise and better on lying down and which, on occasion, may become quite sharp. They suffer from dysmenorrhoea, and deep pain during intercourse, which tends to continue afterwards. Over half are found to have cysts on their ovaries and it is possible that ovarian dysfunction may contribute to the problem. Another interesting finding has been the apparent association of this condition with emotional and psychological problems. A survey in the United States found that 75 per cent of those women observed to have pelvic venous congestion had been sexually abused when children. Similarly, a specialist in Britain has estimated that some 60 per cent of patients with this problem have emotional troubles at the time of diagnosis.

## Investigation of Dysmenorrhoea and Menorrhagia

The type of treatment offered to patients suffering from dysmenorrhoea or menorrhagia will vary according to the underlying condition. Therefore it is very important that the right diagnosis is made. This may require a number of investigations to be performed.

Primary dysmenorrhoea is usually easily diagnosed from the description of the symptoms and the age of the patient. In the case of secondary dysmenorrhoea or menorrhagia, dilation and curettage (D & C or 'a scrape') may be necessary in order to make a diagnosis. In this, the neck of the womb is stretched slightly, under general anaesthetic, and the endometrium is scraped, the scrapings being examined under the microscope. Laparoscopy may be performed under the same anaesthetic. Here a tiny cut is made in the abdomen, usually just by the navel, and an instrument is inserted through which the gynaecologist can see the ovaries, the tubes, the womb and the interior of the pelvis. Nowadays, it is possible to do a curettage, or scrape, in the GP's surgery, using a small pump or syringe that gently sucks out the endometrium. However, this simplified investigation is only suitable for older patients since it may cause pain in younger women.

Before carrying out any of these surgical techniques, the gynaecologist will have examined the patient through the vagina and, sometimes, through the back passage in order to feel whether the uterus is bulky or out of position, whether the ovaries feel normal and whether there seem to be any deposits of endometriosis around the reproductive organs or the bowel. He may take swabs to see whether there is any sign of infection and will usually take a cervical smear if one has not been done recently. Blood may also be taken to see whether the patient is anaemic and, in some cases, for hormone estimations, since some imbalances (such as lack of thyroid hormone) may cause heavy periods.

At one centre in Britain which specializes in the treatment of pelvic pain, patients are routinely offered screening of the pelvic veins, in order to diagnose pelvic venous congestion. This is done in the out-patients' clinic and takes only ten minutes. A long needle is inserted into the uterus through the vagina and an injection of local anaesthetic is given into its muscle layer. Then a dye is slowly injected. This is taken up into the pelvic veins and can be followed on an X-ray screen, which will show whether the veins are dilated and whether blood flow through them is sluggish.

## Orthodox Treatment

This, of course, will depend upon what is causing the patient's symptoms. Most women with menorrhagia will need supplements of iron and folic acid to prevent them from becoming anaemic. If pelvic inflammatory disease is contributing to the problem, a course of antibiotics may be necessary. Because period problems are commoner in obese patients and in those who smoke, weight loss and giving up smoking will be advised where appropriate.

*Primary Dysmenorrhoea*
Since the discovery of the involvement of prostaglandins in primary dysmenorrhoea, drugs that reduce the level of these substances in the body have been shown to be very helpful in the control of this condition. These include flurbiprofen, mefenamic acid, naproxen, ibuprofen and piroxicam. Such anti-prostaglandins are effective in 75–90 per cent of cases of primary dysmenorrhoea providing they are taken in adequate dosage from the moment bleeding starts and for as long as the pain is likely to occur. Aspirin is also effective but needs to be started a few days before the period is due since it seems to inhibit the

manufacture of prostaglandins rather than having any effect on the formed substance.

Because anti-prostaglandins tablets work in slightly different ways, one may sometimes be effective where another has failed, so it is always worth trying at least two before giving up. Unfortunately, they may have side effects, such as diarrhoea, stomach upsets, headache, drowsiness and dizziness. Although they are well tolerated by most women, in those cases where side effects occur or where the tablets are not helpful, or for women who also need a contraceptive, the Pill can be a useful alternative.

Very rarely, in cases where the pain is severe and fails to respond to any of these treatments, an operation may be performed in which the uterine nerves are cut, preventing the pain from being felt.

### Menorrhagia

In cases where investigations have failed to reveal anything abnormal, hormonal treatment may be helpful. Very often such excessive bleeding is associated with an anovulatory cycle (in which no egg is produced) so that progesterone is not secreted. Taking tablets of a progestogen (a substance with a similar action to the natural hormone, progesterone) such as nor-ethisterone or dydrogesterone during the second half of the cycle may relieve the symptoms. However, these can sometimes cause acne and hairiness, so younger women may prefer to take the Pill, which contains a progestogen combined with oestrogen. But in a number of cases, curettage itself will solve the problem, so some gynaecologists like to observe a patient for a few months following this procedure before prescribing any medication. Menorrhagia may be made worse or even caused by an intra-uterine contraceptive device (IUCD, 'coil' or 'loop') and may settle once the device has been removed.

The prostaglandins-inhibiting drugs described in the section on the treatment of dysmenorrhoea may reduce the amount of blood lost but will not make the period any shorter and so are not helpful for those women whose periods continue for more than seven days. Drugs which actually help to shut down bleeding vessels, such as ethamsylate and tranexamic acid, may sometimes be of value, although the latter may occasionally cause diarrhoea, headache, nausea and weakness. For those patients whose menorrhagia is associated with anovulatory cycles and consequent infertility, clomiphene may not only control the menorrhagia but stimulate ovulation. However, this drug cannot be taken for more than a few months and may produce unpleasant side effects such as depression.

Danazol, which is derived from the male hormone, testosterone, stops the ovaries from functioning and therefore produces a 'pseudo-menopause'. As a result, in addition to stopping or reducing the periods, it may also cause hot flushes, a reduction in sex drive, a decrease in breast size and a dry vagina. Its other side effects include acne, hairiness and weight gain, digestive upsets, tremors, cramp and depression. However, it is well tolerated by most women. But it should never be taken by women who act or sing or whose voices play an important role in their lives, since it may produce a deepening of the voice which is irreversible.

If all else fails, hysterectomy may have to be considered.

_Endometriosis_

Progestogens such as norethisterone or dydrogesterone will reduce the growth of the endometrial deposits and have fewer risks for older patients than the Pill, which may, however, be suitable for the under-thirty-fives. Medroxyprogesterone acetate may also be used either in its oral form or as an injection. Danazol is probably the most effective form of drug treatment but has the problem of the side effects mentioned above.

Surgical treatment may sometimes be necessary for endometriosis, to remove adhesions (patches of fibrous scar tissue) which are distorting the ovaries or tubes and to restore the uterus to its normal position. If pain is severe, cutting the uterine nerves may be helpful. In some cases, hysterectomy with removal of the ovaries and tubes may be necessary. Some specialists feel that the laser may play an important role in treatment in the future, since it can accurately destroy patches of endometriosis as well as removing adhesions. At the time of writing, it is only in use in one centre in England but is more widely used in Europe and the United States.

The treatment offered to patients with endometriosis will depend upon how far advanced the disease is and how severe their symptoms are. In 90 per cent of mild cases, drug therapy or simple surgery will be effective. In rather more advanced cases, however, a 50 per cent recurrence rate can be expected. Severe cases require radical surgery to remove uterus, ovaries, tubes and adhesions.

Although pregnancy doesn't cure the disease, it may delay its progression. Seventy-five per cent of women with mild endometriosis are able to conceive, but this figure drops to 50 per cent of those with more advanced disease and only 35 per cent of those who are severely affected.

### Adenomyosis

Sometimes this will respond to curettage alone. In other cases, progestogens may be used or danazol. If drug treatment fails, hysterectomy, in which the ovaries are not removed, may be necessary.

### Metropathia Haemorrhagica

The choice of treatment is identical to that for adenomyosis, with 60 per cent of patients responding to curettage.

### Pelvic Venous Congestion

Since this condition has only been recognized fairly recently, treatment is still in its infancy. However, it seems that medroxy-progesterone acetate is helpful. Hysterectomy seems only to relieve the symptoms if the ovaries are removed as well. Because of the association with emotional problems, psychotherapy can be very effective but it may be a considerable time before the results are evident.

## Complementary Treatment

### Acupuncture

Dysmenorrhoea is said to be due to invasion by cold which obstructs the flow of energy, or Chi, or to problems in the flow of Chi through the liver. Points are chosen which will eliminate cold, warm the energy channels and restore the flow of Chi to normal. The liver is strengthened, as is the kidney, whose energy is said to control the function of the reproductive system.

Menorrhagia is said to be due to problems with the spleen, which is involved in the control of blood flow round the body. Treatment is given which will strengthen the spleen and return blood flow to normal.

### Aromatherapy

In common with herbalists and homoeopaths, aromatherapists find chamomile useful in the treatment of dysmenorrhoea. Other oils used include tarragon, cypress, marjoram, sage and juniper. Cypress, juniper and geranium are among those used to treat heavy bleeding.

### Herbalism

Many herbs are used to treat the various aspects of menstrual disorders. Chamomile is one of the most useful, especially in the treatment of dysmenorrhoea. Shepherd's purse is used specifically to reduce heavy bleeding and cramp bark to reduce the spasm of the uterine muscle which causes pain. Peppermint, too, is an antispasmodic, as are white deadnettle and thyme. Shepherd's purse and white deadnettle are also used to relieve pelvic congestion.

### Homoeopathy

Belladonna may be given to a patient who has cramp-like pain which begins on the day before the period, a heavy bright red flow, loss of appetite and pain when passing stools during the period.

Sepia on the other hand, may be appropriate if the period is late, and produces fatigue, irritability and depression, together with dragging pains which are eased by crossing the legs.

A very heavy period associated with a tearing pain in the lower abdomen and back, loss of appetite, diarrhoea and a fluctuation in symptoms may be an indication for pulsatilla.

Ipecac. is useful when the patient has pain in the umbilical region, dizziness, nausea and headache. Chamomilla may be chosen for someone with labour-like pains, a flow of brown blood with clots and a desire to pass water frequently. Very heavy bleeding in obese women may be treated with sabina and very heavy painless bleeding with crocus sativus or, if the patient also has ringing in the ears, with china. Many other remedies are also used for individual variations of symptoms.

*Hypnotherapy*
This can be very effective in the treatment of dysmenorrhoea since not only can it help the patient to relax, but it can also teach her how to control the pain when it arises.

*Nutrition*
Dysmenorrhoea may be associated with a calcium deficiency, so a supplement of dolomite (calcium plus magnesium) may be recommended.

## Self-help

Since constipation will make dysmenorrhoea worse, a high fibre diet is advisable. Naturopathic recommendations may include a reduction of salt, sugar and dairy produce in the diet, and a raw food diet for the seven days before the period begins.

A survey of over two thousand women that was carried out in Oxford in 1988 found that women who smoked were more likely to suffer from heavy, prolonged, painful, irregular or frequent periods than women who were non-smokers. Giving up smoking might well help to relieve the symptoms of many women with menstrual problems.

## Organizations

The Endometriosis Society has its headquarters at 65 Holmdene Ave, Herne Hill, London, SE24 9LD (tel. 071-737 4764).

# Migraine

## Definition and Incidence

The cause of migraine is unknown and the symptoms from which patients suffer may be extremely varied, but the word is used to describe attacks of severe recurrent headaches which do not have any underlying physical cause.

Migraine is said to affect about one person in twenty, with women being affected more often than men (in a ratio of six to four). It usually begins between the ages of fifteen and forty-five, although it may start at any age and 25 per cent of patients have had their first attack by the age of ten. Before developing full-blown migraine, some children may suffer from recurrent attacks of vomiting. And some youngsters may grow out of the condition during their teens (one study put the chances of this at between 35 and 50 per cent).

The condition tends to run in families, 46 per cent of patients having a close relative (often their mother) who also suffers from it. Some may have only one or two migraines a year, while others have them far more frequently, the average being between one and four a month. The individual pattern varies and patients may have a number of mild attacks with an occasional severe one, or the occasional mild attack in the midst of a stream of bad ones. In about a quarter of cases, the attack lasts for more than twenty-four hours.

## Theories on the Cause of Migraine

Classical migraine consists of the 'aura' (in which the patient may see flashing lights and experience tingling sensations) followed by a severe headache. The traditional theory, first put forward some thirty years ago, is that migraine is caused by a sudden constriction of the blood vessels in the brain (causing the aura), followed by an over-dilation (causing the headache). However, recently, Danish doctors have shown that the brain may be short of blood for some hours before a migraine attack and that this shortage may continue well into the headache phase when, according to the traditional theory, an excess of blood should be flowing through the brain. Other doctors have come to the conclusion that the primary changes during migraine are concerned with the nervous system and not with the blood vessels at all.

A recent discovery is that an intravenous injection of prostaglandins (the hormone-like substances that are involved in numerous bodily functions including the development of inflammation) will produce many of the symptoms that are associated with migraine. It has therefore been postulated that the primary problem is an over-production of prostaglandins. Other research has suggested that some migraines are allergic in origin. Levels of 5-hydroxy-tryptamine, a substance involved in the allergic response, are found to be higher than normal in the urine of patients during a migraine attack.

## Precipitating Factors

Although migraines can occur for no apparent reason, many patients are aware of factors that will bring on an attack. In one study, 81 per cent of the patients cited emotional stress as an important factor. Others include excitement, missing a meal, taking the contraceptive Pill, heat, exercise, changes in the weather and eating certain foods such as cheese, chocolate, onions, peanuts, beer, citrus fruits, monosodium glutamate and red wine. It is possible that some attacks may be triggered by contact with certain chemicals, such as those used in the production of magazines and newspapers. Women who suffer from migraine tend to be more at risk of an attack during the week leading up to a period, when, it seems, there may be a higher level of prostaglandins in the body.

Doctors are often cautious about giving migraine sufferers the Pill, since this may make them worse. However, occasionally they may improve. Some, who have not had migraine before, may develop it for the first time when taking the Pill. Unfortunately, when they come off it, they may continue to have migraines.

## Symptoms

Migraine is made up of two distinct phases – the early symptoms (known as the prodromal symptoms, or aura) and the headache itself. Some patients may just have the headache with no previous symptoms and, occasionally, some may just have the prodromal symptoms which then fizzle out without a headache developing.

The commonest prodromal symptoms are visual. The patient may suddenly be aware of lights flashing across her field of vision or of brilliant shimmering zigzag lines, which may be of various colours. Or the symptoms may be less specific, with simply a blurring or a 'heat-haze' effect. Gradually it may become more difficult to see, although total blindness never occurs. Very occasionally, the muscles controlling the eyes stop functioning so that the patient develops a temporary squint.

Other symptoms include tingling or numbness, which often starts in one hand and spreads slowly up the arm to the face, where it involves the mouth and the tongue. Very occasionally, both arms or the legs are affected. The muscles in the affected area may lose some of their function so that the patient may have difficulty performing fine movements or, rarely, may have problems in speaking. Dizziness or confusion may also occur and, in a few cases, severe dizziness may be the first symptom.

Occasionally there may be changes in mood or behaviour. A child may be pale and unusually irritable for several hours before an attack.

Most patients have one or two of these symptoms (usually the same ones each time) and these last for anything up to twenty minutes, after which the headache begins. In 60 per cent of cases, the pain is only on one side of the head but it may spread to affect the eyes, neck, face and jaws. With the onset of the headache, most patients prefer to lie in a darkened room, since in 80 per cent of cases, the light hurts their eyes and makes the pain worse. Nearly all feel sick and children may complain of abdominal pain. Ten per cent of patients vomit and, sometimes, the headache begins to decrease once they have done so. Occasionally diarrhoea may occur. Fluid retention is common during an attack and the end of the migraine may be heralded by a need to pass water. As patients get older, the headache tends to become less severe, although the prodromal symptoms may remain the same.

# Orthodox Treatment

In the treatment of migraine two types of drugs are used – those that prevent an attack (prophylactic drugs) and those that treat individual attacks when they occur. Prophylactic drugs are not usually recommended unless the patient is having more than two attacks a month. They are thought to work by preventing the abnormal contraction and dilation of blood vessels that is said to cause migraine. However, if one of the other theories of causation proves to be correct. another explanation of how these drugs work will have to be postulated.

*Prophylactic Drugs*
BETA BLOCKERS
This class of drugs, which includes propranolol, metoprolol, nadolol and timolol, is also used extensively in the treatment of high blood pressure. Propranolol is the most commonly used to treat migraine but, as explained in the section on high blood pressure, it is not suitable for asthmatics. More than 50 per cent

of patients who have moderate or severe attacks more than twice a month will obtain relief by taking beta blockers.

PIZOTIFEN

This drug has an antihistamine action and may be appropriate for those patients in whom migraine seems to be part of an allergic reaction. Some 50 per cent of patients will find that their headaches become much less severe while, for another 10 per cent, they will disappear completely. However, pizotifen may have side effects, such as weight gain due to an increase in appetite and, occasionally, nausea, dizziness and pain in the muscles.

METHYSERGIDE MALEATE

This is an extremely effective drug but, unfortunately, may have potentially dangerous side effects. However, used under close hospital supervision, it may be the only orthodox answer for patients whose migraine fails to respond to any other drug treatment.

OTHER DRUGS

Other drugs used as prophylactics include cyproheptadine, naproxen (an anti-inflammatory, anti-prostaglandins drug) and clonidine. Recent research has shown that the calcium-blocking drugs used in the treatment of high blood pressure may also be of value.

_Drugs Used During the Migraine Attack_

In line with the theory that migraine may be associated with an excess of prostaglandins in the body, drugs that inhibit their production may be very helpful in the treatment of the complaint. These include aspirin and paracetamol. Certain experts consider aspirin to be the drug of choice in the treatment of migraine, as long as it produces no side effects (such as indigestion). However, the reason why it probably fails to work in many cases is that it is not taken early enough in the attack. In addition, the stomach is inclined to lose its mobility during a migraine, so that its

contents are not passed into the gut to be absorbed. It is suggested, therefore, that patients should take aspirin right at the
start of an attack and, preferably, in a soluble form which will
allow it to be absorbed more easily. Taking a tablet of metoclopramide which speeds up the emptying of the stomach, followed
ten minutes later by three tablets of aspirin or paracetamol may
be a very effective way of cutting short the attack.

A drug which has, perhaps, become less popular in recent
years for the treatment of migraine is ergotamine. This is believed
to act by constricting the over-dilated blood vessels of the brain.
Here again, if another theory of causation is proved to be
correct, a different explanation of how this drug works will have
to be put forward. Its effectiveness may be considerably reduced
by a failure to absorb it, so it is available in combination with
cyclizine (a drug similar to metoclopramide) as Migril, in suppository form as Cafergot, in tablets that dissolve under the
tongue as Lingraine and in inhaler form as Medihaler-Ergotam-
ine. It may produce side effects which include nausea, vomiting,
abdominal pain, diarrhoea and cramp, and high doses may in
fact cause a headache. Like other migraine medication, it should
be taken early in the attack. Because there are risks associated
with high dosage and with constant use, stated doses should
never be exceeded and the drug should never be taken as a
prophylactic.

## Recent Advances

Dentists at the Glasgow Dental Hospital have shown that, in
some cases, a mal-alignment of the upper and lower teeth may
be instrumental in causing migraine. They found nineteen
patients who suffered from migraine attacks every two to three
weeks, some of whom had been having attacks for many years
and all of whom developed symptoms either on waking or
shortly afterwards. Each was fitted with an acrylic splint which
was worn at night to bring the teeth into the correct position.
During a year in which the patients wore the splints every night,
the incidence of migraine attacks fell dramatically. The dentists

suggested that the malpositioning of the teeth was putting certain muscles in the jaw into spasm and that this was triggering off the migraine. A larger study is now under way.

Meanwhile, a new drug is being developed which has an anti-allergic action, reducing the levels of 5-hydroxy-tryptamine, which are known to rise during a migraine attack. So far, trials of the drug have been encouraging and there appear to be no side effects. The manufacturers, Glaxo, hope to apply for a licence to produce the drug commercially in 1990.

# Complementary Treatment

*Acupuncture*
Very often the pain of migraine is exactly located to the distribution of the Gallbladder channel, which, on each side, runs from a point next to the eye, back towards the ear, then around the ear to the neck, forward to the forehead, and finally back again, down the neck and, passing under the arm, over the abdomen and down the leg to the little toe. Thus it is located over the jaw, whose spasm may precipitate migraine, next to the eyes, which are associated with the prodromal symptoms, on the forehead and crown of the head where the pain is often felt, and in the abdomen which may be affected by nausea. In such cases, the cause of the migraine may be seen as stagnation of energy, or Chi, in the Gallbladder channel and treatment to restore normal flow of Chi may be very effective in preventing further attacks.

*Aromatherapy*
In common with the herbalists, aromatherapists find rosemary and lavender useful in the treatment of migraine. Marjoram, basil, melissa, rose, aniseed, chamomile, eucalyptus and peppermint may also be recommended.

*Herbalism*
Feverfew has been a popular migraine remedy for many years. However, recently, doctors have carried out a scientific trial of feverfew – and have proved that it works. Like some of the orthodox drugs used, it dilates constricted blood vessels. Its one drawback is that in a few patients it may cause mouth ulcers.

Other herbs used to treat migraine include lemon balm (which relaxes the nervous system), rosemary (which stimulates the circulation and strengthens the functions of the nervous system), motherwort (which is particularly useful when attacks are brought on by nervous tension) and vervain and lavender which are relaxant and antispasmodic.

*Homoeopathy*
Iris is a commonly used remedy for migraine and is appropriate when the patient complains of a sick headache associated with diarrhoea and preceded by blurred vision.

Silica may be helpful for someone who suffers from recurrent severe headaches that start in the back of the neck, move forward to the eyes and are associated with nausea and vomiting. When temporary loss of vision heralds a severe throbbing pain which is often on the top of the head or above the eyes and is worse for warmth or movement, natrum mur. may be effective. When a right-sided headache is associated with pain in the shoulder, sanguinaria may help. If the pain is on the left and the patient feels weak and faint and has palpitations, spigelia may be prescribed.

*Hypnotherapy*
This can be remarkably effective in the treatment of migraine. Under hypnosis, the patient is taught a technique which can be used at the start of an attack to prevent the migraine from developing. This may consist, for example, of a visualization where she pictures the blood vessels in her brain contracting and then, as she clenches and relaxes her fists or as she counts slowly to twenty, she sees them returning to normal. (The fact that this may be physiologically inaccurate doesn't matter at all in a visualization.) She is told that what she pictures will actually occur and that by performing this technique she will be able to control her migraine and prevent the symptoms from developing any further. When patients have used this method for a while and have gained confidence in its effectiveness, they will often find that they are having to use it less often, as the attacks become less frequent.

*Manipulation*
Patients who suffer from migraine often have excessive muscle tension in their necks and shoulders which may spark off attacks. Chiropractic or osteopathy may help to remove this tension and restore mobility to the neck joints. Manipulation of the jaw to reduce muscle tension caused by faulty bite, together with dental treatment as described above, may also be of value.

*Nutrition*
Vitamin B$_3$ in the form of nicotinic acid (niacin) has the effect of dilating blood vessels and, if taken in the early stage of a migraine, can stop or reduce the severity of the attack. The only side effect is flushing of the face. To begin with, 100 mg should be taken but if this is not fully effective, the dose may be gradually increased to a maximum of 500 mg until the attacks are being controlled.

# Organizations

The British Migraine Association, 178a High Rd, Byfleet, Weybridge, Surrey, KT14 7ED (tel. 09323 52468), is a self-help organization run by migraine sufferers for migraine sufferers.

# Mouth
# Ulcers
# *and*
# Bad Breath

## (Halitosis)

Mouth ulcers and bad breath (halitosis) warrant only a few lines in most medical textbooks but many people find them a considerable problem.

## Mouth Ulcers

DESCRIPTION AND CAUSES

Known medically as aphthous ulcers, these are small, painful erosions of the lining of the mouth which usually appear in groups, last several days and tend to recur frequently. Attacks often start in adolescence and, as the patient gets older, diminish in frequency until, finally, they stop altogether. The cause is unknown. Patients who suffer from intestinal conditions, such as Crohn's disease, ulcerative colitis and coeliac disease, are more likely to get mouth ulcers than other people, but here again the reason is unknown.

Sometimes mouth ulcers can result from a viral infection and be associated with fever and headache. Tiny blisters develop in the mouth and throat which then become ulcers. Usually the infection lasts only a few days and the patient recovers rapidly.

Soreness of the mouth, without ulceration, may be due to poorly fitting dentures or to a vitamin deficiency, particularly of the B complex or folic acid. A doctor's advice should always be sought concerning a painless ulcer or one that fails to heal as, occasionally, cancer of the mouth may begin like this. However, there are other reasons why ulcers may not heal, one of which is the constant chewing of gum.

## ORTHODOX TREATMENT

Various preparations are available for the treatment of mouth ulcers. These include carbenoxolone sodium, local anaesthetics such as benzocaine or lignocaine in the form of lozenges or gels, and salicylates (aspirin-like compounds). Some of these are available over the counter. Mouth washes such as chlorhexidine may also be helpful. In some cases, steroid pastes or lozenges may be prescribed.

## COMPLEMENTARY TREATMENT

*Aromatherapy*
Myrrh, lemon, tea tree and geranium may be used.

*Herbalism*
A number of herbal mouthwashes may be effective in the treatment of ulcers. They include marigold, myrrh, red sage and thyme, all of which have healing and antiseptic properties.

*Homoeopathy*
For ulcers under the tongue associated with a metallic taste in the mouth, a swollen tongue and bad breath, merc. sol. may be effective. Borax may be prescribed for ulcers that are worse when acid or salty foods are eaten. Ulcers inside the lower lip associated with cold sores may respond to hydrastis.

*Naturopathy*
A cleansing programme in which the patient takes only fruit, vegetables and fruit juices for two to three days may be recommended.

*Nutrition*
Patients who suffer from recurrent mouth ulcers may have an allergy to something in their diet (such as wheat or another

grain) or a vitamin A deficiency. A nutrition therapist will inquire for other evidence of vitamin A deficiency and may suggest an elimination diet in order to pinpoint any allergy before recommending treatment – either in the form of a special diet or by vitamin supplements.

# Bad Breath (Halitosis)

Human beings are very sensitive creatures and are inclined to think themselves smelly when they aren't. This is particularly so among young people. Many people who fear that they have bad breath do not, in fact, smell bad to other people. The best person to consult is the dentist, who is in a very good position to judge while, at the same time, having no reason to tell anything other than the truth. In addition, when bad breath occurs, it is often a dental problem rather than a medical one, being due to decaying teeth or gingivitis (infection of the gums).

Undoubtedly the commonest cause of bad breath is smoking. Other causes include spicy foods, garlic and alcohol.

ORTHODOX TREATMENT
If halitosis is due to infection or decay in the mouth, treatment is the province of the dentist. Once the mouth is healthy again, the smell should disappear.

COMPLEMENTARY TREATMENT
*Aromatherapy*
Myrrh and peppermint may be recommended as mouthwashes.

*Herbalism*
Lavender or vervain mouthwash may be an effective treatment for halitosis. Vervain is also useful for patients undergoing dental treatment as it encourages healing of disease in the teeth and gums.

*Homoeopathy*
If bad breath results from digestive problems, nux vomica or pulsatilla may be helpful. If it is associated with flatulence or

infected gums, carbo veg. may be appropriate. Bad breath after eating may respond to chamomilla and if the breath smells like onions, allium cepa may help.

SELF-HELP
For smokers, the best remedy is to give up smoking. Changes in the diet may also be helpful. Meat and fats tend to slow down the passage of food through the intestines, so that food spends longer in the stomach. Sometimes, changing to a vegetarian diet with a reduced intake of fat may get rid of halitosis. A diet that includes a lot of natural chlorophyll (in other words, raw green, leafy vegetables) may also be beneficial.

# Nosebleeds

## Causes and Symptoms

Nosebleeds are common, especially in children, and often entail only a slight loss of blood. However, bleeding may be recurrent and, occasionally, profuse.

The lining of the nose has many small blood vessels in it and the section covering the front part of the nasal septum (the sheet of cartilage that lies between the nostrils) is particularly rich in vessels. This section is known as Little's area and it is from here that most bleeds occur. Perhaps the commonest cause is injury – often from nose picking. Other causes are a broken nose, local infections such as a heavy cold or sinusitis and general infections including glandular fever and tuberculosis. Patients with hay fever or chronic rhinitis may suffer from nosebleeds, as may those with high blood pressure, leukaemia and benign or malignant growths within the nose itself. Abnormalities of the blood vessels in the nose or of the clotting mechanism of the blood (such as occur in haemophilia) may also be involved.

Usually some blood trickles down the back of the throat. Heavy bleeding may result in the patient swallowing a lot of blood which, because it irritates the stomach lining, may cause vomiting. Very occasionally, vomiting of blood may be the first sign of a nosebleed.

# Investigations

Older patients are usually checked for high blood pressure. When someone has been having heavy nosebleeds, blood tests may be needed to see whether he has become anaemic and whether an abnormality of the blood may be to blame. A nose swab will detect any infection that may have caused the bleed.

# Orthodox Treatment

If the bleeding is coming from Little's area it will often stop if the area is compressed, by squeezing the end of the nose between the fingers for about five minutes. If this fails to work, treatment consists of gently opening up the nostril with a small instrument (speculum) and removing any clots. The doctor can then see whether or not the bleeding is coming from Little's area. If it is, the insertion into the nose of a small piece of cotton wool soaked in adrenaline followed by another five minutes' squeezing will often stop it by helping the blood vessels to contract. However, bleeding may begin again once the effect of the adrenaline has worn off, so some doctors like to follow up this procedure by cauterizing the area using, for example, a cotton bud soaked in silver nitrate solution.

Particularly resistant bleeds may require the nose to be packed, although this is not usually necessary. A narrow ribbon gauze which has been lubricated with Vaseline or a similar substance is introduced into each nostril in layers. This produces a firm, constant pressure on the bleeding area. The ends of the gauze are left hanging out of the nostrils and are secured with a safety-pin in order to avoid their disappearing back into the nose. Some doctors like to give antibiotics to patients who have nose packs, as, theoretically, they could act as a focus for infection.

Patients who have recurrent bleeds from Little's area may need admission to hospital to have the area cauterized under anaesthetic.

Bleeds from the back of the nose are less common than those from the front and are less easy to treat because pressure cannot be exerted on the bleeding point from outside and the point itself cannot be seen. If the bleed doesn't stop of its own accord, the nose has to be packed. However, because the back of the nose is encased in bone, it is only necessary to pack one nostril in order to produce the required pressure. The pack is inserted in the same way as a pack for the front part of the nose and is left for at least twenty-four hours. If bleeding continues after this, it may be necessary to re-pack the nostril or to insert a post-nasal pack. The latter consists of a narrow tube (catheter) with a deflated balloon on its end which is passed through the nose to the back of the throat. The balloon is then inflated until it fits snugly into the back of the nose, blocking it off. The other end of the tube is taped to the patient's face and the nostril is packed with gauze. Some doctors give antibiotics to patients being treated in this way since, in theory, the blood retained within the nose could promote the growth of bacteria.

Very occasionally, surgery is necessary to stop further bleeding. The artery that supplies blood to the affected area is tied off and this may be done via an incision in the neck, through the maxillary sinus in the upper jaw or through the upper part of the nose itself. In other cases, where there is an underlying cause for the bleeding, such as high blood pressure, this will be treated in the appropriate manner.

All patients who are suffering from nosebleeds should be put to bed and propped up in a sitting position so that blood does not run down the back of the throat. If the nose has been packed, the patient will have to breathe through the mouth and will therefore need frequent mouth washes and plenty to drink to prevent the mouth from becoming dry. (Patients with packed noses often find it easier to drink through a straw.) Those who have lost a lot of blood may need admission to hospital for a blood transfusion.

Occasionally drugs are prescribed. For patients who have recurrent nosebleeds and are waiting for admission to hospital for definitive treatment, a preparation which helps to stop bleeding from small blood vessels, such as tranexamic acid or ethamsylate may be used. Sometimes patients become quite anxious about their recurrent bleeds and, in such a case, phenobarbitone may be prescribed as a sedative.

# Complementary Treatment

*Acupuncture*
Nosebleeds are said to be due to an excess of heat in the lung and stomach and a lack of yin (the feminine negative aspect of Chi). The aim of treatment is to eliminate heat, stimulate yin and restore energy flow to normal.

*Aromatherapy*
Essence of cypress on a piece of cotton wool held under the nose may help to stop a bleed.

*Herbalism*
A piece of cotton wook soaked in an infusion of St John's wort or witch hazel may help to stop bleeding if pressed against the nose. Shepherd's purse or yarrow may be prescribed for their anti-haemorrhagic properties.

*Homoeopathy*
If a nosebleed has resulted from an injury, arnica will be helpful, particularly if the bleeding is heavy. Profuse bleeding that occurs after the nose has been blown vigorously may respond to phosphorus. For the irritable, fearful patient, aconite may be appropriate. Belladonna may be prescribed if the bleed is associated with a throbbing headache, and hamamelis if the blood oozes rather than flows. Many other remedies may be used as well.

*Nutrition*
For a patient who suffers from recurrent nosebleeds, rutin tablets may be helpful since they will strengthen the blood vessels.

# Osteoporosis

## Definition, Mechanism and Incidence

Osteoporosis is a condition in which the bones become thin. It is commonest in post-menopausal women and is not so much a disease as an extreme form of a normal bodily process.

Bones are made up from a framework of living cells which, to achieve rigidity, are impregnated with various minerals – primarily calcium phosphate, but also quantities of magnesium and sodium. Like the rest of the body, the bones are continually changing, with cells dying and being replaced. In addition, two types of cells are constantly at work within the bones, one removing bone and the other laying it down again. As a result, a small amount of calcium is lost into the bloodstream each day and fresh calcium is laid down. During childhood and adolescence, the bones become increasingly dense as more minerals are deposited than are lost, and a maximum density is reached during the twenties and thirties. After the age of about thirty-five, more minerals are lost than are replaced and the bones become thinner with advancing age.

In osteoporosis, excessive amounts of minerals are lost and the bones become brittle. The condition probably affects some five million people in the UK and is responsible for some 200,000–300,000 fractures a year. It is estimated that 75 per cent of all women will develop some degree of osteoporosis and, as a result, two thirds of these will have at least one major fracture.

## Causes

Why some people develop osteoporosis and others don't remains a mystery but there is a tendency for the condition to run in families. Recently a group of 'fast calcium losers' has been identified in the population and this natural tendency can be diagnosed by urine and blood tests. These fast losers have a high risk of developing osteoporosis, as do people suffering from certain diseases in which calcium loss is increased, such as thyrotoxicosis, diabetes, chronic malnutrition (for example, in alcoholism), inflammatory bowel disease (such as Crohn's disease or ulcerative colitis, in which absorption of calcium may be reduced), hyperparathyroidism (in which the calcium-regulating parathyroid glands are over-active), Cushing's syndrome (in which there is excessive secretion of steroid hormones from the adrenal glands) and rheumatoid arthritis. Certain types of medication also have the effect of promoting calcium loss from the body. These include steroids taken over a long period of time, diuretics (taken, for example, in the treatment of high blood pressure) and thyroid hormones.

Osteoporosis is four times as common in women as in men but rarely starts before the menopause. There is no evidence that a lack of female hormones actually causes the condition but these hormones do seem to promote the retention of calcium within the body so that it is only when their levels drop that osteoporosis will develop in a susceptible patient. Even after the menopause, the ovaries continue to produce a small amount of oestrogen, so women who have had their ovaries removed have an increased risk of osteoporosis. So too do women who have an early menopause (before the age of forty to forty-five), because they are likely to spend more years of their lives in a post-menopausal, calcium-losing, state. Other women who may be at risk are those whose ovaries functioned imperfectly even before the menopause and who may, as a result, have had infrequent periods. These women are likely to have thinner bones than normal when they reach the menopause, since their premenopausal hormone levels will have been too low to offer them protection. However, women who have been pregnant or who have taken the contraceptive Pill are likely to have more calcium in their bones than others.

People who have larger bones to begin with have more calcium to lose and therefore are less likely to develop osteoporosis. Normally men's bones are larger than women's and those of black people are larger than those of whites or Asians. Plump people seem to be less at risk than those who are thin. Men do develop osteoporosis but it usually occurs at a later age than in women.

Smoking increases the risk of osteoporosis, probably because it breaks down the protective hormones, and heavy smokers are more likely to break bones than other people.

Immobilizing a part of the body can result in considerable loss of calcium from that part and elderly people who remain in bed for periods even as short as a week are likely to start losing calcium at an increased rate from all their bones.

## Course of the Disease

Frequently, the first indication that a patient has osteoporosis is when she breaks a bone, perhaps as the result of a fairly trivial injury. Occasionally symptoms of back pain and tiredness may occur soon after the menopause. However, no changes can be seen on an X-ray until about one third of the total bone density has been lost and this may take another ten to fifteen years. Bone loss is most rapid in the first five years after the menopause and then slows to a steady rate. For some reason the skull is very rarely affected, although the jaw, especially the part holding the lower teeth, may become thin.

The commonest fractures that result from osteoporosis are those of the wrist, the hip (upper end of the femur or thigh bone) and the individual bones of the spine (the vertebrae). A vertebra can collapse and lose its shape simply as a result of the weight of the body pressing down on the thinned bone. This is quite common and is known as a compression fracture. Vertebral fractures can also be caused by minor injury or by the strain of heavy lifting. Such fractures affect the shape of the spine and, as a result. the patient becomes stooped over and loses height.

A compression fracture of a vertebra may cause sudden severe pain in the back which gradually wears off after 4–8 weeks. A patient with osteoporosis may also suffer from a more long-term ache in the back, either in the midline or to either side of the spine. It usually comes on when she has been standing for some time or sitting in one position and can be relieved by rest. Such a pain may be due to arthritis, which will be made worse by the misshapen vertebrae. The bones themselves are not tender in osteoporosis, except at the site of fractures.

As the patient becomes more stooped over, the movement of her chest becomes limited so that her breathing may become shallower and coughing may be difficult. It is not unknown for the trunk to tip so far forward that the base of the ribs touches the top of the hip bones. Even in less extreme cases, there is often a horizontal crease visible in the skin of the abdomen.

## Diagnosis

When a post-menopausal woman breaks a bone, it is usually unnecessary to do a large number of tests in order to diagnose osteoporosis. All that is needed is an X-ray of the spine which will show thinning of the bone and, possibly, compression fractures of the vertebrae.

However, if the doctor is uncertain about the diagnosis or if he feels that there may be some underlying condition which needs treatment (such as thyrotoxicosis), he will take some blood or urine tests as well. The level of calcium in the urine is normal in most cases of osteoporosis but may be raised when the condition is due to thyrotoxicosis or to treatment with steroids.

Urine and blood tests may also be helpful in detecting 'fast losers' early on, so that osteoporosis may be prevented in these high-risk patients. Therefore women whose mothers have suffered from severe osteoporosis may be offered tests involving the collection of all the urine passed over twenty-four hours plus a single specimen of blood.

# Orthodox Treatment

*Hormone Replacement Therapy*

Although osteoporosis is not caused by a hormone deficiency, taking hormones after the menopause can prevent it from occurring, because oestrogen enables the body to retain calcium. Hormone replacement therapy (HRT) starting as soon as possible after the menopause can prevent osteoporosis but, started later, will only stop it from getting worse. Some doctors think all women should be offered HRT post-menopausally and, certainly, it is advisable for those who are particularly at risk. Its benefits probably last only for as long as it is taken, with bone loss beginning once the treatment has been discontinued. Since some ten to fifteen years of bone loss is usual before fractures occur, it seems sensible for women to continue taking HRT until they are at least seventy but, in 70 per cent of cases, this has the drawback that they will continue to have periods.

In 1987, a new form of hormone replacement therapy became available in Britain and other countries. Instead of taking tablets, the woman has a 'patch', rather like a sticking plaster, attached to her skin. The hormones are contained within the patch and are slowly absorbed into the body through the skin. This has the advantage that they travel directly into the bloodstream without having to pass through the digestive system, and therefore are likely to produce fewer side effects than hormones that have to be taken by mouth.

Oestrogen, which also controls menopausal symptoms, needs to be taken continuously but causes a build-up of the lining of the womb (endometrium), a factor which may predispose the patient to develop cancer of the womb. To prevent this build-up a progestogen, which acts in the same way as the natural hormone progesterone, is always given with oestrogen unless the patient has had a hysterectomy. The progestogen is given for only twelve days each month. Each time it is stopped. 70 per cent of women will have a small withdrawal bleed. However, protection from abnormal endometrial thickening does not depend upon the occurrence of bleeding and progestogen is protective in all cases.

Side effects of HRT include breast tenderness, nausea and swelling of the abdomen but these frequently disappear after the first few months. If they don't, changing to a different preparation may help. On the plus side, HRT often gives a woman a sense of well-being and may protect the heart and blood vessels against disease.

Although HRT encourages the retention of calcium within the body, it cannot make up for a poor diet and it is essential that the patient has an adequate calcium intake.

*Calcium*
Many people nowadays seem to eat diets that are deficient in vitamins and minerals. Older women need at least 2 g of calcium a day to try to replace some of that which is being lost. Vitamin D supplements are only necessary if the patient does not absorb enough calcium from the intestines.

*Treatment of Fractures*
Although the bones are thin, osteoporosis does not prevent fractures from healing normally. However, because they can easily break again, problems may occur when it is necessary to pin the two parts of the bone together or to insert a replacement metal hip bone.

A vertebral compression fracture may need two or three weeks of bed rest. After this, an orthopaedic support for the spine may encourage the patient to move around. However, a rigid spinal brace should be used as little as possible because, by restricting movement, it promotes greater bone loss.

A hard mattress will help to relieve back pain following a fracture, and simple painkillers can be taken.

# Recent Advances

Recently doctors in Denmark, the USA and New Zealand have been investigating a drug which is used in the treatment of another bone disorder, Paget's disease. Called etidronate disodium, it seems that this drug may have the effect of enabling the patient to build up her bone again. It is taken for two weeks, after which calcium and vitamin D are given for three months and then the cycle is repeated. Results have been very promising but use of etidronate is still at the research stage and, even if it proves to be successful, it could be some time before it is available for general use.

Another drug that is under investigation is the hormone calcitonin. This is very safe and has been shown to be effective when used with oestrogen but, until recently, has had the disadvantage that it needed to be injected three times a week. It is also expensive. However, a calcitonin nasal spray has been developed which, when it was tried out in Denmark, was shown to increase bone mass. Similar research has been done in Belgium, where women who were given calcitonin for five days a week, together with calcium, were shown to lose significantly less bone over the course of a year than women who were given only calcium.

Research done recently at King's College Hospital, London, suggests that hormone implants can increase bone density whereas oral HRT just serves to maintain it. However, this, too, is still in the experimental stage.

# Prevention

Because immobility promotes bone loss, it is very important that the elderly should be kept mobile. It is also vital that their homes should be safe so that accidents, and possible fractures, are less likely.

Some doctors believe that exercise in the premenopausal years can be protective against osteoporosis, but this has yet to be proved.

Steroids can counteract the effect of vitamin D, so anyone who has to take these should also take 1500 i.u. vitamin D a day plus a calcium supplement of 1 g a day.

An adequate diet and a good calcium intake is important, especially during the years when the bones are still being built up. An American study showed that women who had less than 405 mg of calcium a day in their diets lost bone density at a significantly faster rate than those who were having over 775 mg.

It has been noticed that osteoporosis occurs less frequently in areas where there is a high fluoride level in the drinking water. However, there is little evidence that fluoride supplements are an effective prevention and, indeed, the side effects of such supplements would probably outweigh any benefit they conferred.

## Complementary Treatment

Women who, for reasons of illness or family history, are particularly at risk of developing osteoporosis may find nutrition counselling beneficial. Herbalism, homoeopathy and acupuncture may be indicated for the treatment of diseases such as arthritis or thyroid disease which predispose patients to osteoporosis (see individual sections), and, by raising the patient's level of health, may reduce the risk of the bones becoming abnormally thin. These therapies may also help to speed the healing of fractures.

## Organizations

The National Osteoporosis Society, Barton Meade House, PO Box 10, Radstock, Bath, BA3 3YB (tel. 0761 32472), provides information and advice and has published a booklet about HRT.

# Peptic Ulcer

## Types of Ulcer and Cause

Peptic ulcers can be divided into two types – the gastric ulcer (situated in the stomach) and the duodenal ulcer (in the first part of the small bowel). Both the stomach and duodenum contain acid which is secreted by cells situated in the stomach lining and which is neutralized, further down the intestinal tract, by bile from the liver and by the alkaline fluids produced by the pancreas (see diagram of the digestive system on p. 257). Peptic ulcers are traditionally thought to occur either when excessive amounts of acid are secreted or when the resistance of the stomach and duodenal lining (the mucosa) is reduced, or when both of these happen together. Recently, the discovery that the bacteria *Campylobacter pylori* (abbreviated to *C. pylori*) is commonly present in peptic ulcers has led to theories that it may, in some way, be a factor in their formation. At the time of writing, this has not been proved but it has been shown that *C. pylori* is present in between 70 and 100 per cent of all patients with duodenal ulcers and in two thirds of those with gastric ulcers.

# Gastric Ulcer (GU)

This may occur in either sex and at any age, although it tends to be more common in the decade between fifty-five and sixty-five. Most patients seem to secrete normal or less than normal amounts of acid, suggesting that the fault lies in the resistance of the stomach lining.

# Duodenal Ulcer (DU)

Duodenal ulcer is more common in men than in women and tends to affect younger people than gastric ulcer, having a peak in the 45–55 age group, although it may also occur in the elderly. It affects some 10 per cent of the population but in recent years the number of cases seems to have been diminishing. One third of patients are found to secrete excessive amounts of acid into the stomach, while the secretions of the rest seem normal. DU seems to run in families and, for a reason as yet unknown, is three times more likely to occur in people with blood group O than in those with other blood groups.

# Symptoms

*Gastric Ulcer*
The commonest symptom is pain, occurring in the upper abdomen, below the V of the ribs. It often occurs after eating and may be associated with pain in the back. It is usually relieved by lying flat and is very seldom felt at night.

Vomiting occurs in over 50 per cent of cases and may be self-induced, as it often relieves the pain for a while. Weight loss is common, not because the appetite is affected, but because eating (particularly fried foods and spices) causes pain and is therefore avoided. Bloating and nausea may also occur after food. Bleeding from the ulcer occurs in 30 per cent of patients and the blood may be vomited or passed in the stools. In the latter case (known as melaena) the blood may not be recognizable as such because it has been altered during its passage through the bowel and the stools appear black and sticky.

Attacks, which seem to be commoner in the spring and autumn, usually last between two and six weeks, after which patients are free of symptoms for a few months. However, absence of symptoms does not mean that the ulcer has healed and recurrences are likely to occur if the condition is untreated.

*Duodenal Ulcer*
In some respects, the symptoms of DU are very similar to those of GU. The pain is felt in the same place in the upper abdomen and may go through to the back. Attacks are commonest in the spring and autumn and last up to six weeks, with symptom-free intervals of up to six months in between. However, there the similarity ends. Unlike gastric ulcer pain, that caused by a duodenal ulcer is eased by food and patients are inclined to put on weight as a result. Milk and antacids also relieve the pain and, because patients tend to be woken by the pain in the early hours of the morning, many will keep milk and biscuits beside the bed. Like patients with GU, those with a DU may suffer from bloating, but vomiting is far less common. They may also experience heartburn, water brash (a sour, burning fluid rising up from the stomach into the mouth) and diarrhoea or constipation. Duodenal ulcers bleed more commonly than gastric ulcers so melaena and vomiting of blood occur more often.

# Complications

The most common complications of a peptic ulcer are bleeding and perforation. In the latter, the wall of the stomach or duodenum is completely pierced by the ulcer so that its contents can enter the abdominal cavity. This is an emergency requiring immediate medical care. It is more common in DU than in GU and in men than in women.

When perforation occurs, the patient experiences severe abdominal pain, which is made worse by movement. Fifty per cent also complain of pain in the shoulder. Usually the pulse is raised, the temperature drops, the patient appears pale and sweaty and he may vomit. After three to six hours he may start to feel better but this is only a temporary improvement and without treatment the condition is fatal.

Occasionally, haemorrhage may be the first sign that a patient has developed an ulcer. Although it may settle down of its own accord, there is a high risk that the ulcer will bleed again and so, like perforation, this requires immediate treatment.

A less common complication is known as gastric outflow obstruction – that is, obstruction to the section of stomach that leads into the duodenum. Normally the passage of food from the stomach into the duodenum is controlled by a ring of muscle lying between the two which opens when the stomach's digestive processes are complete. However, if an ulcer occurs in this position, it may cause scarring so that the muscle is no longer able to open fully and the passage of food from the stomach to the duodenum is obstructed. If this occurs, the patient will start to vomit and will bring up food that he may have eaten many hours or days before. He will also be aware of a constant feeling of fullness or pain, particularly after eating. Vomiting rarely occurs more than two or three times a day but, because very little food gets through to the bowel from which it is normally absorbed, weight loss and constipation are likely to occur.

## Diagnosis

The standard method by which an ulcer is diagnosed is X-ray but in many places this has now been superseded by the use of the endoscope. X-ray diagnosis entails the patient drinking a quanity of fluid containing barium, which is opaque to X-rays (a 'barium meal') and pictures are then taken which demonstrate the shape of the stomach and intestines. This method has two drawbacks – firstly, very small ulcers may be missed and, secondly, a stomach cancer may, very rarely, look like, and be diagnosed as, an ulcer. The endoscope is a tube containing a tiny telescope and, sometimes, a camera; this is passed down the patient's oesophagus (gullet) into the stomach and duodenum, and enables the doctor to inspect every part of the stomach and duodenal lining (mucosa), making it far less likely that an ulcer will be missed. In addition, it enables him to take a biopsy from an ulcer in the stomach, which can then be examined to ensure that it is not malignant. The disadvantages of endoscopy are that the patient has to be sedated for the procedure and that it can only be carried out by a specialist.

The patient's stools may be tested to see whether there is any evidence of bleeding and a full blood count may be done to check for anaemia.

Although the diagnoses of perforation or haemorrhage are usually fairly obvious, these must be confirmed. In the case of perforation, air passes through the hole in the stomach or intestine and into the abdominal cavity. This can be seen on an X-ray of the abdomen, taken with the patient in an upright position, as black patches under the diaphragm. In the case of haemorrhage, endoscopy will locate the postion of the bleeding point. Both these techniques can be used to confirm the diagnosis of gastric outflow obstruction – an X-ray will show a greatly dilated stomach and endoscopy (done after the stomach contents have been aspirated) will show the position of the scarring. A barium meal will demonstrate that stomach contents are retained for more than the normal four hours.

## Orthodox Treatment

Treatment of peptic ulcers has been revolutionized in the last decade by the development of the group of drugs known as histamine $H_2$ receptor antagonists. The first of these was cimetidine and others such as ranitidine, famotidine and nizatidine have been developed since. They work by reducing the secretion of gastric acid so that symptoms are relieved very quickly and the ulcer heals in 80 per cent of cases. However, once the treatment has been discontinued there may be a relapse – between 50 and 85 per cent recur within a year – so that a proportion of patients need either to continue to take a small dose of the medication on a long-term basis or to take repeated courses each time the symptoms recur.

Another medication, tripotassium dicitratobismuthate or bismuth chelate, has not achieved the popularity of the $H_2$ receptor antagonists. This is partly because, when it was first introduced, it was unpleasant to take, although some years ago its formulation was changed so that it is now no more unpleasant than its rivals. In addition, it does not relieve ulcer symptoms quite as rapidly as $H_2$ receptor antagonists so that patients often need to take antacids as well. However, bismuth chelate has recently been shown to wipe out the bacteria *Campylobacter pylori* whose presence, it seems, can promote the recurrence of a healed ulcer. It also increases the healing ability of the mucosa of the stomach and duodenum, by stimulating their mucus production. Various studies have shown that, while relapses do occur in patients who are prescribed bismuth chelate (usually when *C. pylori* has not been totally eradicated) these are less likely than in patients who are treated with $H_2$ receptor antagonists. Although more and more specialists are prescribing bismuth chelate, some are still reluctant to use it because the long-term effects of bismuth are as yet unknown, while the action of the $H_2$ receptor antagonists is fairly thoroughly understood.

Sucralfate is another agent which helps to promote the healing ability of the mucosa. It seems to have no effect on *C. pylori* but still has a low relapse rate.

A new drug, misoprostol, has recently been introduced which works in a different way from those mentioned above, being a prostaglandins derivative. Prostaglandins are hormone-like substances produced by the body that appear to play an important role in inflammatory processes. Misoprostol has the dual effect of reducing gastric acid secretion and protecting the mucosa from erosion. Between 10 and 15 per cent of patients who take it develop diarrhoea but this usually clears up in due course, without the patient having to stop the medication.

Despite the efficacy of modern drugs, surgery is sometimes inevitable for the ulcer patient. Nowadays this is usually only performed for patients who fail to respond to medical treatment or for those who have developed complications. For gastric ulcers, it is usual to remove part of the stomach, taking the ulcer together with some of the acid-secreting cells. For duodenal ulcers, the ulcer itself is left intact and the aim of the operation is to reduce the amount of acid secreted by the stomach. This is done by cutting the vagus nerve, one of whose functions is to stimulate the cells lining the stomach. Because the vagus also supplies the muscle that closes off the stomach from the duodenum, cutting it prevents the stomach from emptying efficiently. Therefore the opening into the duodenum (the pylorus) has to be widened (pyloroplasty) to ensure that there is no obstruction. In recent years, some surgeons have been performing the operation known as highly selective vagotomy, in which only the nerve fibres running to the stomach wall are cut and the rest of the vagus is left intact. However, this is a very difficult operation and has a higher ulcer recurrence rate than does the straightforward vagotomy and pyloroplasty.

Surgery may be required as an emergency when an ulcer bleeds. A few surgeons are now using lasers, introduced into the stomach or duodenum through an endoscope, to seal off bleeding ulcers but, as yet, this technique is not generally available.

When a gastric ulcer perforates, the part of the stomach that is involved is removed. However, when it is a duodenal ulcer that has perforated, a patch of membrane taken from inside the abdominal cavity is sewn over the hole, and a vagotomy and pyloroplasty is done at a later date when the patient has recovered from the perforation. In both cases, the abdominal cavity is thoroughly cleaned out and, following the operation, the patient is given antibiotics in order to avoid the risk of infection within the abdomen.

Gastric outlet obstruction is treated in a similar way to a duodenal ulcer but even if a highly selective vagotomy is performed, additional surgery is necessary to enlarge the outlet from the stomach.

# Complementary Treatment

*Acupuncture*
The symptoms associated with peptic ulcer are said to be due to a dysfunction of the spleen, liver or stomach resulting from either an excess or a deficiency of energy (Chi). Treatment consists of balancing the energy and getting it to flow freely again, while strengthening the affected organs in order to restore their function to normal.

*Aromatherapy*
Among the oils used are chamomile, geranium and marjoram.

*Herbalism*
A number of herbs may be prescribed which promote the healing of ulcers, reduce gastric acidity and relieve pain. These include comfrey, marshmallow root, meadowsweet and slippery elm. Liquorice is also used. Some years ago liquorice derivatives were popular with orthodox practitioners for the treatment of peptic ulcers but these have rather fallen out of favour with the introduction of the $H_2$ receptor antagonists.

*Homoeopathy*
The choice of remedy will depend, among other things, upon when the pain occurs and what makes it better or worse. For example, pain occurring after food may be treated with uranium nitricum, kali bich. or arg. nit. Atropinum and anacardium are both used to treat patients whose pain is relieved by eating.

*Hypnotherapy*
Patients whose life-style causes a great deal of stress, which may be preventing the ulcer from healing, can be taught how to relax and to cope more effectively with stress.

*Nutrition*
The amino acids glutamine and glutamic acid in doses of 50–100 mg a day may be recommended in order to promote the healing of a peptic ulcer.

# Piles

## (Haemorrhoids)

---

## Definition and Symptoms

Piles are varicose veins that occur in the anal canal (the lowest part of the back passage). Here there is a network of veins which forms a soft pad inside the canal. Pressure inside the abdomen, such as may be caused by pregnancy, a tumour or chronic constipation, may impair the blood flow out of these veins so that they swell up, forming piles. However, in many cases no specific underlying cause can be found.

Piles are usually classified as first, second or third degree. First-degree piles are usually painless but cause bleeding. This is slight at first, and may remain so for months or years, just a small amount of bright red blood being seen when the patient passes a stool. Later on, the condition may progress to second degree, in which defecation (passing a stool) brings the piles down through the anus so that the patient is aware of soft swellings protruding out of his back passage. These prolapsed piles usually slip back by themselves, or the patient may have to give them a gentle push. Eventually, they begin to prolapse at other times, such as on exertion or when the patient is tired and, finally, they become third-degree piles, which are permanently prolapsed. These may cause great discomfort together with a

329

feeling of heaviness in the back passage and may be associated with a discharge and itching around the anus.

Excessive bleeding from piles may result in anaemia. The other major complication is thrombosis, in which the blood inside a prolapsed pile clots. The pile becomes swollen, purple and very painful. Without treatment it may become infected or may ulcerate, but usually starts to shrivel up after two or three weeks.

## Investigations

Because bleeding from the back passage can sometimes be a sign that there is a serious disorder in the bowels, a doctor should always be consulted when this occurs. He will examine the patient's abdomen to see whether he can feel any abnormal masses and will also examine the back passage. A small instrument called a proctoscope can be inserted into the back passage to enable piles to be inspected. Usually there are three prominent ones, situated at three, seven and eleven o'clock when the patient is lying on his back. In order to rule out any other problems, the doctor may use a flexible telescope (sigmoidoscope) to see higher up the bowel or may send the patient to have a barium enema (described in the section on irritable bowel syndrome).

## Orthodox Treatment

Because piles may be associated with constipation and the resultant straining that is necessary to pass a stool, a high fibre diet and avoidance of straining are effective preventive measures which will also help to stop first-degree piles from getting any worse.

The treatment of choice for troublesome first-degree piles is injection. This is done in the out-patients' department, since it is painless and fairly quick. Phenol in oil is injected into the area above each pile and this shuts down the blood vessel, cutting the vein off and allowing it to shrivel up. This treatment controls bleeding in about 90 per cent of patients but up to a third of these may find that their symptoms return after a while. Sometimes several injections are needed, at monthly intervals. Injections may also be used for more advanced piles if the patient is frail, elderly or otherwise unfit for an operation.

If the patient is young and fit, stretching (dilatation) of the muscle band inside the anus (the anal sphincter) under general anaesthetic is a quick, simple procedure which has very good results. It can be used in the treatment of all degrees of piles, although prolapsed piles may not respond well. Afterwards, some patients find that they are unable to control their bowels completely but this is a short-term side effect which rights itself fairly soon.

Other treatments include drying the piles up with heat (infra-red photocoagulation) or with cold (cryosurgery). The former, used for first-degree piles, is effective and painless but about 18 per cent of patients need further treatment. The latter is less often used since, although it is useful in the treatment of prolapsed piles, it may cause discomfort and a discharge for up to two weeks afterwards.

The treatment of choice for second-degree piles is to tie them off (ligation). Sometimes the piles are injected at the same time. The results are good and up to two thirds of patients with third-degree piles may also be helped by this procedure. Four per cent of those treated develop pain as a result and 1 per cent may have bleeding which, occasionally, is bad enough to warrant readmission to hospital.

For third-degree piles, the usual course of action is haemorrhoidectomy in which the piles are actually removed. The results are excellent, with symptoms recurring in only 5 per cent of patients over a period of five years. Occasionally patients may have problems such as pain, bleeding or acute retention of urine after the operation. Urinary retention is treated with catheterization (insertion of a tube into the bladder to drain it until it regains its function). If the bleeding is severe, it may be necessary to take the patient back to theatre and pack the bowel with gauze around a large rubber tube. This is then removed after forty-eight hours.

Specialists differ on the correct way to treat thrombosed prolapsed piles. Some put the patient to bed with the foot of the bed raised, give painkillers and put ice-packs on the pile and allow the condition to settle by itself. Others prefer to do an immediate haemorrhoidectomy or anal dilatation.

# Perianal Haematoma (Thrombosed External Pile)

Strictly speaking, this is not a true pile but a ruptured vein at the edge of the anus. It develops suddenly, often after the patient has been straining to pass a stool. There is pain and a lump which, if untreated, either subsides over the course of a few days or else bursts and releases a small amount of clotted blood.

Treatment consists of opening the haematoma under a local anaesthetic and removing the clotted blood inside. If, however, it has already started to resolve, frequent hot baths are all that is necessary.

# Complementary Treatment

*Aromatherapy*
Myrrh and cypress are among the oils that may be recommended.

*Herbalism*
Witch-hazel ointment or lotion will relieve itching and soothe inflammation round the anus. The appropriately named pilewort in ointment form will relieve pain and reduce inflammation. Chamomile suppositories, which are pushed into the back passage, may be soothing. A number of other herbs are also used.

*Homoeopathy*
Nux vomica may be prescribed for patients who have large piles that prolapse during defecation and who suffer from constipation and from burning pains which are worse at night. Burning and itching at night which are relieved by lying down, associated with hard stools and, sometimes, diarrhoea in the early morning,

may respond well to sulphur. Patients with very large prolapsed piles which bleed and burn and feel better when bathed with cold water may benefit from aloes. Hamamelis is helpful if there is profuse bleeding. Various other remedies may also be appropriate.

# Premenstrual Syndrome

## Definition and Incidence

A syndrome is a condition in which a number of symptoms occur together. It does not necessarily imply that all cases of the syndrome are due to the same cause. In premenstrual syndrome, the actual cause of the symptoms is, as yet, unknown, although a number of theories have been put forward.

Many women become slightly irritable just before a period or experience some breast tenderness. But when these symptoms become severe and are associated with others, a diagnosis of premenstrual syndrome can be made. The condition affects up to 40 per cent of all women, 5 per cent severely, and is most apparent in the 18–35 age group. Because it is something in the monthly hormonal cycle that brings it about, it is possible for a woman who has had a hysterectomy to continue to suffer from PMS as long as she still has her ovaries. (PMS is sometimes also known as the cyclical ovarian syndrome.)

PMS seems to affect certain types of women more frequently than others. Those suffering from irregular periods are more at risk. So too are those who have sexual or emotional problems, or who are separated or divorced; indeed, it is well known that any kind of stress can make the syndrome worse. Women who take the contraceptive Pill are less likely to have PMS.

# Symptoms

Symptoms may begin anywhere between day 15 and day 26 of a twenty-eight-day cycle and usually disappear by the second day of the period. Sometimes they may vanish quite dramatically once the bleeding has started. The commonest symptoms are depression, tension, swelling and fatigue.

Many of the symptoms seem to be associated with water retention. These include swelling (of the abdomen, legs, ankles and fingers), a feeling of bloatedness, weight gain (sometimes of several pounds), tender swelling of the breasts (sometimes with increased nodularity or pain), sinus-type headaches and stuffy nose (due to swelling of the lining of the nasal passages) and a reduced output of urine.

Slight swelling of the brain cells as a result of water retention is thought to be the cause of the mental symptoms, which include irritability, anxiety, depression, tension, fits of anger, poor control over the emotions, loss of self-confidence and problems with the concentration and memory. Occasionally these symptoms are very severe and are associated with violence or suicide attempts.

Lethargy and fatigue, added to the mental problems, often mean that the patient is less efficient than at other times of the month.

Other symptoms include tension headaches, clumsiness, muscular pain, cramping pains in the lower abdomen, skin problems and changes in the appetite and in sleeping patterns. Patients who suffer from hay fever, asthma, migraine and epilepsy may find that these conditions are worse premenstrually.

# Orthodox Treatment

Several treatments have been devised for PMS, all of which seem successful for certain women. Since these treatments work in quite different ways, it is possible that PMS is due to different causes in different patients and that response to a particular treatment therefore depends on whether or not it is the correct one for that individual. This would explain why, for example, despite the great success claimed for progesterone treatment, controlled trials have been unable to show that it has any significant effect.

Because a number of the symptoms seem to be due to water retention, many doctors recommend a reduction in salt intake (since salt encourages water retention) and prescribe diuretics such as spironolactone. These tablets enable the patient to pass more water and so they relieve swelling and some of the other symptoms. Spironolactone, unlike some diuretics, is also able to get through to the brain and it is suggested that the reduction in mental symptoms that it can produce is because it prevents swelling of the brain cells. However, diuretics only treat symptoms and, although helpful in mild cases, may not be the best treatment for patients with more severe problems.

Those doctors who maintain that PMS is due to a relative lack of the hormone progesterone give progesterone supplements in the form of injections or suppositories. These are given for one or two weeks before the period is expected. Some doctors prescribe synthetic derivatives of progesterone, such as norethisterone or dydrogesterone, which can be taken in tablet form. However, others say that the best effects are to be gained only by using natural progesterone. Unfortunately progesterone and its derivatives may cause side effects such as fatigue, lethargy and depression. Some patients respond very well to this treatment but for others it is ineffective. Some women find that taking the contraceptive Pill relieves their symptoms.

In a few cases, PMS appears to be due to excessive secretion of the hormone prolactin by the pituitary gland. For such patients, bromocriptine will be helpful. However, this, too, has side effects including nausea, dizziness, headache and constipation.

One of the most useful forms of treatment seems to be pyridoxine (vitamin $B_6$). A series of 630 women with PMS were treated with this at the St Thomas's group of hospitals over a period of eight years and about 80 per cent reported a great improvement in mental symptoms, breast problems and headache. Other symptoms were also helped. There are various reasons for thinking that pyridoxine is needed in PMS. First, it reduces the production of prolactin. Secondly, it is vital for the production of the chemical serotonin, a deficiency of which may cause depression. Pyridoxine itself is inhibited by oestrogen, which is why larger amounts may be necessary at those times of the month when the oestrogen level rises. The usual dose is 40 mg twice a day, rising to 75 mg twice a day by gradual steps if necessary, starting three days before symptoms are expected and stopping on the third day of the period. (The patients at St Thomas's were actually taking up to 200 mg a day.) A supplement of 10–15 mg of zinc a day should always be taken when one takes pyridoxine because the two substances work together in the body. Large doses of pyridoxine without a zinc 'chaser' may produce unpleasant side effects.

The most recent treatment to be acclaimed for PMS is evening primrose oil. This is being used by some doctors and the results seem to be very satisfactory. It is suggested that the true deficiency in PMS is one of the essential fatty acids (EFAs), a component of the diet which is vital for the formation of certain chemical compounds involved in bodily function. Evening primrose oil contains all these EFAs. The recommended dose is 1000 mg three times a day for two months, then 500 mg two or three times a day for as long as necessary. One doctor claims a 90 per cent success rate using this regime. It may be beneficial for those who take evening primrose oil to take a supplement of pyridoxine and zinc as well, since this increases the body's efficiency in its use of EFAs.

# Complementary Treatment

*Aromatherapy*
Parsley, neroli or juniper are among the oils that may be prescribed.

*Herbalism*
Herbs such as agnus castus and false unicorn (helonias) root help to balance the patient's hormones. Motherwort and scullcap are among the herbs that may be prescribed to treat anxiety or stress. Dandelion, parsley, couch grass and wild carrot are diuretics.

*Homoeopathy*

A patient who has swollen tender breasts, loss of libido and a bearing-down sensation in her lower abdomen which is relieved by crossing her legs may be helped by sepia. A swollen abdomen associated with swollen tender breasts and irritability may be relieved by natrum mur. Lachesis may be appropriate when the hands swell and the patient complains that her clothes feel tight.

*Nutrition*

PMS may be aggravated by excessive sugar and coffee so patients may be advised to reduce their intake of these items. Tension, irritability, anxiety, bloatedness, weight gain and breast tenderness may be due to a deficiency of B vitamins or magnesium. Magnesium is also necessary to maintain a normal hormone balance. Therefore supplements of this mineral and of B complex may be recommended. To ensure that the body uses vitamin $B_6$ efficiently, zinc will be given as well.

## Self-help

The PMT Advisory Service found that its patients were helped by taking a high-dose multivitamin/multimineral tablet and by adjusting their diet, reducing their intake of fat (especially animal fat), sugar, salt, junk food, tea and coffee, and increasing their intake of fibre, fruit and vegetables.

## Organizations

Advice is available from the National Association for PMS, Box 74, Sevenoaks, Kent, TN13 3PS (tel. 0732 459378) and from the Women's Nutritional Advisory Service, PO Box 268, Hove, East Sussex, BN3 1RW.

## Further Reading

*The Premenstrual Syndrome* by Dr Caroline Shreeve (Thorsons) is a useful and informative book.

# Prolapse

## Types of Prolapse, Causes and Symptoms

The organs in the lower part of the female abdomen are supported by the muscular layer known as the pelvic floor, above which they lie, and by various ligaments and fibrous bands which hold them in place. Damage to, or weakness of, any of these may result in the organs dropping down and bulging into the vagina.

If the anterior (front) part of the vaginal wall becomes weak, the urethra (the tube leading from the bladder, through which urine is passed) or the bladder may sag into it. These conditions are known as a urethrocoele and a cystocoele respectively. Descent of the rectum (back passage) into the posterior vaginal wall is known as a rectocoele; this is usually due to weakness of the pelvic floor. If the uterus (womb) drops down, this is known as uterine prolapse.

There are three degrees of uterine prolapse. In the first, the cervix, or neck, of the womb remains within the vagina. In the second, the cervix protrudes out of the vaginal opening. In the third, the entire uterus, pushing the vaginal lining before it, drops down and out of the vaginal opening. A third-degree prolapse is also known as procidentia.

A few women have an inborn weakness in the muscles and ligaments that hold up the uterus and may develop a minor

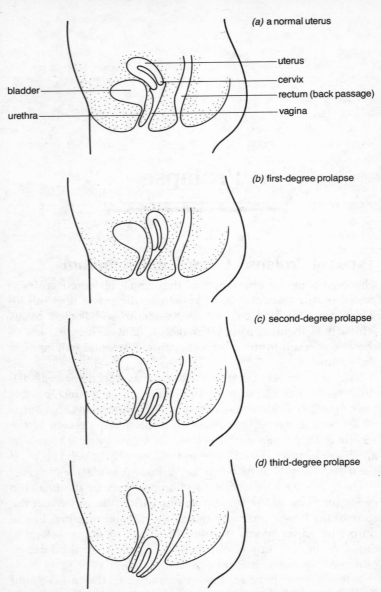

*(a) a normal uterus*

uterus
cervix
rectum (back passage)
vagina

bladder
urethra

*(b) first-degree prolapse*

*(c) second-degree prolapse*

*(d) third-degree prolapse*

*Prolapse of the uterus*

degree of prolapse. However, the majority of cases are due to injury or acquired weakness affecting these supports. This often occurs as a result of childbirth and is particularly likely in women who have had a number of children. Other causes include conditions, such as constipation, recurrent heavy lifting, chronic cough and obesity, which raise the pressure inside the abdomen and therefore put additional strain on the supporting structures. Symptoms may suddenly get worse at the time of the menopause, since the loss of circulating oestrogen in the body may lead to a rapid thinning of the uterine ligaments and of the muscles that support the vaginal wall.

The symptoms of prolapse are variable and it is possible to remain symptom-free even with a second-degree uterine prolapse. One of the commonest symptoms is low back ache and patients also frequently complain of a sense of fullness in the vagina or a dragging discomfort, which is worse after they have been standing for a long time. They may also be aware of a lump which protrudes from the vagina and which is worse when they stand or strain but which disappears when they lie down. If the bladder is pulled out of shape, urinary symptoms may occur, such as urgency, stress incontinence, frequency and pain on passing water. Discomfort or pain may also occur during intercourse. Patients who have second- or third-degree uterine prolapses often have a discharge, which may be blood-stained. Ultimately, ulceration may cause a haemorrhage.

If the angle at which the urethra leaves the bladder is distorted, as may occur in a urethrocoele or cystocoele, it may be impossible for the patient to empty her bladder completely. As a result she may feel that she wants to pass water again as soon as she has finished doing so ('double micturition') and may be troubled by recurrent urinary infections. Patients with rectocoeles may have difficulty in passing stools.

## Investigations

In most cases, a prolapse is easily identifiable on examination. The patient lies on her side and a curved metal instrument known as a Sims speculum is used to hold the walls of the vagina open. She is asked to cough or strain and the doctor can usually see the prolapse coming down. Normally a cervical smear is taken if she has not had one recently and a urine specimen is examined for any indication of infection. In patients with a third-degree prolapse, further investigations of the urinary tract (such as an X-ray of the kidneys) may be undertaken, since damage can occur as the result of long-term pressure on the bladder, leading to incomplete emptying.

## Orthodox Treatment

Because conditions such as obesity, chronic cough and constipation can weaken the supports of the uterus and vagina, patients are advised to lose weight, stop smoking or eat a diet with more fibre in it whenever these measures are appropriate.

Minor degrees of prolapse are common immediately after childbirth and usually all that is needed in such cases is a course of special exercises to strengthen the muscles of the pelvic floor. Spontaneous improvement is likely during the six months following childbirth and it is only if the prolapse continues after this that further treatment will be considered.

For those patients whose prolapse has been exacerbated by the onset of the menopause, hormone replacement therapy may be very helpful.

The use of pessaries, which are pushed into the vagina to hold it in shape, has been standard practice in the treatment of prolapse for many years. However, in recent times, it has become customary to reserve them only for those who are unfit for, are waiting for or have refused surgery, and for patients who are pregnant or have recently given birth to a child.

The ring pessary consists of a ring of flexible plastic which is pushed high up into the vagina and which holds its walls up and apart. The Hodge pessary is similar but more rectangular, while the Gelhorn pessary, which is used for the more severe degrees of prolapse, is shaped like a collar-stud. Long-term use of pessaries may result in ulceration, so patients need to be seen every three or four months and may need to use an anti-bacterial cream to prevent infection. Post-menopausal patients may also need an oestrogen cream to prevent undue thinning of the vaginal tissues.

If the patient is treated surgically, the actual operation used will depend upon the form of prolapse from which she is suffering. For a urethrocoele or cystocoele, the operation is an anterior colporrhaphy in which the sagging part of the vaginal wall is removed and all the tissues are tightened up. A similar technique is used for a rectocoele – a posterior colporrhaphy – and, here, the muscles of the pelvic floor will be repaired as well.

The treatment of choice for a uterine prolapse is hysterectomy. However, some women will not want to lose their wombs and, for them, a Manchester or Fothergill repair is performed in which part of the cervix is removed and the surrounding tissues tightened so that the uterus is pulled up into position again.

After a repair, whichever type has been performed, the patient may need to have a catheter draining her bladder for between two and five days, since urinary retention is common. In addition, she may have had a pack of gauze soaked in antiseptic solution placed in her vagina, which will need to be removed after twenty-four hours. This pack helps to prevent bleeding and infection, and stops the raw tissues from sticking to each other.

If a woman who has had a prolapse repair then has another pregnancy, she will need to have a Caesarean section, since a normal delivery could easily undo all the surgeon's good work.

## Complementary Treatment

Treatment by an acupuncturist, homoeopath or herbalist, combined with pelvic-floor exercises, may prevent a mild degree of prolapse from getting any worse and may help to strengthen the supporting tissues.

# Prostate
# Problems

## Description

The prostate gland lies just below the base of the male bladder, surrounding the urethra – the tube through which urine is passed – and is responsible for producing some of the fluid which, together with the sperm, makes up the semen (see diagram on p. 244). Because of its position, diseases affecting the prostate are likely to cause urinary symptoms. The gland itself has five lobes – anterior, median (or middle), posterior and two lateral – and the symptoms that occur depend primarily upon which lobe is most affected by the disease.

## Benign Enlargement (Benign Hypertrophy)

INCIDENCE

This is an extremely common condition, affecting all men over the age of forty to some extent. Why the prostate enlarges no one knows, and why it should do so more in some men than in others is also a mystery. Only about 10 per cent of those affected actually need treatment and, of these, the majority are between the ages of sixty and seventy. Europeans are more likely to develop benign enlargement than Indians, in whom the condition, when it occurs, tends to affect a younger age group. In black men it is unusual while in oriental men it is very rare.

## THE EFFECTS OF AN ENLARGED PROSTATE ON THE SURROUNDING TISSUES

The prostate may enlarge until it is up to ten times its normal size and it is usually the lateral and median lobes that are primarily affected. The result of this is that the urethra, which lies between them, becomes squashed and distorted. In order to pass urine down this flattened, twisting tube, the bladder has to work harder, so the muscular bands in its wall become thicker. However, the areas lying between the thickened muscles may become weaker as a result, and start to bulge, forming little pockets, or diverticula. Urine can collect in these pockets, acting as a focus for infection, or stones may form in the stagnant urine. The increased pressure within the bladder, produced by the thickened muscles, may also cause dilation of the ureters (the tubes that lead from the kidneys into the bladder) and may encourage urine to flow backwards towards the kidneys. This makes it easier for any bacteria within the bladder to infect the kidneys and, ultimately, renal failure may occur.

If the middle lobe of the prostate is enlarged, this may add to the stagnation within the bladder, since it pushes up into it and acts as a dam. A small pool of urine is therefore always present in the bladder.

The muscles of the bladder can only enlarge to a certain degree. When the obstruction to the flow of urine becomes too great for them to cope with, they give up and become loose and flaccid, causing total retention of urine.

The enlarged prostate may also press on the veins that run round the base of the bladder, causing congestion within them. Occasionally one of these dilated veins may leak, so that blood is passed in the urine.

## SYMPTOMS

Not all men who have enlarged prostates have symptoms and, among those who do, the severity of the symptoms does not necessarily correlate with the size of the gland. Nor are the

345

symptoms always progressive – it is possible for them to reach a certain stage and then get no worse. Indeed, once the patient has had symptoms for about ten years, it is unusual for them to worsen.

The earliest symptom is usually frequency – the patient finds first that he has to get up during the night to pass water (nocturia) and then that he has to go more often during the day. The band of muscle that controls the exit from the bladder may become stretched as it is distorted by the enlarged prostate and, as a result, a small amount of urine may, now and again, leak into the urethra. This automatically causes a desire to urinate so that the patient suffers from urgency – a need to rush to the toilet as soon as he feels that he needs to go.

As the condition worsens, the patient may become aware that his urinary stream is poor. Even when he wants to go, he may have to wait for the stream to start and, when it does so, it is often weak and may stop and start and tend to dribble towards the end. It may take a long time for the patient to empty his bladder and he may be left with the feeling that he has not emptied it completely.

The appearance of a drop of blood either at the beginning or the end of the stream occurs in 20 per cent of cases and, sometimes, may be the only symptom of prostatic enlargement.

Other symptoms include impotence (although, early on, an increase in sex drive may occur), urinary tract infections, stones in the bladder or the kidneys, a feeling of weight in the perineum (the area between the legs) or a feeling of fullness in the back passage.

Retention of urine may be acute or chronic. In the acute condition, the patient feels an urgent need to urinate but finds that he is unable to do so. The bladder is swollen and tender and rapidly becomes extremely painful. Acute retention may be precipitated by the patient having to delay passing water when he feels the need (for example, when driving down a motorway or on a long bus journey), by an excess of alcohol (especially when this is combined with going out on a cold night) or by being confined to bed for a few days.

Unlike acute retention, chronic retention is usually painless.

Each time the patient passes water, some urine is left behind and the bladder gradually distends. He becomes incontinent because small amounts constantly leak out of the over-full bladder, and kidney failure may occur. Occasionally, a patient suffering from chronic retention may develop acute retention as well.

Kidney failure prevents the body from getting rid of many of its waste products. These toxic materials circulate in the bloodstream and cause drowsiness, headache and behavioural and intellectual changes. Occasionally, an elderly man who develops what seem to be psychiatric problems may be found to be suffering from renal failure due to an enlarged prostate.

## INVESTIGATIONS

When a man goes to his GP complaining of a mixture of the symptoms listed above, it is usually quite simple to diagnose that he has a benign enlargement of his prostate. This can usually be confirmed if the GP examines the back passage, through which he will be able to feel the enlarged gland. He may also examine the patient's abdomen and kidneys, looking for signs of retention or of renal failure. A urine test may be taken to see whether it is infected and blood may be taken to check for kidney failure (when this occurs, the level of urea in the blood is higher than normal and the blood cell count may be reduced).

A plain X-ray of the abdomen may be requested if there is any suggestion that the patient has stones in the bladder or the kidneys. And the patient may be given a measuring jug and asked to record the number of times that he passes water over a period of seven days, together with the amount passed each time.

If he has noticed blood in his urine, the kidneys may be screened by giving an injection into a vein of a substance which, when excreted by the kidneys, shows up on X-ray. This test (an intravenous pyelogram or IVP) may also be requested if the doctor suspects that the kidneys have been damaged by back pressure from the bladder or as a result of chronic retention.

If the patient is referred to hospital as a potential candidate for surgery, other tests may be done. The amount of urine left in the bladder after he has passed water can be measured by ultrasound, and the flow rate may be measured by a special machine into which he urinates. A cystoscopy may be performed in which a special instrument is inserted, under general anaesthetic, through the urethra and into the bladder, enabling the surgeon to look for pockets in the bladder wall, stones or tumours.

ORTHODOX TREATMENT

If a patient develops acute retention, a catheter is passed into the bladder, allowing the urine to flow out. This will give immediate relief from the severe pain. Catheterization for the relief of chronic retention has to be a more leisurely affair, since bleeding may occur from the kidneys if it is done too quickly. In such cases, the bladder is drained gradually over a few hours.

Early in 1988 it was announced that prazosin, a drug which has been used in the treatment of high blood pressure, had been approved for treating patients with benign prostatic hypertrophy. Trials in Sweden, Italy and the UK had shown that 75 per cent of patients had a significant improvement in their symptoms when given this drug. Although surgical removal of the prostate is the only treatment which will permanently and completely relieve the symptoms of benign hypertrophy, prazosin is likely to prove very useful for those patients who, because of long waiting-lists, have to wait a considerable time before they can have their operation.

For those whose symptoms are disabling, prostatectomy will be recommended. In this, the enlarged inner section of the gland will be removed, leaving behind the outer 'false capsule' consisting of normal prostatic tissue which has become compressed by the swollen segments. Prostatectomy is a very safe operation and the results are usually very good, especially if performed before complications such as infection, retention or renal failure have occurred. There are several ways of doing it, of which trans-urethral resection (TUR) is the most popular. In this, an instrument is inserted into the prostate through the urethra and the gland is removed piecemeal. Over 90 per cent of patients are suitable for this operation, which has the advantage that no skin incision is necessary. However, exceptionally large prostates cannot be treated by TUR and have to be removed in another way. The oldest type of operation is a transvesical prostatectomy, in which an incision is made horizontally, low down on the abdomen, just above the hair line. The prostate is then approached via an incision in the bladder. Nowadays this operation is used mainly for those patients who, in addition to prostatectomy, need some operative treatment on the bladder, such as the removal of a diverticulum, or pocket. For other patients who are not suitable for TUR, retropubic prostatectomy can be performed. This is done through the same low abdominal incision as a transvesical prostatectomy, but the bladder is not opened.

*Complications of Operation*
In 3 per cent of cases, the prostate regrows, the symptoms return and the operation may have to be repeated.

Some 10–14 days after the operation, haemorrhage may occur. This is often associated with an infection. Since clots may form in the bladder, causing an obstruction to the flow of urine, readmission to hospital is usually necessary so that the bladder can be washed out. Because of the risk of infection, it is usual to do a urine test some two to four weeks after the operation.

Occasionally a patient may be unable to pass urine after the operation, because the muscles of the bladder have become flaccid. However, a short period of catheterization usually resolves this problem.

Two per cent of patients develop a stricture (narrowing) in the urethra or at the neck of the bladder in the first year following the operation. This results in an increasingly poor stream of urine but can be treated surgically.

Very occasionally patients complain of impotence following a prostatectomy, although there appears to be no physical reason for this. Incontinence, too, may occur but this is usually slight and resolves within a short time with the help of special exercises, bladder training and, if necessary, drugs. It is more likely to occur when patients have developed severe symptoms (such as retention) before having the operation.

All these complications, however, are quite uncommon. One which occurs more frequently, especially when a retropubic prostatectomy has been performed, is retrograde ejaculation.

349

Because one of the two bands of muscle that controls the opening of the bladder is destroyed in this operation, the ejaculate, instead of passing down the urethra, passes up into the bladder. Therefore the patient may not be impotent but is likely to be sterile. Another complication that may occur after a retropubic prostatectomy is acute epididymitis – infection of the epididymus, the little gland that sits on the top of each testis. In order to reduce the risk of this occurring, some surgeons do a vasectomy before performing the prostatectomy, thus making it harder for infection to reach the epididymus.

# Acute Prostatitis

This is a fairly common condition that usually affects young men. It may be caused by bacteria that have been carried in the bloodstream from another area of infection in the body, such as the tonsils, the teeth or a crop of boils on the skin. In a few cases, it may be secondary to an infection in the bladder or kidneys.

SYMPTOMS
The onset of the illness is sudden, with the patient complaining of flu-like symptoms and a raised temperature. He may develop frequency and dysuria (pain on passing water) and may pass some blood. Pain or discomfort may be experienced in the back, the perineum, the lower abdomen or the back passage and, if it is severe, retention of urine may occur.

INVESTIGATIONS
The doctor may ask the patient to urinate, catching the urine in three containers in turn. The middle specimen is sent for culture while the first is examined for 'threads', tiny thread-like structures which, although not diagnostic of prostatitis, are often associated with it. Very often, the urine has no bacteria in it. A diagnosis is usually made primarily on the patient's symptoms.

ORTHODOX TREATMENT AND COURSE
Most cases of prostatitis clear up quickly when treated with

antibiotics. However, delayed or inadequate treatment may result in the formation of an abscess (this is rare) or the development of chronic prostatitis. If an abscess forms, the pain becomes throbbing and the patient's other symptoms may worsen. However, once the abscess has been drained surgically, it seldom causes any further trouble.

# Chronic Prostatitis

The symptoms of this condition are rather more vague than those of actue prostatitis and are probably due to small areas of chronic infection within the prostate. It tends to affect men between the ages of thirty and fifty but may be a complication of benign hypertrophy of the prostate.

SYMPTOMS
The patient may be aware of a dull ache or a feeling of fullness in the perineum or the back passage, which is made worse if he sits on a hard chair. Often he has low back pain which may travel down his legs. Usually he will also have urinary symptoms such as frequency, urgency and pain on passing water, and he may develop retention. Some patients have a recurrent fever and feel generally unwell. Premature ejaculation or impotence may occur. Some men find that ejaculating relieves their symptoms, while for others this makes them worse.

INVESTIGATIONS
By inserting a finger into the patient's back passage, the doctor can massage the prostate, causing a few drops of prostatic fluid to run down the urethra. This fluid can be collected and examined for bacterial growth and cells. Often no bacteria can be cultivated although pus cells are evident. The three-container urine test used for acute prostatitis may also be helpful in diagnosis since, as in the acute condition, the first glass may contain 'threads'.

ORTHODOX TREATMENT
Although antibiotics may help to relieve the urinary symptoms,

their ability to wipe out an infection deep within the prostate seems to be limited. If the flow of urine becomes obstructed because the urethra is constricted, a prostatectomy may be necessary.

# Cancer of the Prostate

This is one of the commonest tumours occurring in men and is the most common in men over the age of sixty-five. About 5000 new cases are diagnosed in the UK each year. It is rare before the age of forty and uncommon before fifty, but the incidence rises steeply in the 65–75 age group. However, many elderly men with prostatic cancer die from other causes – up to 60 per cent of men who die in their seventies are found to have the disease on post-mortem, although less than one sixth of them have had any prostatic symptoms.

SYMPTOMS
In 75 per cent of cases, the cancer begins in the posterior lobe of the prostate and so, at first, produces none of the symptoms that are associated with benign hypertrophy of the lateral lobes. The first symptom in 20 per cent of cases is pain in the hip bones or back, or sciatica, due to the cancer spreading in the blood to the bones. About 50 per cent of patients develop urinary symptoms, such as frequency or a poor stream, and retention is not uncommon. Only 10 per cent, however, will pass blood in the water. Some patients may have pain in the perineum or in the lower abdomen and some may become anaemic.

INVESTIGATIONS
The doctor will examine the patient through the back passage. A prostate gland which is affected by cancer may feel hard and uneven, unlike the smooth outline of a normal gland or of one with benign hypertrophy.

The blood tests that are done are the same as those performed in cases of benign hypertrophy. In addition, blood is taken to measure the enzyme acid phosphatase, which will be raised above normal in 50 per cent of cases of cancer of the prostate.

X-rays of the bones, especially those of the pelvis, lower back, thighs and chest, may indicate whether or not the cancer has spread to other parts of the body.

A cystoscopy will enable a biopsy to be taken of the prostate, and the specimen will be examined under a microscope.

ORTHODOX TREATMENT

In many cases, the diagnosis of cancer of the prostate is only made when a TUR (see above) is performed to treat acute or chronic retention. In such cases, if the cancer is small, it may be possible to remove it completely. In some countries, total prosta-tectomy, in which the entire gland is removed, is performed, but this is not done in the UK. The disadvantage of total prostatec-tomy is that the patient is always impotent and usually inconti-nent after the operation.

Radiotherapy is a useful treatment, especially for younger patients in whom the cancer shows no evidence of having spread to other parts of the body. It may be given as an external therapy, with an X-ray beam directed at the prostate, or radio-active iodine or gold may be implanted into the prostate during the operation. Radiotherapy is also helpful for those patients whose cancer has spread only to a single site and can often give instant pain relief.

When the cancer has begun to spread, hormone therapy can be very effective, since the cancer seems to need the male hormone, testosterone, in order to survive. The aim of treatment is to remove or suppress the patient's hormone output and this can be done by orchidectomy (removal of the testes), which may produce a dramatic remission in the disease. However, some doctors feel that the psychological problems that may be as-sociated with orchidectomy make this a less valuable therapy and many prefer to treat patients by using female hormones which suppress the patient's male hormones.

When female hormones are given, it is usually in the form of stilboestrol. This, unfortunately, may have side effects which include enlargement of the breasts, pigmentation of the nipples and scrotum, and shrivelling of the testes. It may also cause fluid retention. This is a problem for a patient who has heart disease, because the increased blood volume which the heart has to

353

pump due to the presence of the excess fluid may overtax it and precipitate him into heart failure. Until recently, orchidectomy was the best form of treatment for such patients. However, a new class of drugs has been developed which blocks the production of testosterone by the testes. These are known as LHRH analogues – LHRH standing for luteinizing-hormone releasing hormone. Luteinizing hormone (LH) is the hormone that stimulates the production of testosterone, and LHRH stimulates the production of LH. An LHRH analogue replaces the patient's own LHRH and prevents it from acting – rather like an incorrect key which, although it will not open the lock, will prevent another key being inserted. At the start of treatment with these drugs, the production of testosterone may be temporarily increased, so the patient is usually given another drug such as cyproterone acetate to counteract this. Cyproterone is also used in treatment on its own to block the action of the male hormones.

The adrenal glands, too, produce a small quantity of male hormones. This can usually be suppressed by using cyproterone or an LHRH analogue but sometimes removal of the adrenals may become necessary. This can be very effective for patients who are suffering from pain in the bones due to cancer deposits and whose pain is not relieved by other measures. The drug ketoconazole has been used to suppress the action of the adrenals but can cause damage to the liver.

## Prostatic Calculi (Stones)

Occasionally these may cause symptoms similar to those of chronic prostatitis or benign enlargement, but generally they are symptomless and are discovered on X-ray or at prostatectomy. They usually occur in men over the age of fifty.

If they are small, prostatic massage through the back passage, plus a course of antibiotics, is likely to relieve any symptoms. Otherwise a prostatectomy may be necessary.

## Recent Advances

In Israel, doctors have been using microwaves to treat benign enlargement, prostatitis and prostatic cancer. The treatment is given via a rod which is inserted into the back passage and which heats the prostate, but not the surrounding tissues, to a higher temperature than normal. For benign enlargement, one or two hour-long sessions of treatment are given a week, up to a maximum of ten. In the treatment of cancer it is used together with radiotherapy. How it works is unknown but it seems to be effective and to have no side effects. The doctors using it are claiming a success rate of around 60 per cent. However, at present, the equipment necessary is very expensive and, at the time of writing, the treatment is not yet available in Britain, although one London hospital is reported to be considering giving it a trial. If the large-scale studies now under way prove successful, this could be a great step forward in the treatment of prostate problems. Every year over 50,000 prostates are removed in the UK, each patient needing up to ten days in hospital and four weeks off work.

# Complementary Treatment

*Aromatherapy*
Oils containing essence of onion or pine may be recommended.

*Herbalism*
Various herbs which act as urinary antiseptics may be helpful in prostatitis. These include horsetail, sea holly (eryngo) and gravel root, all of which also act to reduce inflammation. Herbs with hormonal effects, such as damiana may be useful in the treatment of benign enlargement. Saw palmetto, horsetail and couch grass may also help to control symptoms in this condition.

*Nutrition*
Gama aminobutyric acid (GABA) may help to reduce an enlarged prostate by stimulating the release of the hormone prolactin from the pituitary.

# Psoriasis

## Incidence and Cause

Psoriasis is a fairly common, chronic, scaly condition of the skin that affects about 2 per cent of the white European and North American population but occurs less frequently in black and Japanese people. It tends to run in families and about one third of patients have a blood relative who also has psoriasis. A child who has one parent with psoriasis has a 20–30 per cent chance of developing the disease, but if both parents are affected, the risk to the child is nearer 50 per cent.

Although psoriasis can cause serious problems for some patients, many have only a few small areas of skin affected at any one time. Some may have a single severe attack which clears up and does not recur, although it is more usual for the disease to come and go throughout the patient's life.

Psoriasis usually makes its first appearance between the ages of fifteen and thirty. It is very rare under the age of five and uncommon between the ages of five and ten. When it does occur in childhood, the attacks are usually mild. There is no upper age limit after which it will not develop, and people have been known to have a first attack in their eighties. The sexes are equally affected, but in men the condition causes fewer cosmetic problems, since the rash can be covered by trousers and the long sleeves of a shirt.

The cause of psoriasis is unknown but there are probably several factors involved, one of which may be an inherited defect in the skin. Attacks can occur quite suddenly and seem to be precipitated by mental stress, injury to the skin and some drugs, such as the anti-malarial chloroquine. They also tend to occur two to three weeks after streptococcal infections.

# Types of Psoriasis

## PLAQUE PSORIASIS

Psoriasis may take a number of different forms, the commonest of which is known as plaque, discoid or scaly psoriasis. In this chronic form the patient has one or more dark red, scaly, circular or oval plaques, raised above the surface of the normal skin. Each plaque has a well-defined border and has the appearance of having been stuck on. The upper surface is covered with silvery or white crumbly-looking scales, although occasionally these are absent. Plaques may be as small as 1 cm across but may grow larger; sometimes smaller plaques merge together to form one large plaque with a scalloped edge.

Although plaques can occur anywhere, the commonest sites are the knees, elbows, lower part of the back, and the scalp, especially behind the ears. They also tend to appear wherever the skin has been injured and so may be precipitated by hard manual work. Affected skin is brittle and therefore prone to injury, which may be a problem for young people whose knees and elbows may get knocked when they are playing sports. The rash can also become worse if it is constantly being rubbed (for example, by a waistband or bra strap).

Sometimes this type of psoriasis can affect skin folds (known as the intertriginous areas) – in the groins, the armpits, under the breasts, between the toes, and around the umbilicus and the anus. In these areas, where the skin tends to be moist and the touching skin surfaces rub each other, the plaques are often smooth and red without any scale on them. Intertriginous psoriasis is more common in older age groups and may cause considerable soreness, which can make it difficult for the patient to move comfortably.

Itching is an unusual symptom in psoriasis but may occur when it affects the intertriginous areas or the scalp.

## GUTTATE PSORIASIS

This form usually occurs in children under the age of sixteen and often follows a streptococcal throat infection. The spots, which are small and scattered over the trunk and limbs, are smoother than those of plaque psoriasis but scratching them will reveal the classic silvery scale. They usually appear suddenly and often clear spontaneously within three months. In most cases the only treatment needed is ultraviolet light (see below) and the majority of patients will be free of the rash within six weeks if treated three times a week. A few, however, will go on to develop chronic plaque psoriasis.

## PUSTULAR PSORIASIS (VON ZUMBUSCH'S DISEASE)

This condition, which is rare, starts suddenly with the appearance of tiny pustules (pus-filled spots) all over the body. The skin may be red and usually the patient has a high temperature, which may precede the appearance of the spots. The pustules themselves are sterile (that is, they do not contain bacteria) but the patient is often quite ill and needs admission to hospital. Absorption of food from the intestines may become abnormal, making intravenous drip-feeding necessary.

## PSORIASIS OF THE HANDS AND FEET

This has a quite different appearance from plaque psoriasis. The skin may be red, scaly and cracked, and the affected areas often have a sharp border. The cracks may become inflamed and very painful and may prevent the patient from using his hands normally or from walking.

The hands and feet may also be affected by a localized form of pustula psoriasis, which is sometimes known as persistent palmar and plantar pustulosis or recalcitrant eruption of the palms and soles. Small red scaly areas with sterile pustules develop on the palms and soles and may last for years. Occasionally only one palm or sole is affected but usually both are involved. However, less than 20 per cent of patients affected by this type of psoriasis have plaques on other parts of their bodies.

## PSORIASIS OF THE NAILS
The nails are commonly involved in cases of chronic plaque psoriasis. The first sign is usually the appearance of tiny pits on the nail surface. The nails may then become discoloured, thickened and distorted and may separate from the underlying nail bed (a condition known as onycholysis) so that the end of the nail looks white. This may interfere with the patient's dexterity, making fine manual work, needlework and even typing difficult to perform. Bacteria that produce a coloured pigment may breed under the detached part of the nail so that it appears green or black.

## PSORIASIS OF THE FACE AND SCALP
One of the few good things about psoriasis is that it rarely affects the face. On the odd occasion that it does so, it produces a rash which looks like seborrhoeic dermatitis (see the section on eczema). However, the scalp is often involved, occasionally without the rash being apparent anywhere else on the body. It may involve the whole scalp or just small areas, and affected parts feel lumpy and irregular where the scales shed from the surface of the rash have piled up. The shed scales also produce very severe dandruff. Usually the rash stops at the hair line and doesn't spread on to the neck.

## ERYTHRODERMIC PSORIASIS (ERUPTING ACTIVE PSORIASIS)
This is a fairly rare complication of chronic psoriasis. The rash suddenly becomes worse, with redness and scaling spreading all over the body, particularly over areas of skin that have been injured or scratched. The increased blood flow to the skin surface causes the patient to lose heat and, particularly in cold weather, hypothermia may result. Fluid can also be lost through the

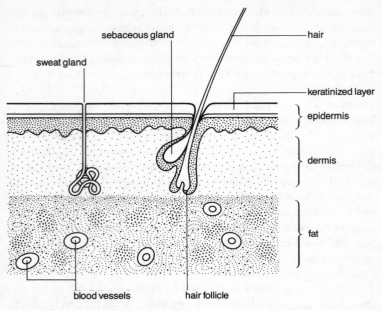

*A section through the skin*

damaged skin. Patients with erythrodermic psoriasis need immediate hospital care.

NAPKIN PSORIASIS
This occurs in babies, starting in the napkin area, and looks somewhat like plaque psoriasis, being a rash of dull red patches with well-defined borders and, sometimes, large silvery scales. However, experts are uncertain whether this really is a form of psoriasis. It may spread to other parts of the body but it responds well to simple treatment and does not recur.

## Mechanics of Psoriasis

In normal skin the cells of the epidermis are replaced every 50–60 days but in psoriasis the process is enormously speeded up and the turnover occurs every 5–6 days. When the intertriginous areas are affected, the sweat glands may become blocked so that sweating is reduced and heat stroke can occur if the patient works in a hot atmosphere.

Although the skin around the psoriatic plaques usually appears normal, examination under the microscope shows that changes have occurred here too; one of these is a tendency to speed up production of skin cells if it becomes injured. Thus injury can precipitate the production of another plaque.

# Prognosis

Most people who have psoriasis will have it for life. However, its course is very variable and sometimes it may disappear spontaneously for periods of months or years. The less severe the condition, the more likely these remissions are to occur. Most patients will be able to find some form of treatment that will either get rid of their rash or dramatically improve it.

Women usually find that psoriasis improves during pregnancy, probably as a result of the increased hormones that their bodies are producing.

About 5 per cent of patients with psoriasis develop an associated arthritis. If their blood serum is tested for the 'rheumatoid factor' found in patients with rheumatoid arthritis, it is negative; this form of arthritis is therefore one of those that is known as 'sero-negative'. It often affects the joints of the hands, knees and ankles, and may occasionally occur in a patient whose skin is perfectly normal. In such a case, the diagnosis is difficult and may only be made if all other forms of arthritis have been excluded and if the patient has a family history of psoriasis. The treatment of psoriatic arthritis is similar to that of rheumatoid arthritis (see separate section), and the condition usually responds well to anti-inflammatory drugs. However, steroids, which are useful in other forms of arthritis, are not recommended because, when the dose is reduced, the patient's psoriasis may become worse.

# Diagnosis

When a patient develops the classic scaly plaques, diagnosis is not difficult. However, sometimes the advice of a skin specialist is necessary before a firm diagnosis can be made.

In some cases the plaques look smooth, but if the doctor gently scrapes one of them with a wooden spatula the typical silvery scales will appear. If he removes all the scale, a red, smooth, slightly moist area will be left with a few tiny bleeding points.

The scaly type of psoriasis which affects the hands and feet may be hard to distinguish from chronic eczema if there is no rash on other parts of the body. And, occasionally, psoriasis affects the nails without there being any skin rash. In such cases it may be very hard to tell it from a fungal infection of the nails. One helpful point is that a fungal infection usually begins in only one nail and rarely affects more than a few, whereas in psoriasis all the nails may be involved. However, in order to make the diagnosis, the doctor will need to take some nail clippings. These will be sent to the laboratory and examined under a microscope. Absence of fungal disease suggests that psoriasis is the cause.

# Orthodox Treatment

Many cases of psoriasis can be controlled with simple ointments or creams. However, the GP may refer a patient to hospital if the rash is extensive, if it doesn't respond to simple treatments or if it is causing problems because of its situation (a rash on the feet, for example). Types of medication available can be divided into topical (applied to the skin) and systemic (taken by mouth or injected). Most of the systemic treatments mentioned below are available only from hospital consultants.

TOPICAL TREATMENT
*Emollients*
Emollients are used to reduce dryness in the skin. They work by leaving an oily film over the skin surface which allows moisture to build up underneath it. They often come in the form of bath

oils or as emulsifying ointments which can be used instead of soap. Unfortunately, the effects start to wear off after three or four hours so, for the best results, they need to be applied several times a day.

For patients with just a few small plaques, Vaseline can be useful, rubbed in once or twice a day.

### Keratolytics

Keratolytics smooth the skin surface by promoting the shedding of scales. One which is commonly used is salicylic acid (a relative of aspirin) in a dilution of 1–6 per cent. However, it is unsafe to use this on large areas of skin since it may be absorbed into the body and produce the same effects as an overdose of aspirin.

### Tar

Tar is an end product of the distillation of coal or wood and contains thousands of different organic compounds. It is often helpful in the treatment of psoriasis although the way in which it acts isn't clear. The main problem with tar is that the more effective the preparation, the messier it is to use, crude coal tar preparations giving better results than tar-containing creams. Various bath additives and shampoos and a somewhat less messy tar stick are also available. In order to keep messiness and staining of clothes to a minimum, tar preparations should be applied sparingly and should be covered with a light dressing. However, they need only be applied once a day.

Tar is especially useful in the treatment of psoriasis situated in the groin, around the navel or under the breasts. It is also very helpful for areas where the skin has become thickened or itchy. Its action is improved by ultraviolet light. Used by itself it will usually take three weeks before any improvement is noticeable and may take as long as eight. Unfortunately, some patients are unable to use it because it irritates the skin and, occasionally, it can produce an acne-like rash.

### Steroids

Steroid creams can produce a dramatic improvement in a psoriasis rash but, unfortunately, the effect is often short-lived and only lasts for as long as the cream is used. Once it is stopped, the patient relapses and the rash may become worse than it was originally. In addition, it is thought that using steroids on plaque psoriasis may occasionally precipitate an attack of pustular psoriasis.

It is impossible for a patient to continue to use steroid creams long term, in order to prevent relapses, because of the risk of serious side effects. Not only is there a danger that the steroids may be absorbed into the body but they may result in the local area of skin becoming thin. Thin skin may easily be damaged, may bruise readily and may take several months to return to normal after the steroid cream has been stopped. Stretch marks may also appear in the treated skin and, once formed, these are permanent.

For all these reasons, steroids have only a very limited part to play in the treatment of psoriasis. They can be useful for treating the groin, the navel and the skin under the breasts, which may be oversensitive to other forms of treatment, and they are also used for patients whose psoriasis has become very active, with new patches appearing rapidly. However, strong steroids should not be used for more than two weeks at a time and there should be an interval of at least two months before they are used again.

No topical treatment has been discovered that will restore the nails to normal. Steroid injections have been tried around the nail beds but were found to be painful and relatively ineffective.

*Dithranol*
Dithranol has two things in common with tar. First, it is a complex organic substance (although it is synthesized in the laboratory rather than being distilled). And, second, the way in which it works in the treatment of psoriasis is not understood. It is useful for plaque psoriasis but is not suitable for use on the scalp or the intertriginous areas and should never be used on the face or near the genitalia. Differing concentrations are available but the strongest are reserved for patients who are receiving treatment in hospital. Normally dithranol is prescribed only for people whose rash cannot be controlled by tar preparations.

When it is used in hospital, the patient usually takes a tar bath and is then exposed to ultraviolet light before the preparation is applied to the rash. If this is done five days a week, the plaques will usually disappear within two to three weeks. If dithranol is used without tar and ultraviolet light it usually takes at least three weeks to produce an improvement and may take up to eight weeks. No benefit has been found from applying it more than once a day.

Dithranol is an irritant and may cause redness or even blistering in some patients. A low concentration is usually prescribed at first, stronger preparations being used later if necessary. It stains the clothes and the skin a brownish-violet shade but, once the treatment has stopped, the skin discoloration will peel off within a few days. Treatment must always be stopped as soon as the psoriatic plaques have disappeared in order to avoid irritating normal skin.

*Shampoos*
Patients whose psoriasis affects the scalp need to wash their hair frequently with a special shampoo. If the scalp is thickly encrusted with scales, it is advisable to use a tar and salicylic acid ointment on the scalp every night and a tar-based shampoo every morning.

SYSTEMIC TREATMENT
Because of their potentially serious side effects, systemic preparations are usually only prescribed by hospital dermatologists. In pregnancy, all systemic therapy must be stopped immediately because of the risk that it may cause malformations in the unborn child.

Cytotoxic (cell-killing) drugs such as methotrexate, which prevent cells from dividing rapidly, are used only for very severe cases which respond to nothing else, and for generalized pustular and erythrodermic psoriasis.

*Methotrexate*
This drug is usually taken by mouth once a week, although sometimes injections are given. During the course of treatment, all alcohol is forbidden because, mixed with methotrexate, it can cause severe liver damage. Even without alcohol, there is a risk

to the liver if the drug is taken over a long period. For patients who may be on it for some years, a liver biopsy may be done before the course begins (to ensure that the liver is normal) and then repeated at regular intervals of eighteen months to two years for as long as treatment continues. Any deterioration in the condition of the liver would entail the patient coming off methotrexate immediately.

Other side effects are indigestion, nausea, abdominal pain and an increased susceptibility to infections. In addition, methotrexate can suppress the production of blood cells in the bone marrow, so regular blood counts are necessary. Other cytotoxic drugs used in the treatment of psoriasis have been shown to affect the liver less but are more likely to affect the bone marrow.

### Etretinate

This is a derivative of vitamin A which is taken daily by mouth. It takes four to six weeks to work and is always accompanied by side effects such as dry skin, cracked lips, nosebleeds and, sometimes, temporary hair loss. It can also cause a rise in the level of fats in the blood, making regular blood tests necessary. It can cause malformation in an unborn baby so, because it stays in the body for a long period, it is necessary for women to continue to use contraception for at least a year after stopping treatment. Etretinate is often used to good effect together with PUVA (see below) and is particularly useful in the treatment of generalized pustular psoriasis and erythrodermic psoriasis. The forms affecting the hands and feet also respond well but in cases of chronic plaque psoriasis the response is often quite poor.

### PUVA

PUVA stands for psoralens with ultraviolet light type A. Psoralens are naturally occurring (but now synthetically manufactured) compounds which sensitize the skin to light. In the treatment of psoriasis, the patient takes the preparation by mouth and, two hours later, is exposed to ultraviolet light from special lamps. Treatment is usually given three or four times a week at first but, once the rash has responded, this may be reduced to maintenance therapy once or twice a week. Most patients become quite tanned during the treatment. There are, however, drawbacks. The lamps are contained in a special cabinet in which the patient has to stand and some people are unable to tolerate this without developing claustrophobia. Also some very fat patients may be unable to fit into the cabinets safely and comfortably. Occasionally, excessive treatment may burn the skin and fair-skinned people who are known to be sensitive to sunlight may be unsuitable for PUVA.

Because every part of the body, including the eyes, is sensitized to light by psoralens, the patient has to wear special protective spectacles from the minute she takes the drug until at least twelve hours have elapsed after treatment. The method of action of PUVA, like the other psoriasis treatments, has not been clearly demonstrated but it is thought that, in the presence of ultraviolet light, it acts on the nuclei of the cells to slow down their activity.

Most people need about fifteen treatments in order to clear the rash and, after this, will usually have four or five months without relapsing. Even with maintenance therapy, there is a tendency for the rash to return after a period of several months. However, some 90 per cent of patients with plaque psoriasis find this form of treatment effective. It is also helpful for localized pustular psoriasis of the palms and soles, where the affected areas can be exposed to the light by putting the hands or feet into a little box containing lamps. PUVA may also be used for some patients with generalized pustular or erythrodermic psoriasis.

PUVA is not generally used on patients under eighteen unless the rash is so severe that the alternative is cytotoxic drugs. And even in older patients it is only used if the rash covers 20 per cent or more of the body surface. In the 18–60 age group, PUVA is usually used only if dithranol has failed to produce results or irritates the patient's skin even in low concentrations.

# Recent Advances

In 1987 a group of Japanese doctors reported that they had treated twenty-two psoriatic patients with a vitamin D compound and had found that the results were almost as good as those that could be expected from using a steroid cream. A trial which used vitamin D preparations taken by mouth and used topically over a period of three months resulted in 76 per cent of patients reporting at least a moderate improvement of their psoriasis with practically no side effects.

. Doctors at the Royal Hallamshire Hospital in Sheffield have found that ten capsules a day of the fish-oil extract Maxepa significantly reduced itching, redness and scaling in patients with psoriasis.

Meanwhile, some patients have found their condition becoming worse when they have been put on drugs for other complaints. This has resulted in doctors suggesting that the antihistamine terfenadine, the anti-inflammatory drug indomethacin and the blood-lipid-lowering drug gemfibrozil should not be prescribed for those with psoriasis.

# Complementary Treatment

*Aromatherapy*
Lavender and bergamot may be prescribed.

*Herbalism*
Herbalists often equate chronic conditions with toxicity, the accumulation of toxins resulting from and contributing to a malfunction of the tissues affected. The aim of treatment is to cleanse the system and promote normal function in the tissues. Herbs that are often used in toxic skin conditions to cleanse the tissues and restore healthy function are burdock root, red clover and sarsaparilla.

*Homoeopathy*
The choice of remedy will depend, among other things, on where the rash is worst (for example, behind the ears or on the hands), whether it is itchy, and on the appearance of the rash itself. For example, arsenicum album may be used for a patient whose rash is burning and itching but whose symptoms are relieved by warmth, while sulphur may be suitable for one whose rash is itchy, sore and made worse by contact with water.

*Hypnosis*

For those patients whose psoriasis is made worse by stress or emotional upset, hypnosis is a very valuable therapy. First the patient will be taught how to relax and then how to hypnotize herself. During her sessions of hypnosis with the therapist she will be given the suggestion that, as she becomes more relaxed, her psoriasis will disappear. She may be given a visualization as well; for example, she may be told to imagine that she is swimming in a clear blue stream and that, as she swims, her rash is being gently washed away. She can then use the visualization when she practises her self-hypnosis. The improvement in the patient's skin is usually slow but steady and she develops confidence in her own ability to keep the rash under control in stressful situations.

*Nutrition Therapy*

High-dose vitamin A derivatives are used in orthodox medicine as a treatment for psoriasis, but patients who are not being prescribed these may find a daily supplement of vitamin A helpful, together with zinc which is important for the maintenance of healthy skin.

## Self-help

People with widespread psoriasis, particularly if it affects the intertriginous areas, should avoid working in overheated or badly ventilated places, as their sweating mechanism may be defective.

Humidifiers may be helpful at home, since dry air will make the rash worse.

Baths should be tepid rather than hot and an emulsifying ointment or soap substitute should be used for washing, rather than soap, which has a drying effect on the skin. Once out of the bath, the patient should gently pat her skin dry rather than rubbing vigorously, as damaging the rash may make it worse.

Sunlight often makes the rash better but an excessive amount may make it worse.

A naturopathic diet may help, in which the patient reduces

her intake of meat, refined carbohydrates, dairy produce, coffee, tea and sugar, and increases her intake of nuts, seeds, whole grains and pulses.

## Organizations

The Alternative Centre, College House, Wrights Lane, Kensington, London, w8 5sh, runs a psoriasis helpline (tel. 071-351 2726) offering emotional support and advice on how to live with and treat psoriasis.

The Psoriasis Association, 7 Milton St, Northampton, nn2 7jg (tel. 0604 711129), which promotes research into the condition, publishes a newsletter for sufferers three times a year – entitled *Beyond the Ointment*.

## Further Reading

*Living with Psoriasis* (Alternative Centre Publications) is by Sandra Gibbons who, having suffered from the condition for many years, was co-founder of the Alternative Centre (see above). Described as a practical self-help guide, it gives information and advice about psoriasis.

*Psoriasis, the Rowland Remedy* (Javelin) contains details of the regime prescribed by naturopath John Rowland for the treatment of psoriasis. It is based on the idea that the body needs detoxification and consists mainly of changing the diet and taking vitamin and mineral supplements and herbal remedies. John Rowland claims to have cured hundreds of patients with this treatment.

# Rhinitis

## Definition

Rhinitis is defined as a condition in which the patient suffers from sneezing and a running or blocked nose for more than an hour on most days. If it occurs only at certain times of the year it is known as seasonal rhinitis but if it occurs all year round, it is perennial rhinitis.

## Seasonal Rhinitis (Hay Fever)

This allergic condition is commonly known as hay fever, although patients are rarely allergic to hay and fever is not one of the symptoms. It is the commonest allergic disease known and most frequently affects boys and girls in their teens – up to one fifth of teenagers will have symptoms during June and July. It can begin at any age but is rare in children under four. Often, those who develop hay fever will have had eczema when they were younger. Males and females are equally affected but the condition seems to run in families.

Symptoms include itching in the nose, eyes and soft palate (the back of the roof of the mouth), sneezing and a running nose. The eyes, too, may water profusely. Patients may become 'bunged up' with catarrh and lose their sense of taste or smell,

371

and may develop a cough because of the catarrh flowing down the back of the throat from the nose (post-nasal drip). Occasionally they may have nosebleeds or develop polyps in the nose (see below). Some have sinusitis and about 20 per cent (mainly children) have asthma. Children with hay fever frequently have dark rings under their eyes, known as 'allergic shiners'.

In March, April and May hay fever is due to an allergy to pollen from trees. From June to the beginning of August, grass pollen causes symptoms and, overlapping with this, from the end of June to September, hay fever may be due to spores released from moulds that grow on a number of cultivated plants and on compost heaps. One of these moulds grows round the roots of grass and its spores are released by mowing the lawn. Patients who are allergic to this will find that their symptoms are the same whatever the pollen count but that they may decrease during wet weather when the lawns remain uncut. The majority of patients with hay fever are allergic to grass pollens, with nearly 80 per cent having symptoms during June and nearly 70 per cent during July. By comparison, only 15 per cent have hay fever during September and less than 10 per cent in April.

# Perennial Rhinitis

*Symptoms*
The main symptoms of perennial rhinitis are sneezing and either a running or a blocked nose. The eyes and throat are rarely affected. However, some patients develop sinusitis. The condition is commonest in the teens and twenties, becoming less frequent with age.

*Allergic Perennial Rhinitis*
The commonest cause of this is an allergy to the droppings of house dust mites, tiny insects invisible to the naked eye, that live in their thousands in dust, especially in older, damper buildings. The next commonest cause is an allergy to domestic pets, especially cats. Moulds, fungi, industrial dust and fumes can also cause symptoms, and affected patients are likely to be particularly

sensitive to things such as cigarette smoke, strong perfumes and traffic fumes, although these, in themselves, cannot set up the allergy.

*Non-allergic Perennial Rhinitis*
Some patients have symptoms without any cause being apparent. This is sometimes known as vasomotor rhinitis, although the abnormality of the nasal blood vessels which is implied in the word 'vasomotor' has not been proved. However, in some cases, symptoms may be due to a hormonal imbalance and are seen in pregnant women or at the menopause or in some patients on the contraceptive Pill. When symptoms occur in pregnancy they usually disappear within a few hours of the baby being born.

# Nasal Polyps

Polyps are round, smooth, soft, fleshy structures that grow out of the lining of the nose and are attached to it by a thin stalk. They may occur in association with any type of rhinitis and, by blocking the nose, may result in loss of taste and smell and may make breathing through the nose difficult.

# Investigations

Many patients can work out for themselves what it is that causes their allergy. A skin-prick test is sometimes used to test for allergies but this may be misleading because 20 per cent of people without symptoms will have positive tests. Sometimes a nasal swab can be helpful in differentiating between allergic and non-allergic rhinitis since, in the former, white cells involved in allergic reactions (eosinophils) will be found in the nasal mucus.

# Orthodox Treatment

For allergic patients, antihistamines are particularly effective in controlling sneezing, itching and watering of the eyes. They are less effective in stopping the nose from running and do little to relieve blockage by catarrh. Many of them cause drowsiness, although the newer ones such as astemizole and terfenadine are free from this effect. Antihistamines can also be used as eyedrops for those patients in whom the eyes are badly affected.

Decongestants are useful in the acute attack but must never be used for more than a few days because, otherwise, they can produce a 'rebound' congestion, so that the symptoms are worse at the end than they were to begin with. Such substances include ephedrine, xylometazoline, oxymetazoline and a number of preparations that are available over the counter.

Anti-allergic drugs such as sodium cromoglycate are very effective since they prevent the nasal lining from reacting to the allergen (the substance causing the allergy). Eighty per cent of patients with allergic rhinitis find them helpful, as well as a smaller number with non-specific rhinitis. One, ketotifen, which is taken by mouth, has the disadvantage of causing drowsiness in about 20 per cent of patients. Sodium cromoglycate is also available in the form of eye drops.

A steroid spray such as beclomethasone is very effective in all forms of rhinitis. Only small amounts are used so it is not absorbed into the bloodstream and harmful side effects are therefore avoided. In very severe cases of rhinitis, another steroid, prednisolone, may be given by mouth for very short periods. Continued use of a steroid nasal spray may prevent nasal polyps from recurring after they have been surgically removed.

Desensitizing injections are used only for patients who are known to be allergic to grass pollen or to the house dust mite. Increasingly larger amounts of the allergen are injected over a period of time, until the patient can tolerate contact with quite large amounts without developing symptoms. However, the treatment is not always effective and has the risk of producing a violent, and potentially fatal, allergic reaction (anaphylaxis).

## Complementary Treatment

*Acupuncture*
Chronic rhinitis is said to be due to a deficiency of Chi in the lung. Acute rhinitis is said to be caused by invasion by wind and cold. Depending on the individual symptoms, treatment will

consist of using points to stimulate Chi in the lung or to eliminate wind and cold. In either case, points will also be used which will restore the flow of energy to normal.

*Aromatherapy*
Eucalyptus, peppermint and hyssop are among the oils that may be useful as an inhalation.

*Herbalism*
Many herbs have an anti-catarrhal effect. These include elder-flower, eyebright, golden rod, garlic, yarrow and agrimony. Chamomile and eyebright may also be used by patients with hay fever, to bathe the eyes.

*Homoeopathy*
Arsenicum alb. may be useful if the patient's eyes are running and feel hot, if he has a profuse burning discharge from his nose, sneezes a great deal and feels worse after midnight. A patient whose nasal discharge is worse during the day and whose nose becomes blocked at night, whose eyes feel gritty and who has a headache may respond to euphrasia. When chronic thick catarrh and loss of taste and smell are the symptoms, becoming worse in a warm room and better out of doors in the evening, pulsatilla may be appropriate. Patients whose symptoms are worse in the early hours of the morning and who suffer from chronic catarrh, loss of smell, sore throat and bad breath, may be given kali bich. For someone whose symptoms include a running nose, sore upper lip, itching eyes, tickling cough and sneezing whenever he enters a warm room, allium cepa may be the remedy of choice.

*Manipulation*
Massage and manipulation of the neck may help to drain the sinuses and produce some relief in cases of chronic rhinitis.

*Nutrition*
Dairy products are mucus-promoting and should be avoided by patients with catarrh. Dolomite (calcium and magnesium) helps to stabilize the levels of histamine, which is involved in allergic

reactions, and may therefore be helpful in cases of hay fever. Allergies may also respond to 5000 mg of vitamin C or to supplements of vitamin B$_6$ and zinc.

## Self-help

Patients should try to avoid whatever it is they are allergic to although, in some cases, this is difficult, if not impossible. However, finding another home for domestic pets and avoiding industrial fumes may relieve the condition entirely in some cases. For those who are allergic to pollens, it may be helpful to wear sunglasses, keep the car windows shut when driving, avoid walking in the country, especially in the late afternoon when the air may be thick with pollen, and keep the bedroom window shut at night. Patients often find they are better when at the seaside, since sea breezes tend to blow pollen inland.

The house dust mite is impossible to eradicate. However, putting plastic covers on the mattress and pillows, removing carpets and keeping floors scrupulously clean may help reduce the count considerably. Recently an anti-mite paint, Artilin 3A, has been introduced. Used as an ordinary household paint on interior woodwork, it kills the house dust mite and is effective for a period of three years or more. It is available from GEM Services (UK) Ltd, Harwal Works, Elliott St, Silsden, Keighley, West Yorkshire, BD20 0DP.

# Ringworm

## Definition

Ringworm is the name given to a group of fungal infections that affect the skin. The medical term for this condition is tinea – a Latin word meaning 'gnawing worm'. In actual fact, the infection itself is usually a great deal less unpleasant than the names given to it.

There are various types of fungus that can affect the skin and, depending on which type is involved and which part of the body is affected, the symptoms will differ. The fungi can be divided into those which affect only human beings and those which can also affect (and can therefore be caught from) animals. On the whole, the human-only types tend to produce chronic low-grade infections while those that can affect animals tend to cause more intense and shorter-lived infections. Apart from one type of ringworm of the scalp, these fungal infections are not particularly contagious – indeed, it is well known that a man with ringworm of the feet can share a double bed with his wife for many years and never transfer the infection to her. It seems likely that those people who do develop the infections have some sort of inbuilt susceptibility.

Although ringworm can be, at times, uncomfortable or even painful, and can look very unsightly, it is not capable of doing any real harm to its host because it infects only dead cells. It lives in the uppermost layer of the skin, which is made up of cells that have died and in which keratin, a horn-like substance, has been laid down. It also lives in the hair and the nails, which are composed mainly of keratin. The fungus secretes a chemical which enables it to break down and digest the keratin in these structures. If, as occasionally happens, the body reacts to the infection and inflammation occurs, this may cure the infection, since the upper layer of the skin may be shed rapidly, getting rid of much of the fungus while that which remains is unable to survive in cells which contain little or no keratin.

Ringworm infections are usually divided into categories, according to which part of the body is affected. The feet and the groins are the two commonest sites, probably because the fungus grows more readily in moist areas.

## Ringworm of the Feet (Tinea Pedis)

This is the commonest ringworm infection and accounts for a large number of cases of 'athlete's foot' (which may also be due to other types of infection or just to poor foot care). It occurs mainly in young and middle-aged adults, more often in men than in women, and is rare in children.

Tinea pedis usually begins with peeling and slight maceration of the skin between the toes. Maceration is that condition of the skin which occurs, for example, when a sticking plaster has been left on too long and the skin becomes waterlogged, white and soggy. Usually a fungal infection begins between the fourth and fifth toes and may extend to the other spaces, although it is rarely found between the first and second toes. Between the toes the only symptom may be slight irritation and the infection may never spread any further. However, in some cases it extends to the under-surface of the toes and to the sole and sides of the foot.

Depending on which fungus is causing the infection, the rash may be dry and scaly with thickening and hardening of the affected skin, or it may produce blisters and painful cracks. Sometimes it can be very itchy. A sudden flare-up may occur, with the formation of blisters filled with yellowish fluid, and splits in the skin, associated with itching and pain. In such cases, a bacterial infection may take hold on the inflamed skin, causing further complications.

## Ringworm of the Groin (Tinea Cruris)

This is the second commonest site for ringworm to occur and, like tinea pedis, it is commoner in men than in women. It tends to occur more frequently in warm weather and may appear in patients who already have tinea pedis.

It usually begins with redness and slight maceration in the skin fold of one groin. The infection extends outwards, developing a raised red border which may have tiny blisters on it. The whole area is scaly and usually slightly itchy and it may, in the long term, become darker than the surrounding normal skin. Sometimes the infection remains confined to one groin but it may spread to affect not only the other groin but the genitalia, the buttocks, the thighs and the abdomen. Other 'satellite' patches may develop elsewhere on the trunk, the feet or the hands.

## Ringworm of the Body (Tinea Corporis)

This usually starts as one or more little red spots which extend outwards over the course of the following week or two to form a round or oval plaque with a raised, red border, which may have tiny blisters, and a paler centre. The pale centre is due to the fact that the skin tends to heal as the infection spreads outwards and away from it. Sometimes, however, the entire area remains red, raised and scaly.

The commonest sites for tinea corporis to occur are the face, neck, arms and legs. Usually the patches remain relatively small although extensive infections are quite common in tropical climates.

Sometimes a lump will form in the skin, known as a tinea granuloma, which may be associated with little pus-filled spots.

# Ringworm of the Scalp (Tinea Capitis)

This is the most infectious form of ringworm and can cause outbreaks in schools. Although adults can develop tinea capitis, the most commonly involved fungi tend to attack only children.

The affected area is usually an oval or round patch on which the skin has become scaly and the hairs have broken off, their remnants looking like small black dots. The fungus digests the keratin in the hair, making it brittle, but hair loss is not uniform and usually some can still be seen growing from the infected skin. Most of the scalp may become involved and, in many cases, the patient has patches on the neck, just below the hairline, as well.

Sometimes acute inflammation occurs and the area becomes red and swollen and oozes pus. Although this may look very alarming, it is thought to be due to an immune reaction occurring in the skin. If left untreated, it will heal after about six to eight weeks, usually without any scarring or permanent hair loss.

# Ringworm of the Hands

Ringworm seldom affects the hands. When it does so, it causes slight redness and scaling of the palms. Inflammation with blistering and scaling may occur but this is rare in temperate climates.

# Ringworm of the Nails (Tinea Unguium)

Some patients may have tinea pedis for many years without infection of the nails. Similarly, infection of the hands does not necessarily involve the nails. Other patients, however, may have signs of infection in both the skin and nails. Why the nails become infected in some people but not others is not known.

The first parts of the nail to become infected are usually the sides and the tip, which become yellow and thickened. As the fungus spreads, the whole nail may become distorted. Although, eventually, all the nails may be involved, it is usual for the infection to be confined to one or two at first.

# Investigations

In many cases the diagnosis of ringworm may be obvious simply from its appearance. However, particularly when it occurs on the feet, it may be hard to distinguish from eczema or psoriasis. Nails that are affected by psoriasis, eczema or the thrush organism, monilia, may look very similar to those infected by a fungus.

The investigations necessary for a diagnosis of ringworm are quite straightforward, although it may take some time before the results are available. Normally, when the skin is affected, it is gently scraped and the resulting flakes are sent to the laboratory for examination. If the nails are involved, a small piece is cut off for examination.

Two of the fungi which cause tinea capitis have the peculiar quality of fluorescing when put under a particular type of ultra-violet light known as Wood's light. This is an easy way not only of diagnosing the infection but also of screening classes of schoolchildren who may have become infected. However, tinea capitis can be caused by a fungus that does not fluoresce, so absence of fluorescence does not necessarily rule out the diagnosis, particularly in adults, in whom the condition is usually caused by the non-fluorescent variety.

# Orthodox Treatment

There are numerous products available nowadays for the treatment of fungal infections but one, griseofulvin has proved to be outstandingly useful. It is taken by mouth and is deposited in the skin cells and the growing hair and nail. However, it cannot penetrate the dead keratinized cells but has to wait until the cells which it enters become keratinized in their turn. This means that it takes a long time to work – up to a month for skin infections, two to three months for hair infections and up to two years for infections of the toe-nails. Because of this, and because there are a number of effective ointments, creams and paints available, only those patients with particularly troublesome skin infections are offered griseofulvin. However, it is invaluable in the treatment of tinea capitis and tinea unguium, since topically applied preparations cannot penetrate the hair or the nails. It has the advantage of having few side effects although, occasionally, it may cause nausea, headaches or rashes. Ringworm of the skin responds well, although that occurring between the toes tends to relapse. The relapse rate is also high for the toenails but there is a much greater chance of a permanent cure when treating the finger-nails. Patients with tinea capitis should trim down any remaining hair in the area after two to three weeks on griseofulvin, to remove a potential source of re-infection. Because tinea capitis is quite infectious, it is usually advisable for children to stay away from school after the diagnosis has been made. They can return three or four weeks after they have started to take griseofulvin.

Topical agents come as creams, ointments, lotions and paints. One of the oldest is Whitfield's ointment which has the advantage of being cheap and effective and the disadvantage of being greasy so that it may be unpleasant to use. Equally effective but more pleasant and more expensive are substances such as clotrimazole, econazole, miconazole and sulconazole, all of which come as creams. Econazole is also available as a lotion, which is useful in the treatment of a rash which has become moist, blistered or weepy. Another anti-fungal agent is salicylic acid, which is available in a cream or a paint, the latter having the property of drying up moist skin, although it cannot be used on areas that are cracked. For skin that has become particularly inflamed and weepy, potassium permanganate soaks are helpful in the early stages of treatment.

Although several of these preparations are available over the counter, it is advisable to have the condition correctly diagnosed before trying to treat yourself. It is also important that the treatment is continued for several weeks after the infection seems to have disappeared completely in order to prevent a relapse. Medicated dusting powders should be avoided as these may irritate the skin. Griseofulvin is only available on prescription.

# Complementary Treatment

Herbs can be used in the treatment of ringworm, particularly marigold and myrrh, both of which have a healing action on the skin. Aromatherapists may recommend tea tree for tinea pedis and other forms of athlete's foot. Homoeopathy may also be helpful.

## Self-help

Because tinea cruris and tinea pedis prefer moist conditions, avoiding tight underwear and close-fitting unventilated shoes will help to speed recovery. After bathing, it is very important to dry carefully between the toes.

Patients who are being treated for tinea capitis would be well advised to throw away their brushes, combs, hair slides and hats, or else to clean them very thoroughly before using them again.

# Schizophrenia

## Definition and Incidence

Although, nowadays, mental illness is no longer a taboo subject, being openly discussed in the press and on television and radio, there is still confusion in the minds of many people as to what constitutes schizophrenia. The old, incorrect, notion that it is a condition in which the mind is 'split' and in which the patient exhibits multiple personalities is still fairly widely accepted. In fact, the condition of multiple personalities is extremely rare, whereas schizophrenia, which is characterized by bizarre delusions, hallucinations, illogical thinking and, often, inappropriate emotions, is not uncommon.

Schizophrenia affects between two and four people in every thousand. The majority of cases begin between the ages of fifteen and twenty-five, and it is unusual for the condition to develop in people over the age of forty. It tends to run in families – the brother or sister of a patient is sixteen times more likely to develop schizophrenia than the average person, the son or daughter of a patient is nineteen times more likely and the grandchild of a patient four times more likely. In the case of identical twins, if one develops schizophrenia, the other is also likely to be affected in between 50 and 90 per cent of cases.

# Symptoms

Patients who develop schizophrenia have often had strange personality traits before any indication of illness becomes apparent. They may have been introspective and unsociable, cold and aloof – although, of course, by no means all people with this so-called 'schizoid' personality develop schizophrenia. A little while before the onset of overt symptoms, the patient may have been inclined to have headaches or attacks of anxiety or depression, and may have lost his appetite or become absent-minded. The onset may occur soon after an infection or an operation, or at a time when the patient is worried about something, such as important examinations.

Most specialists now agree that there is an organic basis to schizophrenia – in other words, that it is caused by a disturbance in the chemicals of the brain. However, the exact mechanism has not been discovered and it seems likely that it is not a single disease but a number of conditions in which the symptoms are similar. Although it has been customary to divide schizophrenia into certain fairly well-defined types, these may overlap in the individual patient.

There are some symptoms which are common to several of these types, such as an inability to relate to the real world, a lack of insight into what is happening (although occasionally a schizophrenic patient may realize that he is ill, particularly at the start of an attack), a reduction in emotional response and thought disorder.

Thought disorder comprises a number of symptoms. The patient is not confused but his thought processes become irrational. He may jump from subject to subject in conversation, use words of his own invention and be unable to concentrate, even on what he himself is saying. He may be unable to think in abstract terms and may exhibit 'concrete thinking' – for example, if asked to explain a proverb, such as 'half a loaf is better than no bread', he may say it means that if the baker has run out of large loaves, you have to buy a small one.

The patient may complain that he has lost control over his thinking and that thoughts that are not his own suddenly

385

appear in his mind. Or he might say that his thoughts are broadcast to other people or that they are removed, so that his mind goes blank. He may attribute these effects to hypnosis or telepathy on the part of others or to the use of radio, television or electronic instruments.

Delusions are defined as false unshakeable beliefs. First of all, the patient may become convinced that an everyday event has a special meaning specifically for him. For example, he may believe that there is a message coded into how many people get on and off a bus at each stop. This 'message' is then elaborated on, forming a basis for further delusions. Hypochondriacal delusions, in which the patient believes that part of his body is withering away or is grossly diseased, may sometimes be present for some years before there is any other evidence of schizophrenia or may appear once the disease has become established. The patient may also come to believe that people are talking about him and doing certain things specifically to annoy him or, at the other extreme, that he does not exist, or that the world around him does not exist. Paranoid delusions may occur in which he believes himself to be very important and thinks that he is being persecuted by those who are jealous of his success.

Hallucinations are defined as false perceptions – in other words, the patient sees, hears, tastes, smells or feels something that is not there. When they occur in schizophrenia, they usually take the form of voices (auditory hallucinations). Some patients hear them only when they are relaxing but, for others, they are there all the time, to the extent that they are unable to concentrate on even the simplest task. They may believe that the voices are being transmitted by machines or are being sent out by other people around them. Occasionally patients see visual hallucinations but they are usually aware that these are unreal and they may refer to them as visions. They may also have hallucinations of taste and smell and of bodily sensations such as pain or pressure.

Emotional abnormalities may occur, particularly at the start of the illness. The patient may begin to hate someone whom he has previously loved and may have outbursts of anxiety, rage or misery. Or his emotions may appear shallow and may fluctuate rapidly.

# Types of Schizophrenia

## PARANOID

This form of the disease is more likely to occur in someone who is over the age of thirty when he becomes schizophrenic. His first symptom is often fear, which is associated with a delusion that he is being persecuted. This may be reinforced by auditory hallucinations. As time goes on, although he still believes that 'people are after him', the patient exhibits far less anxiety about it and may appear quite complacent. However, he may become aggressive and attack anyone whom he believes to be his enemy. In some cases there is a religious element to the delusion – the patient believing that he has a special relationship with God and so constitutes a threat to people of a certain religion who are 'out to get him'.

## CATATONIC

Catatonic schizophrenia affects not just the mind but also the body and is most common in teenagers and young adults. Patients may develop a stiff, rigid way of walking and may have periods during which they lie totally immobile and uncommunicative. If allowed to, they may sit or stand in one position for hours on end. They don't eat, drink or voluntarily empty their bladders or bowels, and may be incontinent as a result. If someone tries to move them, they may resist, and if they are asked to do something they may do the opposite. They may also develop the strange condition known as waxy flexibility in which they allow their limbs to be moved into positions which they then hold for minutes at a time. As well as these attacks of stupor, patients may have episodes of over-excitement in which they suffer from delusions and hallucinations.

Rapid recovery from attacks is not unusual and patients may remain free from symptoms for several years. In some cases, after one attack, the condition never recurs.

## HEBEPHRENIA

This is the least common form of schizophrenia. It affects teenagers and young adults, usually developing slowly and taking a chronic course. The patient has delusions and hallucinations and his thinking is disturbed. His emotional response to situations is shallow and inappropriate – for example, he may laugh or remain unmoved when told of some disaster or of the death of a near relative – and he behaves in a silly way. The disease may progress steadily or may be interspersed with periods of excitement that can result in a sharp deterioration in the patient's condition.

## SIMPLE SCHIZOPHRENIA

In this type, there is a general deterioration of the patient's personality, with blunting of the emotions and disorders of thinking but no delusions or hallucinations. The patient becomes apathetic and withdraws from social contact with other people. The condition often begins in adolescence and may develop insidiously.

## CHRONIC SCHIZOPHRENIA

Eventually, after many years, the patient ceases to have acute attacks and is left dull and apathetic, with hallucinations, delusions and, sometimes, disorders of thinking. He is unable to look after himself and may become anxious about his health and the world around him.

## PARAPHRENIA

This is a condition in which a patient in his forties or fifties develops paranoid delusions and hallucinations but none of the other symptoms of schizophrenia.

# Course of the Disease

In the past a diagnosis of schizophrenia usually meant that the patient would be shut up in a mental institution for life. Just before the Second World War, two thirds of all schizophrenics who were admitted to hospital would stay there for two years or more. Nowadays, thanks to modern medication, only 10 per cent of schizophrenic patients need long-term hospital care. Forty per cent have frequent relapses but 30 per cent are able to adapt to life in the community. The final 20 per cent recover completely after a single attack.

In some cases the progress of the disease is a steady downhill course. In others, new symptoms appear in acute attacks; they then die down after some months leaving the patient worse than he was before. Those who suffer from hallucinations are more likely to become chronically ill and hebephrenia, on the whole, has a poor outlook.

Patients who are depressed or excited and who do not demonstrate emotional blunting have a better chance of recovery. Early diagnosis and treatment also improves the prognosis. Other pointers associated with a good prognosis are a sudden onset, a previously normal personality, above-average intelligence, a stable home environment, a good work record and a short first attack. Patients who have no family history of schizophrenia, who were under stress at the time of the first attack, who are married and are over the age of thirty are also likely to do better, as are those whose symptoms are mainly catatonic.

Poor prognosis is associated with an insidious onset, a previously unsociable (schizoid) personality, an absence of precipitating events (such as stress), blunting of the emotions, onset at an early age and a family history of schizophrenia.

## Orthodox Treatment

Strong sedatives are used to reduce the symptoms of an acute attack. These include chlorpromazine, thioridazine, trifluoperazine and haloperidol. Trifluoperazine is usually the drug of choice for the more apathetic patient since it also has stimulant properties. All of these drugs have some side effects, such as drowsiness and dryness of the mouth. They can also produce disturbances of the nervous system so that symptoms similar to the tremor and muscle rigidity of Parkinson's disease may occur, although these can be controlled by using drugs such as procyclidine, benzhexol or orphenadrine in addition. Patients who relapse after recovering from a first attack are usually put on long-term treatment, which may consist of one of the drugs mentioned above or a long-acting injection, such as fluphenazine, which needs only to be repeated every two to three weeks. It is usual to give an anti-Parkinson's drug as well.

Most patients respond well to drug treatment but occasionally ECT (electroconvulsive therapy) may be required for someone who is severely depressed or who cannot be roused from a catatonic stupor. Very rarely it may be necessary to operate on a chronically ill patient who fails to respond to other forms of treatment. The operation, known as a leucotomy, consists of making a tiny cut in the brain, and can produce a considerable improvement in the patient's symptoms.

All patients need to be followed up for life. As well as medication, they need support which will help them to adjust to living in the community, and family psychotherapy may be helpful.

## Complementary Treatment

Treatment by a herbalist or homoeopath may help to stabilize the patient's condition so that less medication is needed.

However, some of the most important work on schizophrenia that has been done recently is in the field of nutrition. Dr Carl Pfeiffer of the Brain Bio Centre in Princeton, New Jersey, USA, has found that most patients with psychoses (severe mental illness in which insight is lost) have either high or low levels of histamine in their bodies. Histamine is usually thought of as the body chemical involved in allergic reactions but it also plays an important role in the functioning of the nervous system. Patients who are severely histapenic (that is, low in histamine) tend to have disorders of thinking, hallucinations and paranoia. They are also inclined to have a lot of fillings in their teeth, few colds and few allergies. Associated with the lack of histamine is an excess of copper and a deficiency of zinc. Dr Pfeiffer and his colleagues have found that treating schizophrenic patients with supplements of zinc and manganese (to raise the zinc levels and bring down the copper), vitamin C (to prevent the uptake of more copper) and the amino acid methionine (to detoxify the excessive histamine in the brain) can have remarkable results.

# Organizations

The National Schizophrenia Fellowship, 78 Victoria Rd, Surbiton, Surrey, KT6 4NS (tel. 081-390 3651), offers information and help to sufferers and their families.

The North West Fellowship, 46 Allen St, Warrington, Cheshire, WA2 7JB (tel. 0925 571680), runs self-help groups and promotes community care (hostels, flats and day care) for schizophrenic patients in the north-west.

The Schizophrenia Association of Great Britain, International Schizophrenia Centre, Bryn Hyfryd, The Crescent, Bangor, Gwynedd, LL57 2AG (tel. 0248 354048), offers information on the latest forms of treatment and advice on the management of the disease.

# Shingles

(Herpes Zoster)

## Cause

Shingles and chicken pox are caused by the same virus – the varicella/zoster virus or VZV. But whereas chicken pox is caught from someone else who has the disease, shingles is due to a re-emergence of the virus which has lain dormant in the patient's body, sometimes for many years, since she had chicken pox. If her resistance to infection is lowered, the virus may become active again, producing an attack of shingles. This is why shingles is most common in the elderly population, whose resistance is often less than robust, and rare in children, many of whom have not yet had chicken pox.

The virus seems to lie dormant in the nervous system. Inside the spinal column, or backbone, is the spinal cord from which all the nerves that supply the body originate. The backbone itself is made up of a series of bones called vertebrae and, between each pair of vertebrae, a pair of spinal nerves runs to each side of the body. Clumps of nerve cells known as the root ganglia are situated on the nerves soon after they leave the spinal cord and it is here that the dormant VZV seems to lie. Because the virus is usually activated only in one root ganglion, the area affected is normally confined to one side of the body and to skin supplied by a single spinal nerve (this area is known as a dermatome).

Sometimes shingles involves areas of the head and neck which are supplied by the cranial nerves that run directly from the brain. Here, too, the rash is confined to the area supplied by a single nerve.

## Symptoms

Shingles often begins with pain, a bruised feeling or itching over the area of skin where the rash will develop. The patient may also feel unwell and have a slight fever. After two or three days a crop of blisters appears, usually with some redness of the surrounding skin. The blisters are often in groups and new groups may continue to appear over the next few days. As the disease progresses, the blisters may become purplish due to the presence of blood in them. Eventually they crust over and the rash usually clears up within two weeks although, occasionally, it may last twice that time. It can be both painful and itchy, and these symptoms sometimes continue after the rash itself has gone. Because the rash contains the virus, it is possible for someone who has not had chicken pox to catch it by coming into close contact with a patient suffering from shingles.

The most usual area of the body to be affected is the chest, with the rash extending in a sweep from the spine round to the centre of the chest in the front. If the arm is involved, there may be weakness and wasting of the muscles, which may persist after the infection is over.

Shingles affecting the lower spinal nerves which supply the bowel and bladder may cause problems with emptying the bowels or with passing water. Such complications usually resolve completely within four months.

Involvement of the facial nerve causes paralysis of the facial muscles that it supplies. Fifty per cent of patients recover fully from this and another 39 per cent have a good, if not complete, recovery, but it may take over a year. In the Ramsay Hunt syndrome, facial paralysis is associated with a shingles rash on the ear and in the throat and, sometimes, deafness may occur.

Perhaps the most troublesome form of shingles is that affecting the ophthalmic nerve, in which the rash can affect the eye. Conjunctivitis, ulceration and inflammation of the whole eye can occur. Scarring may result in reduced vision or blindness. In about a third of patients, the muscles that move the eye become paralysed but this usually resolves within three months.

Occasionally a patient whose immunity is greatly reduced (such as the very elderly or someone suffering from another, serious, disease) may develop generalized shingles in which the rash covers the entire body.

While the patient has the rash, there is a risk of secondary bacterial infection which may need treatment with antibiotics. Once the rash has subsided, the greatest problem is post-herpetic neuralgia, a condition that affects about 10 per cent of patients, being commonest in those over the age of sixty-five and those who had a rash involving the ophthalmic nerve. The patient has a burning, continuous pain that does not respond well to painkillers. Usually it disappears after a period of weeks or months and most patients have recovered after about two years, but in some cases it continues indefinitely.

## Orthodox Treatment

Many cases of shingles can be treated simply with painkillers and rest. Because of the distressing nature of the pain, some patients need mild tranquillizers. Antihistamine tablets may be useful to reduce the itching, but these can make the patient drowsy.

In recent years the discovery of anti-viral agents has made possible the treatment of shingles on more than just a symptomatic level. Dressings soaked in idoxuridine applied to the rash for the first three or four days of the illness help to reduce pain and accelerate healing. However, acyclovir (ACV) seems to be emerging as the treatment of choice. Given orally five times a day for seven days it has the effect of reducing the severity of the attack and promoting healing. If the eye is involved, ACV ointment can be used in addition. Patients with generalized shingles or serious complications may need to be given ACV intravenously.

ACV does not seem to reduce the risk of post-herpetic neuralgia. However, the steroid prednisolone, given in gradually decreasing doses over a period of three weeks may prevent this complication in patients over sixty if given early enough in the illness.

# Complementary Treatment

*Acupuncture*
A red rash with blistering is said to be due to heat in the channel which it overlies. The aim of treatment is to eliminate heat and restore energy flow to normal.

*Aromatherapy*
Clary sage, eucalyptus, geranium and lavender are among the oils that may be beneficial.

*Herbalism*
A preparation of oats may be used, as this is a nervous restorative which will strengthen the nervous system as a whole. Scullcap works in a similar way and marigold is used to promote healing of the rash.

*Homoeopathy*
If the patient has large blisters and the skin is red, swollen, burning and feels better if something cold is put on it, apis may be helpful. If, however, the symptoms are relieved by a warm application and itching is severe, arsenicum alb. may be the remedy of choice. For a patient who has a hot itchy rash of small blisters which is better for warmth, rhus tox. may be appropriate.

*Hypnotherapy*
Hypnosis may be useful in some cases of post-herpetic neuralgia to teach patients how to control their pain.

# Sinusitis

## The Sinuses

'Sinus' means a hollow or cavity and doctors, when referring to 'the sinuses' mean the cavities within the bones of the skull. They are also known as the paranasal sinuses, because they lie alongside and communicate with the nasal passages. Whether they have any function other than that of making the skull lighter and the voice more resonant is doubtful.

The two maxillary sinuses lie in the cheekbones, the two frontal sinuses in the forehead and the two sphenoidal sinuses behind the nose. The ethmoidal sinuses vary in number and may consist of as few as three large cavities or as many as eighteen small ones situated between the eyes. These are the only sinuses to be fully developed at birth; the others grow during childhood, the maxillary sinuses becoming evident after the age of eighteen months and the frontal and sphenoidal sinuses after the age of ten. For this reason, infection of the frontal and sphenoidal sinuses is rare in children.

The sinuses are lined with mucous membrane, similar to that which lines the nose. The individual cells of this lining have tiny projections (cilia) which sweep the mucus secreted within the sinus out into the nasal passages.

# Acute Sinusitis

Inflammation of the lining of the sinuses usually occurs as the result of a heavy cold. The exits of the sinuses, through which mucus drains, become blocked and there is a build-up of fluid which may become infected with bacteria. Other circumstances that can bring on sinusitis include foreign bodies in the nose (which also prevent adequate drainage), injury to the sinus involved, infection of the teeth and jumping into cold water without first holding the nose.

When, as is usual, sinusitis is preceded by a cold, the patient will find that on the third or fourth day, just when the symptoms should be getting better, they suddenly get worse. The nose is more blocked and any nasal discharge becomes heavier. The patient loses his sense of smell, is feverish and may feel quite unwell. A heavy feeling in the face and head is made worse by bending forward and the patient may awake in the morning with a headache which takes some time to wear off.

The exact location of the pain depends on which sinuses are inflamed. Usually the maxillary sinuses are involved, resulting in pain and tenderness in the cheekbones. The ethmoidal sinuses, too, are frequently affected, producing pain between and behind the eyes. There may be swelling of the overlying skin, particularly in children.

Inflammation of the frontal sinuses may be one-sided and often produces a severe headache over one eye which is there when the patient wakes in the morning and lasts until late afternoon. It may also cause pain around the eye and, if severe, swelling of the eyelids. Specific infection of the sphenoidal sinuses is hard to diagnose but it may produce pain in the centre of the head which radiates to the temples and may occasionally be mistaken for earache. There may be a thick green discharge from the nose but the patient doesn't usually complain of a blocked nose.

Very occasionally, the maxillary sinuses become infected as a result of an infection in the teeth. In such cases, the nasal discharge is likely to be very foul-smelling.

## INVESTIGATIONS

The diagnosis is often clear from the history, but a nasal swab is usually taken to try to determine which bacteria are involved in the infection. An X-ray of the skull may show clouding in the normally clear sinuses, an indication that fluid has accumulated there. A full blood count may also be taken and later repeated, the number of white cells reflecting the course of the infection.

## ORTHODOX TREATMENT

The patient needs to be put to bed in a room that has an even temperature and even humidity. The nasal lining contains a network of blood vessels whose job is to warm the inhaled air, while its cells secrete mucus to moisten the air before it enters the lungs. By keeping the temperature and humidity constant, the nasal lining is allowed to rest as it does not have to keep adapting to changes.

The patient should drink plenty of fluids, which not only allows the mouth to remain moist and helps to combat the fever but also helps to prevent the nasal mucus from becoming too sticky.

Painkillers are usually prescribed together with antibiotics, which should be taken until at least forty-eight hours after the symptoms have subsided. For adults, steam inhalations may be very helpful but, because there may be a risk of scalding, these are not recommended for children. Menthol or Friars Balsam in the steaming water may help to clear the nasal passages.

Usually the condition settles quite quickly if treated in this way. However, occasionally the symptoms may persist and in such cases it may be necessary to wash out the appropriate sinuses. Depending on the sinuses involved, it may be possible to do this through the nose under a local anaesthetic, or a larger operation may be necessary.

## COMPLICATIONS

It is essential that acute sinusitis be treated promptly and cleared up completely since there are a number of complications that can occur. Not least of these is progression to chronic sinusitis.

Other complications are uncommon. They include a spread of the infection to the eye socket, causing swelling of the eyelid and eye and resulting in double vision. Failure to treat at this stage may result in blindness. Antibiotics and draining of the collected pus from both the eye socket and the infected sinus will usually resolve the condition.

Infection may also spread to the bone of the forehead from the frontal sinuses. This usually occurs in children and young adults (more often boys) and there may be a history of injury to the area. The patient is quite ill and often drowsy, although initially the only symptoms may be swelling of the eyelid and of the forehead. Urgent treatment is required to prevent the infection from spreading to the brain. An X-ray will usually confirm the diagnosis by showing a 'moth-eaten' appearance of the bones of the forehead, and a blood culture will enable the doctor to determine the bacteria involved. The patient is admitted to hospital and given large doses of antibiotics. If abscesses form, these will need to be drained.

The bone of the upper jaw may become infected, particularly if maxillary sinusitis is the result of a dental infection. This is a rare condition, usually occurring in children. The patient is quite ill, with extensive swelling of the cheek. Urgent treatment is necessary to prevent damage to the jaw and teeth. The infection usually responds rapidly to large doses of antibiotics and drainage of any abscesses. Once the patient has recovered, it may be necessary to wash out the sinuses.

Infection spreading to the brain causes drowsiness, headache, fits, vomiting and weakness. After X-rays and blood cultures, treatment consists of large doses of antibiotics and drainage of abscesses.

## Chronic Sinusitis

Although many cases of chronic sinusitis seem to result from acute sinusitis that has not completely resolved, other factors may be important. Allergies, such as hay fever, that cause swelling of the lining of the nasal passages may reduce the drainage from the sinuses and encourage stagnation of mucus within them. Smoking may act in the same way, as may living in a polluted atmosphere and the consumption of large amounts of alcohol. Dental infection is often associated with chronic sinusitis but it is often not clear which condition came first.

The patient suffers from discomfort in the nose and face, catarrh, headache and a poor sense of taste and smell. The nose may be blocked or constantly running. The nasal discharge is often greenish-yellow or brown. Sudden onset of pain suggests that an acute infection has taken hold on top of the chronic condition. Some patients have recurrent attacks of tonsillitis, sore throat or laryngitis.

INVESTIGATIONS
A nose swab will show whether bacteria are contributing to the problem. An X-ray of the skull will often show that the lining of the sinuses has become thickened.

ORTHODOX TREATMENT
Adequate treatment will help to prevent attacks of acute sinusitis from occurring and will prevent the condition from getting any worse. It is difficult to resolve chronic sinusitis completely, however.

Life-style is an important part of the treatment, so the patient may be advised to stop smoking, eat a more nutritious diet, avoid alcohol and have regular dental check-ups. If an active infection is detected, antibiotics will be given. Steam inhalations are very helpful. However, the use of decongestants may be counter-productive since, although these will help to clear the nasal passages initially, they usually cause a 'rebound' congestion if used for more than two or three days and, in the long-term, make the condition worse. For those patients in whom there seems to be an allergic component, a steroid nasal spray may be prescribed.

For those patients in whom chronic sinusitis causes intolerable long-term symptoms, operation may be necessary. This usually consists of opening up the exit from the sinus into the nose or forming a new one so that the mucus from the sinus can drain away more readily.

# Complementary Treatment

*Acupuncture*
Sinusitis is said to be due to a deficiency of Chi in the lung which leads to the accumulation of harmful factors in the respiratory system. Points are chosen which have the specific properties of eliminating these harmful factors, strengthening the Chi of the lung and promoting normal flow of Chi through the system.

*Aromatherapy*
Niaouli, eucalyptus, pine or thyme may be recommended as inhalants.

*Herbalism*
Herbs such as elderflower, eyebright, marshmallow and golden rod are used to combat excessive mucus production. The last two also have anti-inflammatory properties. Echinacea may be prescribed for patients with chronic sinusitis, since it increases resistance to infection and is valuable in the treatment of chronic infections.

*Homoeopathy*
Patients with frontal sinusitis may benefit from kali bich., natrum mur. or pulsatilla. Other remedies that may be prescribed for sinusitis include hepar sulph. and silica.

# Self-help

A naturopathic cleansing diet consisting of fresh fruit and fruit juice for a few days followed by a further few days on a restricted diet of mainly salads and vegetables with a reduced quantity of starch may be helpful.

# Styes

## Definition, Causes and Symptoms

A stye (or hordeolum) is a type of boil which occurs on the upper or lower eyelid. It is caused by an infection in the root of one of the eyelashes and produces a firm, painful, red swelling, which usually lasts several days before finally bursting and then subsiding.

The infection itself is caused by bacteria called staphylococci which are fairly widespread and are responsible for a number of skin diseases, such as impetigo and boils. However, it is possible for them to live on the human body without causing illness and 30–40 per cent of normal people are nasal carriers, having staphylococci living in their noses without it doing them any harm. But it may be only in the nose that this harmony between man and bacteria can be maintained. If carriers blow, pick or rub their noses and then rub their eyes, they run the risk of transferring the bug to the eyelids where it may cause an infection.

Although most styes are fairly short-lived affairs, some persist, gradually become smaller, without bursting. This type is known as an internal stye and is caused by an infection of one of the tiny Meibomian glands which are situated in the eyelids. The glands have tough walls, so pus from an infection

402

remains contained within them and is not discharged to the surface. Once the infection has died down, the stye may disappear completely or it may leave a small cyst behind.

# Orthodox Treatment

Styes clear up by themselves, so normally no treatment is necessary. However, a doctor may prescribe an antibiotic cream to be applied to the eyelid. This will not speed healing but will prevent the bacteria contained in the discharging pus from infecting another eyelash root.

If a patient has recurrent styes, a nasal swab will show whether or not the nose is harbouring staphylococci. If the swab is positive, an antibiotic cream inserted into the nostrils for a few days may clear the bacteria and thus stop them from spreading to the eyelids.

A Meibomian cyst resulting from an internal stye can be cut open under anaesthetic and its sticky contents removed, after which it is likely to heal very well.

# Complementary Treatment

*Acupuncture*
Traditional Chinese medicine ascribes boils of any kind to an invasion by heat. In an acute attack needles are inserted into points which have the specific function of dissipating heat. One of these, which is situated on the side of the nose, is particularly appropriate for conditions affecting the region of the eye. If the patient has recurrent styes, this suggests that the protective body energy, or Chi, is deficient, so points are used to stimulate this energy in order to increase the body's resistance.

*Herbalism*
Burdock is used for toxic conditions which affect the skin and may be prescribed for a patient with styes. A lotion of eyebright may help to reduce pain and inflammation.

*Homoeopathy*

Remedies need to be taken early in the development of the stye if any benefit is going to be felt. They may prevent an internal stye from turning into a cyst.

The choice of remedy will depend upon the position of the stye, the symptoms and whether or not the condition is recurrent. Recurrent styes on the upper lids associated with redness of the eyes may need sulphur, whereas phosphorus or staphysagria might be used for styes on the lower lids. If the eyelids are swollen, itchy, burning and sticky, and the whole eye seems inflamed, pulsatilla may be prescribed. Often this is the first remedy to be tried. Aconite may be given to a feverish patient with a very painful stye.

*Nutrition*

Healthy skin depends on vitamins A and C, so patients with recurrent styes may be advised to take supplements of these.

During the attack itself (and, indeed, during a bacterial infection of any kind) extra vitamin B should be avoided since bacteria thrive on this.

# Self-help

Sometimes, when the stye seems ready to burst, pulling out the eyelash in whose root it has formed will help the discharge of pus. Before this, bathing the eyelid with warm water can relieve some of the pain.

The naturopathic treatment of recurrent styes may include a cleansing regime – either a fast or a diet of raw foods only. Fasts should only be undertaken if prescribed by a qualified naturopath, but a raw diet is quite safe to follow without supervision. Nothing but raw fruit and vegetables, yoghurt, fruit juices, mineral water and herb teas are taken for up to a week. A diet of this sort, undertaken at regular intervals, may prevent styes from recurring.

# Thrush

## Definition and Occurrence

Thrush is caused by a yeast-like organism called monilia or candida, which is often to be found living in the mouth and intestines of perfectly healthy people. Usually symptoms only arise when excessive amounts of monilia appear or when it starts to grow in a situation in which it does not normally occur.

Like the fungi that cause ringworm infections, monilia likes moist places. It also seems to thrive on sugar. This is thought to be the reason why it is more likely to affect patients with diabetes, whose blood and urine may contain excessive amounts of sugar. It tends to grow in the vagina of pregnant women, possibly because the cells lining the vagina have a high glycogen content during pregnancy. (Glycogen is the form in which glucose is stored within the body.) Other patients who are at risk of getting monilial infections are the very young and the very old, debilitated patients (especially those suffering from leukaemia and some forms of cancer), those whose parathyroid glands (which control calcium metabolism) function inadequately, those with iron-deficiency anaemia, patients taking steroids or the oral contraceptive Pill, and anyone who takes antibiotics. One of the side effects of antibiotics is to kill off the useful bacteria that normally inhabit the large bowel. Since monilia is kept in check by these bacteria, their destruction may allow monilia to multiply to such a degree that it begins to cause problems.

## Oral Thrush

Babies, especially if they are premature, are prone to develop thrush in the mouth. The infection can be seen as white patches that look rather like milk curds, usually on the tongue, the palate, the gums, the inside of the cheeks and the back of the throat. It may be confined to a small area of the mouth or may be quite widespread and cause the infant to go off its feed. If the patches are rubbed off, they come away quite easily, leaving a red, raw area. Sometimes the infection spreads down the oesophagus (the gullet) and can cause vomiting, which may be blood-stained. Because monilia can travel through the digestive system and be passed in the faeces, oral thrush is often associated with a monilial skin infection around the anus.

It has been suggested that infants pick up monilia from the mother's birth canal while being born or that it is a contaminant of feeding bottles. Whatever the reason, babies who are completely breast-fed are less likely to be affected than those who have bottle feeds.

Oral thrush can also affect adults, particularly those who have been on antibiotics. Here it may cause a smooth, painful, red tongue ('antibiotic tongue'), sometimes associated with inflamed lips and cracks at the angles of the mouth (cheilosis). Occasionally thrush may affect denture wearers, causing redness of the palate against which the denture lies. Usually this is symptomless but some patients develop cheilosis.

## Vaginal Thrush

This is a common condition affecting some 15–20 per cent of all pregnant women and a considerable number of those who take the contraceptive Pill. Women who have recurrent infections find that they seem to occur just before a period is due.

Monilia is not normally found in the vagina and, once there, can cause a thick white discharge with intense irritation and soreness. Intercourse may become painful and the infection may spread to the surrounding skin, making it red and sore. Occasionally, however, a monilial infection in the vagina causes no symptoms and is discovered by chance when the patient has a cervical smear.

## Infections of the Hands

Unlike ringworm, monilial infections of the hands are far more common than infections of the feet. Occasionally there may be redness, peeling and maceration (soggy white skin) between two fingers but, more commonly, monilia infects the nails. The commonest infection of the hands is a paronychia – infection of the nail fold, the area from which the nail grows. This tends to occur in people who spend a lot of the time with their hands in water and, among children, is most common among thumb-suckers, the infection probably getting in through a damaged cuticle.

At first there is pain and swelling of the nail fold, which may become red and exude a small amount of pus. Later, the condition tends to become chronic, with the nail fold remaining swollen and slightly red, but not painful, and the cuticle disappearing. If the nail itself is infected, it may turn a brownish-green in colour and become distorted. Ultimately all the nails may be involved.

## Infection of the Skin Folds (Intertrigo)

This is more common in women than in men. Because the skin folds tend to be moist places, monilia is more likely to take hold in the groins, between the buttocks, around the vagina and below the breasts. From here the infection may spread outwards. The rash often looks shiny and pink, has an irregular scaly edge which may show tiny blisters and tends to itch or burn. The skin fold itself may be macerated and the skin cracked. Satellite patches often occur around the original rash, starting as small spots that burst, leaving red areas.

In babies, a monilial infection of the bowel may be associated with a monilial napkin rash which is red, often macerated, and slightly swollen and weeping. Often it takes advantage of skin that is already affected by eczema.

# Urethritis (Infection of the Urethra)

Monilia may invade the urinary tract, but this is much commoner in men than in women. It may cause an acute infection with a profuse greenish-white discharge, which may contain some blood. The opening of the urethra at the end of the penis becomes red, itchy and swollen, and passing water may cause pain. Sometimes the infection is subacute, in which case the patient is aware only of a very small amount of discharge, usually early in the day, associated with itching at the opening of the urethra and a burning sensation when passing urine first thing in the morning.

# Balanitis

This is an infection of the end of the penis and the foreskin. When due to monilia it occurs mainly in young men, although it may affect boys and older men. Red patches with blisters appear, often associated with intense burning and itching. The area where the foreskin is attached to the penis may become swollen and the infection may spread to the surrounding skin.

# Investigations

A swab will usually be taken of the affected area and this will be examined under a microscope and cultured in the hospital laboratory. However, some 5 per cent of vaginal infections may produce negative swabs. If the doctor strongly suspects that monilia is present despite a normal swab result, he may wish to repeat the test. He may also take a urine test to check that the patient is not developing diabetes, since, occasionally, a monilial infection may be the first sign of this.

# Orthodox Treatment

There are several substances that are useful in the treatment of monilia. Nystatin is one of the oldest but some strains of monilia have now become resistant to it. More recently discovered drugs are the imidazole derivatives which include clotrimazole, keto-conazole, econazole and miconazole. A recently introduced medication, flucanazole produced a 93 per cent success rate in trials where it was used to treat vaginal thrush. Normally, suspensions or gels are used for mouth infections, pessaries and creams for vaginal infections and creams for skin infections. Ketoconazole, if taken orally, is absorbed into the bloodstream and is sometimes used for resistant infections which are not responding to topical treatment. Nystatin is not absorbed when taken orally and is therefore useful for treating infections of the large bowel, since it passes straight through.

In some resistant cases of vaginal thrush a gentian violet paint can be useful but has the disadvantage that it stains the under-wear. This, too, is a disadvantage of nystatin pessaries, which leave a yellowish stain.

Unfortunately, vaginal thrush can become recurrent and can seriously disrupt the patient's life. Sometimes, it appears that a woman is being re-infected by her partner and, in such cases, treating both together may be helpful. However, for those who continue to have attacks, recent research has shown promising results. At the Royal West Sussex Hospital in Chichester, it was found that giving the patient clotrimazole a week before her period and again two weeks later and then repeating this every month prevented recurrence in 81 per cent of the patients treated over the course of a year; in the control group which was not offered this treatment regime, 76 per cent of patients had a recurrence within three months. Another trial at St Mary's Hospital, Portsmouth, gave 100 women who had suffered from recurrent thrush a course of two pessaries of miconazole a day for a week followed by one twice a week for three months and then one a week for a further three months. While on this treatment, not one of the patients had a repeat attack.

# Complementary Treatment

*Aromatherapy*
Tea tree or thyme may be recommended.

*Herbalism*
Marigold and myrrh are among the herbs that may be used to treat thrush, since their action is to heal inflamed and infected tissues. Thyme may be used as a douche for vaginal thrush.

*Homoeopathy*
A patient who has an inflamed mouth, a red tongue and bad breath as a result of a monilial infection may respond to arsenicum alb. A sore mouth in a child, associated with blisters inside the cheek and bad breath, may call for merc. sol. If the tongue is white and associated with blisters in the mouth and if the patient complains of excessive salivation and a foul taste, sulphur may be appropriate. Other remedies may be prescribed for vaginal thrush and monilial skin infections.

*Naturopathy*
In order to restore balance to a bowel that has become overgrown with monilia, it is essential to replace the bacteria which usually keep it in control. This can be done by eating live yoghurt or taking capsules of acidophilus or superdophilus (the bacterial element in live yoghurt). These bacteria will also help to vanquish monilia in other sites, and live yoghurt or acidophilus may be used as a douche in cases of vaginal thrush. Garlic is also a valuable anti-monilial agent. If a needle is used to insert a piece of thread through a clove of garlic, it can be used as a tampon. Changed for a fresh clove twice a day, it can have a dramatic effect on vaginal thrush. However, some patients may be sensitive to garlic and, if it seems to be causing inflammation, the treatment should be stopped immediately.

A naturopath may also recommend a special anti-monilial diet.

## Self-help

Because monilia likes moisture, it is important to keep affected areas as dry as possible. Patients with a skin infection or vaginal thrush should avoid tight underwear, especially if it is made of nylon, while those with infections of the hands should wear a pair of cotton gloves inside rubber gloves for all household chores.

## Further Reading

*Candida Albicans* by Leon Chaitow (Thorsons), explains how to conquer thrush using naturopathic methods.

# Thyroid Diseases

## Function of the Thyroid Gland

The thyroid is a butterfly-shaped gland that lies in the front of the neck and is responsible for controlling the body's rate of metabolism – that is, the rate at which it uses up energy. It does this by secreting two hormones, thyroxine or $T_4$ and tri-iodothyronine or $T_3$, both of which contain iodine as an essential ingredient. The rate of secretion of $T_4$ and $T_3$ is controlled by another hormone, thyroid-stimulating hormone or TSH, which is produced by the pituitary gland in the brain. Thyroid problems can therefore be due to a dietary deficiency of iodine (found in sea fish, vegetables, milk and meat) or to disorders of the pituitary gland. However, the vast majority of cases are due to disease within the gland itself.

In many cases of thyroid disease, the gland becomes swollen and this may be accompanied by a disruption of its function. In some cases the patient may develop hypothyroidism – a lack of thyroid hormones; in others hyperthyroidism or thyrotoxicosis – an excess of thyroid hormones – may develop.

## Investigation of Thyroid Disease

If a doctor suspects that a patient is suffering from some form of thyroid disease, he will usually begin by taking a blood sample to measure the levels of $T_4$, $T_3$ and TSH. Some thyroid diseases are auto-immune conditions in which the body manufactures antibodies against itself and, in such cases, these antibodies can be detected in the blood.

Although the thyroid is usually situated in the neck, in a few people it is lower down and part or all of it is retrosternal – that is, lying behind the sternum, or breastbone. An X-ray may show whether or not a retrosternal gland is enlarged. Sometimes the patient is asked to swallow some liquid containing barium (such as is used in X-rays of the intestines to diagnose peptic ulcers). This outlines the oesophagus, or gullet, and shows whether the thyroid is pressing into it.

Ultrasound is sometimes used to assess whether a lump in the thyroid is a cyst or a solid mass. When a sample of thyroid tissue is needed in order to diagnose the cause of a lump or swelling, this is usually taken from the anaesthetized patient with a fine needle.

Because the thyroid takes up iodine from the bloodstream, if the patient is given radioactive iodine (or 'radioiodine'), this will be absorbed into the functioning parts of the gland. A scan can then determine whether any part of the thyroid is either under- or over-active by its concentration of radioiodine.

# Smooth Non-toxic Goitre (Colloid Goitre)

This condition occurs when there is inadequate iodine available to the thyroid, either as a result of a deficiency of iodine in the diet or because the patient is taking something which prevents the thyroid from using iodine correctly. Some drugs may occasionally do this, as may an excess of a natural chemical which is found in vegetables of the cabbage family.

The output of thyroid hormones is reduced, and this results, by a feedback mechanism, in more TSH being secreted by the pituitary. This, in turn, causes a swelling of the thyroid which, in mild cases, will manage to produce enough hormone to keep the patient healthy. However, in severe cases of deficiency, the patient may become hypothyroid.

Smooth non-toxic goitre is, like most thyroid conditions, much commoner in women than men. It usually develops between puberty and the age of thirty. The gland is smooth and some-times large enough to cause symptoms such as shortness of breath when the patient lies in a certain position (due to pressure on the trachea, or windpipe), or redness of the face, giddiness or fainting (due to pressure on the jugular veins). Rarely, it may cause hoarseness because it presses on the nerves that run down the neck to the larynx (voice-box). Occasionally, bleeding may occur into part of the gland, causing a sudden increase in size.

Treatment consists of ensuring that the patient is receiving adequate iodine in the diet and, if necessary, giving $T_4$ to stop the excessive secretion of TSH. Surgery is only rarely necessary.

# Physiological Goitre

Some adolescents (nearly always girls) develop a soft swelling of the thyroid around the time of puberty. This usually disappears of its own accord by the age of twenty or twenty-two and no treatment is necessary.

# Thyroiditis

The suffix -itis usually implies an inflammation of the organ concerned. There are several forms of thyroiditis.

## HASHIMOTO'S THYROIDITIS

This is an auto-immune disease and is the commonest form of thyroiditis. Antibodies which attack the thyroid are found in the blood of about 90 per cent of patients. Within five years, a quarter of those affected have developed hypothyroidism. Eventually, 90 per cent become hypothyroid.

The disease mainly affects women, who are usually between the ages of thirty and sixty. However, it can occur in younger patients and even in children. The thyroid becomes swollen and feels firm and rubbery; distinct lobules can sometimes be detected or the gland may feel smooth. The swelling may only be slight and, often, the first symptoms are those of hypo-thyroidism.

414

Treatment consists of giving T$_4$, which will reduce the size of the gland and remedy the hypothyroidism.

DE QUERVAIN'S THYROIDITIS
This mainly affects middle-aged women and seems to be due to a viral infection. It often follows a head cold or sore throat and may come on suddenly or may be preceded by a few days in which the patient feels unwell and has a slight fever and headache. The symptoms include swelling and tenderness of the thyroid with pain radiating up into the jaw or the ears, together with fever, generalized aching and headache. For four to six weeks, the patient may become hyperthyroid because of an excess of hormones leaking into the bloodstream from the inflamed gland. After that, she may develop hypothyroidism, which gradually recovers after a period of weeks or months. Less than 10 per cent of patients remain hypothyroid. Episodes of inflammation may recur but, each time, these are less severe and, eventually, they peter out.

Treatment consists of rest and anti-inflammatory drugs such as aspirin or NSAIDs (non-steroidal anti-inflammatory drugs). In severe cases steroids may be given to reduce the inflammation. Hypothyroidism is treated with T$_4$.

POST-PARTUM THYROIDITIS
This is said, by some specialists, to affect up to 9 per cent of women after pregnancy. Symptoms are those of mild hyperthyroidism, occurring between two and four months after the birth of the baby. Up to three quarters of those affected have a swelling of the thyroid. One quarter have a close relative who has suffered from thyroid disease. Usually the condition subsides of its own accord although, in a few cases, hypothyroidism may result.

# Hypothyroidism
MYXOEDEMA
This is the adult form of hypothyroidism which affects about one person in 100 in Great Britain. Six out of every seven people

affected are women. The commonest cause is an auto-immune condition, either so-called idiopathic atrophy or, less often, Hashimoto's thyroiditis. It may also occur in patients who have previously been treated for hyperthyroidism with surgery or radioiodine. Idiopathic atrophy usually affects women between the ages of thirty and fifty, particularly around the time of the menopause. Antibodies against the thyroid are found in over 80 per cent of patients.

The condition may come on very gradually so that neither the patient nor her relatives are aware that she is ill until quite a late stage.

The symptoms are very varied and a patient may have a few or many. Often they are vague, particularly at first. The patient may feel unusually tired and may notice that she gets cold very easily. She is likely to put on weight and may become constipated. She may complain of aching muscles, stiffness, deafness, chest pains, unsteadiness when walking and shortness of breath on exertion. Other symptoms include heavy or prolonged periods, infertility, a constantly running or blocked nose and swelling of the ankles.

The patient's appearance also changes. Her face becomes heavy and expressionless and develops a yellowish tinge, with a flush over the cheekbones. Her eyelids become puffy and her skin dry and rough. Her hair becomes thin and dry and often the outer section of the eyebrows is lost.

Her speech becomes hoarse and slurred because the larynx and the tongue are swollen. Her thinking processes slow down and her memory is poor. In severe cases, she may become very confused. Depression is quite common, as is headache.

On examination, the doctor will find that the patient's pulse is slow. In a quarter of cases, the blood pressure will be raised. An X-ray may show that the heart is enlarged because of fluid that has accumulated in the sac (the pericardium) that surrounds it. Blood tests may reveal a mild anaemia that resolves when the myxoedema is treated or an iron-deficiency anaemia resulting from increasingly heavy periods. In 12 per cent of cases, the patient has pernicious anaemia, another auto-immune disease, which has to be treated with regular injections of vitamin $B_{12}$.

There are two serious complications of myxoedema which,

fortunately, are rare. One is so-called 'myxoedema madness', in which the patient may develop schizophrenia-like symptoms, sometimes shortly after starting treatment. This is usually confined to elderly patients with severe hypothyroidism. The other is myxoedema coma, which may be precipitated by a sudden stress such as infection, trauma or coldness, and which is fatal in some 50 per cent of cases.

CRETINISM
Rarely, about once in every 3500 births, a baby develops hypothyroidism as soon as it is born. This is usually because the thyroid gland has failed to develop. The condition affects boys and girls equally and, in some cases, may be mild, only becoming apparent after a few months of life.

In mild cases symptoms may include failure to develop at the normal rate, floppiness, constipation and a hoarse cry. The skin may seem coarse, cool and dry, and the tongue is large and may protrude from the mouth.

In more severe cases, jaundice is often the first symptom. It is not uncommon for newborn babies to be jaundiced but, in the hypothyroid baby, this lasts much longer than the usual few days. The symptoms observed in mild cases are soon apparent and the baby's large tongue may interfere with feeding and may make the breathing sound noisy. The face is characteristic, with a low hair line, wrinkled forehead and broad flat nose, and the eyes are set well apart. The neck is short and thick, and the limbs short with broad hands and feet. The baby may be overweight, has a large abdomen, often with a bulge at the umbilicus caused by a hernia, and tends to lie very still. The danger of cretinism is that it can lead to severe mental retardation. However, if treated early, this can usually be avoided. Treatment will also reverse most of the physical symptoms of the condition.

ORTHODOX TREATMENT OF HYPOTHYROIDISM
The treatment simply consists of replacing the missing hormone, $T_4$ (thyroxine), in tablet form. However, $T_3$ (tri-iodothyronine) is usually given to patients who have angina, since it has a shorter

duration of action than $T_4$ and hence allows greater flexibility should the drug make their angina worse. Once the patient is no longer hypothyroid, it is quite safe to change to $T_4$.

# Hyperthyroidism (Thyrotoxicosis)

Like hypothyroidism, this can be produced by several different conditions and the symptoms vary somewhat according to the cause, but the overall picture will be outlined here before the individual diseases are described. It affects between two and five women in every 100 but only two men in 1000.

The first symptom is often extreme fatigue. The patient may lose a considerable amount of weight, despite the fact that her appetite is increased. She becomes intolerant of heat and sweats a lot.

Anxiety, restlessness and irritability are common and the periods may become scanty. The patient may complain of loss of strength, palpitations, shortness of breath and swollen ankles. On examination, the doctor may find that she has a fine tremor of her outstretched hands and of her tongue, and that her movements are jerky and clumsy. Her skin appears warm, pink and moist and may have a velvety texture, and her hair is fine and silky. A fast pulse rate (over 90 per minute) is common and, in older patients, there may be an irregular heart beat. Sometimes this irregularity may be the only sign of hyperthyroidism in the elderly.

When hyperthyroidism is due to Graves' disease, the eye condition known as exophthalmos is not uncommon. In mild cases, the upper eyelids become retracted and the eyes bulge slightly, making the patient look as though she is staring. The bulging is due to swelling within the eye itself and to an increase in the bulk of the fat and muscles within the eye socket. In more severe cases, the conjunctiva may become thickened and the eyes may water a lot, especially in the morning. Sometimes one eye may seem to bulge more than the other. The muscles that move the eyes may become weak, resulting in double vision or even a noticeable squint. Occasionally the eye symptoms may become temporarily worse after treatment for hyperthyroidism has been started. Rarely, a progressive condition may occur in which the surface of the eye becomes ulcerated, the whole eyeball becomes inflamed and the patient's eyesight is threatened.

Seventy per cent of patients find that their eyes return more or less to normal after they start treatment for hyperthyroidism. In a further 20 per cent the eyes remain unchanged, while, in 10 per cent of cases the symptoms may get somewhat worse.

## GRAVES' DISEASE (SMOOTH TOXIC GOITRE)

This is the commonest cause of hyperthyroidism. It tends to run in families and may occur at any age but mainly in women between the ages of twenty and forty. Like Hashimoto's thyroiditis and idiopathic thyroid atrophy, it is an auto-immune disease. However, in this case the antibodies stimulate the thyroid to produce more hormones, rather than depressing its secretory function.

Usually the thyroid is enlarged, smooth and firm. Eye problems are common, as are anxiety, trembling and other symptoms affecting the nervous system. It is not unusual for symptoms to come and go and, in about 40 per cent of patients, they disappear completely and do not return.

Blood tests will show raised levels of hormones and antibodies.

## SOLITARY TOXIC NODULE (ADENOMA)

This only accounts for some 5 per cent of cases of hyperthyroidism. A little nodule of hyperactive tissue forms within the thyroid and secretes large amounts of hormone, while squashing the normal thyroid tissue around it. The amount of hormone circulating in the blood will prevent the pituitary from secreting TSH (via the feedback mechanism), so that the rest of the thyroid may stop functioning while the nodule, which is independent of TSH, carries on secreting.

This condition occurs mainly in women and at any age over ten. The patient may complain of a swelling in the gland, which may be large enough to cause shortness of breath (from pressure on the trachea) or hoarseness (from pressure on the nerves leading to the larynx). Sometimes a cyst forms within the nodule and bleeding may occur into the cyst cavity, causing sudden pain and an increase in swelling.

Investigations that can be used include a needle biopsy and also a radioiodine scan, in which the injected substance will be shown concentrated within the nodule.

## MULTINODULAR GOITRE

Patients who develop this condition are usually over fifty and have had a non-toxic goitre for some time. Sometimes multinodular goitre runs in families. More women are affected than men but the ratio is not as great as in Graves' disease.

The thyroid is enlarged and individual smooth, rounded swellings can be felt within it. In some patients the gland grows faster than in others and may press on the trachea, oesophagus, laryngeal nerves or the jugular veins, causing a cough, breathing difficulties, discomfort on swallowing, hoarseness or faintness.

Not all patients become hyperthyroid but, in those that do, the symptoms are more likely to be associated with the heart than with the nervous system. An irregular heart beat is common and heart failure may occur, so that the patient may complain of severe shortness of breath, palpitations, fatigue and swollen ankles.

## ORTHODOX TREATMENT OF HYPERTHYROIDISM
*Exophthalmos*
In mild cases, treatment consists of diuretics to reduce water retention within the eyeball and socket plus glasses to protect the over-exposed eyes from foreign bodies and the drying effect of wind. In more severe cases, steroids may be necessary to reduce the swelling. In progressive cases, where there is a danger that the optic nerve may be damaged by swelling or that the surface of the eyeball may become ulcerated, operative treatment may be necessary. This consists of reducing the pressure within the eye and socket and partially sewing the eyelids together. Sometimes this is combined with radiotherapy which may be helpful. Occasionally, surgery is also necessary to improve a squint.

*Graves' Disease*

Although drugs are very effective in controlling 95 per cent of cases, up to 60 per cent recur and then need other treatment. The drugs available are carbimazole and propylthiouracil. Both have side effects and patients who cannot tolerate one are usually switched to the other. Carbimazole is generally tried first. It reduces the production of thyroid hormone and, in most cases, symptoms begin to disappear within two to three weeks. It is customary to prescribe it for a period of 12–18 months but after this, relapses are common, usually within two years of the treatment ending. Side effects of carbimazole include rashes, joint pain and a sudden drop in the numbers of white blood cells produced by the bone marrow. The last of these is very serious, since white blood cells are responsible for the body's immunity. It is always accompanied by a sore throat, so patients are warned that, at the first sign of soreness, they must stop the treatment and report to their doctor immediately.

Beta blockers, which are described more fully in the section on high blood pressure, may be used in the early stages of treatment, to control symptoms associated with the heart and circulatory system while the patient is waiting for surgery or before the full effect of carbimazole or propylthiouracil has been felt.

Radioiodine, as well as being used as a diagnostic tool, can be used in treatment. The patient drinks a glass of water containing the substance, which is then absorbed into the bloodstream and taken up by the over-acting parts of the thyroid gland, where it suppresses the excessive secretion of hormones. It usually takes two to three months before the effect is felt, so drug treatment may be necessary in the interim. Sometimes it may cause discomfort in the neck and a worsening of symptoms in the early stages of treatment. The ultimate success rate is 75 per cent but it is not suitable for all patients. Normally, it is not offered to women who are under forty, or perhaps forty-five, since there is a risk that it might affect an infant's thyroid were the patient to become pregnant. Unfortunately, it often produces hypo-thyroidism, affecting some 30 per cent of those treated within ten years. These patients then have to have supplements of $T_4$ for the rest of their lives.

Surgery is used for those patients who have failed to respond to drugs, who have relapsed more than once or twice on drug treatment, who have large goitres or who, for one reason or another, are not suitable for radioiodine treatment. Complications are rare, although 20 per cent of those treated will eventually become hypothyroid. Carbimazole is given first of all, until the patient is no longer hyperthyroid. Then this is stopped and potassium iodide is given for 10–14 days. This has the effect of making the gland less active and reducing the amount of blood flowing through it. Finally, an operation is performed in which a large section, but not all, of the thyroid is removed. In 5 per cent, the operation doesn't control the condition and the patient relapses. In such cases radioiodine is very effective as a follow-up treatment.

*Toxic Nodule*
Usually the nodule itself is removed and TSH is given to stimulate the rest of the gland back to normal function. Drugs and radio-iodine are less effective.

*Multinodular goitre*
In elderly patients, where the diagnosis is clear, there is no evidence of hyperthyroidism and the patient has no symptoms, it is customary to do nothing. However, if the gland is causing symptoms through pressure on surrounding structures, part of it is surgically removed. In younger patients, a partial thyroid-ectomy is usually done, whether or not there are symptoms, because there is a danger that hyperthyroidism will occur or that bleeding may occur into the gland, and a small risk that one of the nodules may become malignant.

# Thyroid Nodules

The vast majority (85 per cent) of single nodules are adenomas or toxic nodules. The rest are malignant growths.

CANCER OF THE THYROID
This is a rare condition which is two to three times more common in women than in men. Many patients have had

goitres for several years. There are five main types of thyroid cancer, known as papillary, follicular, medullary and anaplastic carcinomas, and lymphoma.

Usually the first sign is a nodule in the thyroid or an enlargement of the gland, which feels firm or hard. There may be a sudden increase in size over a matter of days or weeks, with the patient complaining of a choking sensation or a tightness in the throat. Hoarseness and difficulty in breathing or swallowing may also occur.

Each type of cancer is treated slightly differently from the others but, because most thyroid tumours are under the control of TSH secreted by the pituitary, supplements of $T_4$, which suppress the production of TSH, can cause regression of the tumour. Therefore $T_4$ is given to most patients who are diagnosed as having thyroid cancer.

### Papillary Carcinoma
This accounts for 70 per cent of cases and is commonest in children and young adults. It usually takes the form of a single hard nodule in a previously normal gland. The outlook is excellent, since the cancer is very slow growing.

Treatment consists of removing all the thyroid on the affected side and part of it on the other side. The patient will then have to take $T_4$ supplements for the rest of her life. If the cancer seems to have spread, the whole of the thyroid will be removed, together with the lymph glands in the neck. This is followed up, if necessary, with radioiodine treatment.

### Follicular Carcinoma
This accounts for 20 per cent of cases and it, too, has a good outlook if caught early enough. It mainly affects young and middle-aged adults. Treatment is the same as for papillary carcinoma.

### Medullary Carcinoma
This affects patients of any age, men equally with women, and forms 5 per cent of all cases of thyroid cancer. It may run in families and may be associated with growths in other glands.

423

The outlook is not as good as for papillary and follicular carcinoma but, even so, 60 per cent of patients are still alive five years after the diagnosis was first made.

Treatment usually consists of removal of the entire thyroid gland and the lymph glands of the neck.

### Lymphoma

This is rare and is usually treated with a combination of surgery, radiotherapy and chemotherapy.

### Anaplastic Carcinoma

This, too, is rare, mainly affecting older patients. Treatment is by surgery and radiotherapy but the outlook is poor.

## Complementary Treatment

### Acupuncture

Goitre is said to be due to obstruction of the flow of blood and of energy (Chi) and to accumulation of phlegm in the neck. Treatment uses points which will relieve the obstruction, disperse the phlegm and restore normal flow.

### Herbalism

For those patients who need extra iodine, kelp may be prescribed. This may also help to regulate the function of the thyroid.

### Homoeopathy

Patients with exophthalmic toxic goitre and weight loss may benefit from thyroidinum or natrum mur. Calc. iod. and calc. carb. may be used for simple non-toxic goitre, and iodium and spongia may be helpful in the treatment of either condition.

### Nutrition

Since vitamins C, $B_3$ and $B_5$, and the minerals manganese, calcium and zinc are especially important for the normal function of the pituitary gland and the thyroid, supplements of these may be prescribed.

# Urinary Tract Infections

## Cause of Infections

The urinary tract, which comprises the kidneys, ureters, bladder and urethra is the commonest site of bacterial infection in the human body. (See diagram of the urinary tract p. 212.) Normally, although the end of the urethra closest to the exterior may contain bacteria, these are prevented from spreading further by the antibacterial properties of the lining of the urethra and by the fact that the urinary tract is repeatedly being flushed out by sterile urine. Urinary tract infection (UTI) occurs much more frequently in women than in men because the female urethra is comparatively short, wide and straight, making it easier for bacteria to travel along it.

Although many cases of infection occur in otherwise healthy women, there are certain abnormalities that can predispose patients to UTI. These include obstruction of the urinary tract, which causes pooling of urine (incomplete emptying of the bladder) and encourages the growth of bacteria, stones (which can act as a focus for infection) and diseases, such as diabetes, in which the patient's resistance to infection is lowered. Pregnant women have an increased risk of developing UTIs because the pressure of the foetus on the bladder can lead to pooling of urine.

In addition, the high level of progesterone found in the blood-stream during pregnancy causes dilation of the ureters, which allows this stagnant urine to flow backwards towards the kidneys. Patients who have disorders of the nervous system and are unable to empty the bladder completely are also more prone to infection. Vigorous sexual intercourse is quite a common cause of UTI in women (sometimes known as 'honeymoon cystitis'). It is thought that this results either from injury to the urethra or from bacteria being forced up the urethra and into the bladder.

Vesico-ureteric reflux is a condition in which the one-way valve which leads from the ureter into the bladder ceases to function correctly and, as the bladder contracts, forcing urine out, it also forces some back up the ureters. When the bladder relaxes, this urine flows in again, so that the patient never has a completely empty bladder. When seen in children, it is thought to be associated with the development of chronic pyelonephritis (see below).

## Acute Cystitis

Cystitis, or inflammation of the bladder, is very common, affecting about 50 per cent of all women at some time in their lives. Most have only one or two attacks but a few go on to have frequent recurrences. This is especially likely if there is a predisposing cause.

The attack comes on suddenly, the patient developing pain and tenderness in the bladder area. Passing water causes pain (dysuria) but she feels that she wants to go very frequently (frequency). The urine is likely to be smelly and may be blood-stained (haematuria). Sometimes patients develop abdominal pain, fever or haematuria without frequency or dysuria. In children, especially, the symptoms may be vague and may include fever, abdominal pain, bed-wetting and a general sense of being unwell.

About 5 per cent of schoolgirls have UTI at some time and, of these, 80 per cent will have more than one attack. Thirty-five per cent of affected children are found to have vesico-ureteric reflux – a much higher proportion than in the population as a whole.

## Chronic Cystitis

This is always associated with a predisposing cause and, if that can be successfully treated (for example, removal of a kidney stone) the condition may well be curable. The symptoms are those of frequency and dysuria occurring over a prolonged period of time, sometimes clearing up but never for more than a week.

The symptoms of chronic cystitis can also be caused by other conditions than bacterial infection. Most of these are rare and include tuberculosis (which is always secondary to TB elsewhere in the body, usually the lungs), Hunner's ulcer or interstitial cystitis (ulceration of the lining of the bladder, which tends to affect middle-aged women) and cystitis cystica (in which little glands in the bladder lining enlarge to form nodules or polyps). In men, prostatitis can also cause urinary symptoms.

Fifty per cent or so of women who suffer from persistent or oft-repeated attacks of frequency and dysuria have no bacteria in their urine. The term 'urethral syndrome' is used to cover this group but it is probable that there are a number of causes for their symptoms. In some cases, it seems to be due to an attack of thrush and, in post-menopausal patients, may be associated with a lack of oestrogen, which also causes drying of the lining of the vagina (atrophic vaginitis).

## Acute Pyelonephritis

If an infection travels up the urinary tract to the kidneys, it can cause acute pyelonephritis, a potentially serious disease, which, in nine out of ten cases, affects women. There is a sudden onset, the patient becoming feverish and ill, shivering and vomiting and complaining of pain and tenderness around the kidney area, in the back just below the ribs. Unlike acute cystitis, the urinary symptoms of dysuria and frequency may be only slight or absent altogether. If the infection is untreated, it may spread to the bloodstream, causing septicaemia, in which case the patient becomes very ill with a high fever.

# Chronic, or Atrophic, Pyelonephritis (Reflux Nephropathy)

This is a condition in which the kidneys become scarred and, eventually, cease to function effectively. The patient develops high blood pressure (see section on secondary hypertension) and this may be followed by renal failure. Unlike the other forms of UTI, chronic pyelonephritis affects as many men as women.

It is thought to originate in childhood in patients who have vesico-ureteric reflux due to the incompetent valve mechanism. The constant pool of stale urine in the bladder predisposes the patient to infection and the bacteria may be swept up to the kidneys in the refluxed urine. Usually reflux stops around puberty, as the bladder becomes stronger, but by this time the damage may have been done.

Thirty per cent of those children with reflux who suffer from UTI are at risk of developing scarring of the kidneys. About 10 per cent go on to develop high blood pressure and renal failure. Because vesico-ureteric reflux may run in families, some doctors now recommend screening the children of parents with chronic pyelonephritis, since early detection and treatment can prevent damage to the kidneys.

# Investigations

All patients who are thought to have a UTI will be asked to provide a mid-stream urine specimen, or MSU. A swab is used to clean the area round the urethra. The patient starts to pass water into the toilet, and then introduces a receptacle to catch some of the urine before finishing into the toilet. This means that any bacteria which just happen to be in the urethra, but not in the urine itself, will be flushed out and will not contaminate the specimen. If TB of the urinary tract is suspected, however, the patient will be asked for a specimen of the first urine of the morning (early morning urine or EMU), since this is the most concentrated and is best able to show up the presence of TB.

Only if a patient has recurrent infections, or if there is reason to believe there may be an underlying abnormality, will further investigations be performed. Men and children are always investigated, since they are far more likely than women to have a predisposing cause. An intravenous pyelogram (IVP) consists of an injection of dye into a vein followed by a series of X-rays of the kidneys and bladder as the dye is excreted in the urine. It will show up any stones in the urinary system, scarring of the kidneys and other abnormalities. The patient is asked to pass water and, as he does so, it is possible to detect any vesico-ureteric reflux and to see whether the bladder is emptied completely. Ultrasound investigation can also be used to detect some abnormalities.

Cystoscopy (inspection of the inside of the bladder under general anaesthetic, using a special telescope) is rarely used in the investigation of UTI. However, it may be considered necessary in some cases of haematuria or if a condition such as Hunner's ulcer is suspected.

## Orthodox Treatment

In all cases in which there is an underlying cause, such as stones or diabetes, treatment will be directed at this as well as at the infection itself.

Acute cystitis is treated with antibiotics and an increased fluid intake. If necessary, a preparation such as potassium citrate may be prescribed to make the urine less acidic and therefore reduce the burning. Although potassium citrate can be bought over the counter, it is vital that patients do not rely solely on such symptomatic treatment, but see their doctors in order to have the infection correctly treated. Potassium citrate should be used sparingly since prolonged or excessive use can lead to a dangerous rise of potassium levels in the body. If a patient has a history of thrush infections, she may need to be given some anti-thrush treatment (such as nystatin) to take together with her antibiotics, in order to prevent a recurrence.

Usually antibiotics are given for one to two weeks but, recently, it has been discovered that short courses (one to three days) of certain antibiotics are as successful and have few side effects. Some specialists, however, are still not entirely convinced about the value of short courses and continue to prescribe antibiotics for a longer period. It is very important, because of the way in which antibiotics work, that whatever length the course, all the tablets are taken.

If a first attack does not respond to antibiotic treatment, a longer course, for up to six weeks, may be necessary. For patients who have repeated attacks, a low-dose course of antibiotics given for between six months and a year is often successful in producing a cure.

Acute pyelonephritis, too, is treated with antibacterial drugs (sulphonamides are usually preferred to the newer antibiotics, since 90 per cent of cases will respond to these).

Vesico-ureteric reflux is sometimes treated surgically, the ureters being reimplanted into the bladder in such a way that reflux is less likely to occur. Prompt treatment of UTI in children will also help to prevent scarring of the kidneys. However, a badly damaged non-functioning kidney needs to be removed and, if possible, replaced with a healthy transplant.

Tuberculosis of the bladder is treated with anti-TB drugs given for a period of a year. Sometimes surgery is necessary to relieve constrictions caused by scarring. Surgery may also be helpful in the treatment of Hunner's ulcer. Dilation of the bladder under general anaesthetic will relieve the symptoms for up to six months, and this treatment can be repeated whenever necessary. In severe cases, removal of that part of the bladder affected by the ulcer may be required.

Urethral syndrome may respond to painkillers, antispasmodic drugs or dilation of the urethra. In post-menopausal patients in whom it is associated with atrophic vaginitis, an oestrogen cream applied to the vagina may be helpful.

# Prevention

Patients who are susceptible to UTI should drink at least five pints of fluid a day – more if they are in a hot climate. They should try to avoid constipation, since this may cause pressure on the bladder and prevent complete emptying. They should pass water at least every three hours and should always do so before going to bed.

A woman in whom UTI seems to occur after sexual intercourse should pass water immediately after having sex, thus flushing out any bacteria that may have been forced up into the bladder. Because bath additives – such as bath salts and foam baths – may predispose susceptible patients to UTI, these should be avoided by women who have recurrent attacks. No one should ever use disinfectants in the bath, as these can cause damage to the lining of both the urethra and the vagina.

For children in whom vesico-ureteric reflux is a factor and for other patients in whom bladder emptying is incomplete, a technique known as double micturition is helpful. (Micturition simply means passing water.) The patient passes water, walks around for a few minutes and then tries to go again. This helps to avoid pooling of stale urine in the bladder.

# Complementary Treatment

*Acupuncture*
Treatment will consist of strengthening the kidney and its energy flow.

*Aromatherapy*
Sandalwood, pine and juniper are among the oils that may be helpful.

*Herbalism*
Various herbs have the effect of increasing urinary flow, thus flushing out bacteria from the bladder. Some have an antiseptic action and relieve inflammation and spasm within the bladder. Such herbs include bearberry and buchu (both potent antiseptics), cornsilk, marshmallow and horsetail.

*Homoeopathy*
Cantharis may be helpful if the symptoms are made worse by

standing or walking and if passing water is slow and painful. If the urine is dark and bloody and associated with burning pain and spasm, merc. cor. may be prescribed. Abdominal pain with severe dysuria and a few drops of blood in the urine may indicate a need for sarsaparilla. Aconite is particularly useful for treating children and staphysagria for 'honeymoon cystitis'. Other remedies may also be appropriate in individual cases.

## Self-help

During an attack of cystitis it is advisable to drink plenty of fluid in order to flush out the urinary system frequently. Cranberry juice, garlic (taken in capsule form) and barley-water will all help this flushing out, by increasing the kidneys' output, and they all have a soothing action on inflammation within the bladder and urethra.

Naturopathic advice may include a reduction in intake of animal protein and citrus fruits and avoidance of acidic foods such as tomatoes, rhubarb, gooseberries and pickles.

# Vaginal Discharge

## Causes of Discharge

Large numbers of women suffer from a vaginal discharge at one time or another and many are uncertain whether or not this is abnormal. The normal vagina and cervix (neck of the womb) are covered with fine mucous membrane – very similar to the lining of the mouth – which has cells in it that secrete fluid. This fluid is necessary to keep the vagina lubricated, and the cells that produce it are under the control of the female sex hormones, the amount they secrete being influenced by the hormone levels in the bloodstream. More may be secreted in mid-cycle (halfway between two periods) and by women who are on the contraceptive Pill but after the menopause the vagina may become dry as the cells cease to function. The cells also respond to sexual stimulation, so that the vagina is well-lubricated for intercourse. A slight discharge after intercourse, consisting of vaginal fluid and some of the male ejaculate, is not uncommon.

However, a discharge which occurs regularly and either wets or stains the underwear or which is smelly or irritating is never normal and needs investigation and treatment. There are a number of organisms which may produce a vaginal discharge. One of the commonest is monilia, which causes thrush. This is dealt with in a separate section.

# Trichomonas

This relatively common organism causes a profuse discharge which is often frothy and smelly, may be greyish, yellow or green, and is usually worse after intercourse and following a period. It causes itching and soreness, and intercourse may become very uncomfortable or even painful. In about one quarter of cases the infection spreads to the urinary tract and causes discomfort on passing water and frequency. Occasionally the organism is found on a cervical smear in a woman who has no symptoms. Infected men are often asymptomatic although they may have some discomfort when they urinate.

To diagnose trichomonas samples of the discharge are examined under a microscope and are cultured in the laboratory.

Several drugs can be used in treatment, of which the commonest is metronidazole. Side effects include nausea, vomiting and a metallic taste in the mouth but these can all be minimized by taking the tablets during or immediately after a meal. Drinking alcohol tends to make the side effects worse, so it is advisable to remain teetotal while having treatment. It is important that the patient's partner is treated as well, even if he or she has no symptoms since, otherwise, the couple are likely to keep passing the infection back and forth to each other. About 90 per cent of patients are cured by a single course of tablets and those who fail to respond will usually do so if given a larger dose over a longer period of time.

# Chlamydia

This is a common cause of discharge from the penis in men and they may pass the infection on to their sexual partners. In women it may cause few symptoms. However, a watery or purulent discharge can occur and, if this is untreated, the infection may spread to the tubes and, ultimately, cause a chronic pelvic infection with resulting infertility.

A vaginal swab is necessary for diagnosis and the infection can be treated with the antibiotics tetracycline, co-trimoxazole or erythromycin.

# Gardnerella

This organism is often found in the vagina and there is debate among specialists as to whether it does in fact cause an infection or whether it is one of the several non-harmful bacteria which normally live there.

However, it does seem in many cases to be associated with a vaginal discharge which is often greyish white and profuse and has a distinctly cheesy smell. The discharge is often worse around the time of a period. Other symptoms may include itching, discomfort or pain on intercourse, bleeding after inter-course, pain on passing water and frequency.

Like trichomonas, gardnerella can be treated with metroni-dazole or tinidazole.

# Gonorrhoea

This is a relatively common disease although it is to be hoped that the precautions recommended to reduce the spread of AIDS (fewer sexual partners and the use of condoms) will also help to reduce the spread of gonorrhoea.

It is very contagious, so someone who has sex with an infected partner can expect to be infected themselves within a month. Unfortunately, although over 95 per cent of infected men have symptoms, up to half of all infected women may be symptom-free. Not realizing that they have the disease, they do not request treatment and therefore may spread it still further. This is why anyone who is diagnosed as having gonorrhoea will be asked about his or her sexual contacts within the past month or so, so that others who may be infected can be diagnosed and treated.

Men who have gonorrhoea usually have a purulent discharge from the penis, swelling around the end of the urethra, frequency, and pain on passing urine. In women, however, the discharge may only be slight. It may be any colour between white and green and is sometimes brown or blood-stained. If it is profuse, it is usually because the patient has a trichomonas infection as well – in fact, over half the women who are diagnosed as having gonorrhoea are also infected with trichomonas. There may be urinary symptoms – frequency and discomfort – and pain and swelling in the vulval area caused by infection of the Bartholin's glands, which are situated there. The infection frequently spreads to the anus and back passage but, although discomfort may occur, this is often symptomless.

If gonorrhoea is untreated, it is likely to spread and cause a chronic pelvic infection which may produce constant lower abdominal pain and may result in the tubes becoming blocked, with subsequent infertility. Patients may also experience heavy, painful periods and pain on intercourse.

Investigation of both sexes consists of swabs taken from the urethra and the back passage and, in female patients, additional swabs from the neck of the womb and the vagina. Blood tests are also taken to test for syphilis, which may occur together with gonorrhoea.

There are several antibiotics which can be used to treat gonorrhoea, the choice often depending on whether or not the patient has another infection (such as syphilis or chlamydia) as well. After the treatment is finished, further swabs will be taken to ensure that the infection has been eradicated.

## Complementary Treatment

If there is any chance that a patient with a discharge is suffering from gonorrhoea, she must see a doctor to ensure that a correct diagnosis is made, since this infection must be treated with antibiotics.

However, combined with orthodox medicine, complementary treatment may be used for any form of vaginal discharge to speed recovery. In those cases where the patient continues to have a discharge despite negative swabs and orthodox treatment, complementary therapies may be particularly helpful.

_Acupuncture_
A white discharge is said to be due to a lack of energy (Chi) and the presence of damp in the reproductive system. A yellow discharge is said to be due to damp heat. Specific points are

chosen to restore Chi to normal levels, to eliminate damp and, where appropriate, heat, and to strengthen the kidney, one of whose functions is said to be control of the reproductive system.

*Aromatherapy*
Bergamot may be recommended to treat an irritating discharge; among other oils used are eucalyptus, thyme, geranium, hyssop and juniper.

*Herbalism*
Various herbal preparations may be prescribed which, inserted into the vagina, will help to reduce inflammation and discharge. These include marigold, myrrh, beth root and arbor-vitae.

*Homoeopathy*
A patient who has a smelly yellow discharge which is associated with burning and severe itching and which is worse after a period may benefit from kreosotum, while someone with a smelly brownish discharge, itching and a prickly pain may be helped by nit. ac. Pulsatilla may be appropriate for a woman who has a thick, burning, yellowy-green discharge and sepia for someone whose discharge is white or yellow and jelly-like.

# Self-help

Some people recommend using a tampon soaked in yoghurt and changed several times a day as an additional treatment for gardnerella. It seems that by itself it is not very effective but, in combination with orthodox drug treatment, it may help to clear up the condition more rapidly. It does this by making the secretions of the vagina more acidic and thus less suitable for gardnerella to live in, and by helping to restore the normal bacteria of the vagina which will, themselves, overpower the invaders.

# Varicose Veins

## Definition and Causes

Animals who walk on four legs don't suffer from varicose veins. However, as soon as Man pulled himself upright and started to walk on his two hind legs, he started to put much greater pressure on the veins in those legs. The arteries, through which blood is distributed to the body, have a layer of muscle and a layer of elastic tissue in their walls, and are thus able to respond to the rhythmic pumping of the heart (as felt in the pulses). But once the blood has flowed through the tissues in the tiny capillaries and has been gathered together again into the much thinner-walled veins, the pumping action has been lost. This is why blood spurts from a cut artery but flows from a cut vein.

The blood returns to the heart through a system of veins, assisted by the movement of the surrounding muscles which helps to push it along. To prevent the blood from pooling, the veins contain a series of valves which stop it from flowing backwards. Normal blood flow in the leg runs from superficial to deeper veins through small communicating vessels known as perforators, and these connections are also controlled by valves. The pressure of blood on the valves in the leg veins is much greater than elsewhere in the body because of their position

438

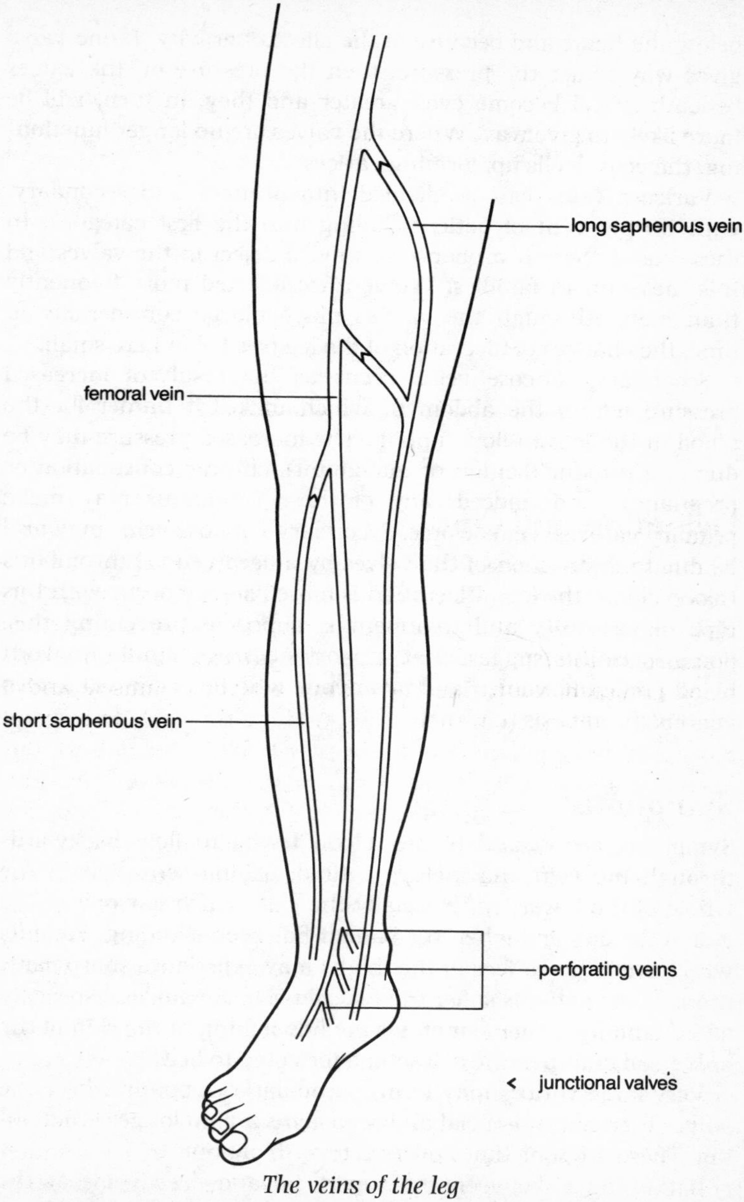

long saphenous vein

femoral vein

short saphenous vein

perforating veins

< junctional valves

*The veins of the leg*

439

below the heart and because of the effect of gravity. If one valve gives way under the pressure, then the pressure on the valves beneath it will become even greater and they, in turn, will be more likely to give way. Where the valves are no longer functioning, the vein swells up, forming varices.

Varicose veins can be divided into primary and secondary, with 80 per cent of patients falling into the first category. In these cases, there is probably an inborn defect in the valves and this may run in families. Women are affected more frequently than men. Although the varices may enlarge considerably in time, the chances of ulceration of the leg (see below) are small.

Secondary varicose veins occur as the result of increased pressure within the abdomen, which makes it harder for the blood in the legs to flow 'uphill'. The increased pressure may be due to a tumour (benign or malignant), chronic constipation or pregnancy, and, indeed, any of these conditions may make primary varicose veins worse. Secondary varicose veins may also be due to destruction of the valves by a deep venous thrombosis (blood clot in the leg). Ulceration is more likely to occur with this type of varicosity and treatment is aimed at preventing this. Some specialists suggest that support stockings should be worn by all pregnant women and by anyone who has ever had a deep venous thrombosis (DVT).

## Symptoms

Symptoms are caused by the blood trying to flow backwards through the vein and include a tired, aching sensation in the whole of the lower leg, especially the calf, which is worst at the end of the day and when the patient has been standing. Patients who have large varices in the thighs may experience sharp pains there. Some patients suffer from swelling of the ankles, especially after standing. Other symptoms include itching in the skin of the ankle and cramp in the calf soon after going to bed.

Very large varices may form, particularly at points where the valves between superficial and deep veins are no longer functioning. These are sometimes referred to as 'blow-outs'.

If the valves between the superficial and deep veins at the

ankle become incompetent, the tiny blood-vessels in the skin become more prominent and may form a fan-shaped flare over the ankle bone. This may be associated with an abnormal firmness and a darkening of the skin, the three signs together being known as lipodermatosclerosis. This is a danger sign that an ulcer is likely to form.

## Complications

A minor injury to a varicose vein may cause haemorrhage which, because of the high back pressure within that vein, may be very profuse and frightening, although easily treated (see below).

Sometimes phlebitis occurs, in which the blood in a varicose vein clots. The vein becomes very tender and hard, the overlying skin is inflamed and the patient may have a fever and be quite unwell. Very occasionally, this occurs as the result of treatment of the veins by injection.

Ulceration is the most worrying complication of varicose veins since, once ulcers have formed, although they heal easily, they tend to recur. They are particularly associated with incompetent valves in the deep veins of the leg, frequently occurring as the result of a DVT. They usually develop around the ankle rather than on the foot itself. Why this should be so is unclear and the actual mechanism of their development is not fully understood. However, it is suggested that fibrinogen, a substance involved with the clotting of blood, leaks out of the veins as a result of the very high pressure within them and forms a barrier in the surrounding tissues. This barrier prevents oxygen and nutrients getting through to the tissues, which therefore start to die. Very rarely, the edge of a long-standing varicose ulcer may become malignant – this is known as Marjolin's ulcer.

## Investigations

Varicose veins can be diagnosed simply by looking at them, but some investigations are necessary to determine which method of treatment will be best.

One method is to tie a rubber tube around the patient's leg while she is lying down (and the veins are comparatively empty), in order to prevent blood flowing backwards. If the tube is applied round the thigh and, when the patient stands up, the lower varices do not fill rapidly, this suggests that it is only the valves in the upper part of the leg which are incompetent and that the Trendelenburg operation described below will give a good result. If, however, the lower varices do fill rapidly, this suggests that there are incompetent valves in the perforating veins lower down the leg. Further experiments in tying the tube at different levels will demonstrate which these are. Just before treatment, these points will be marked so that the perforators can either be injected or tied off.

A large varicosity in the thigh (called a saphena varix) may sometimes be difficult to differentiate from a hernia. In order to make the diagnosis, the doctor will keep one finger on the varix and will tap gently on the dilated veins lower down the leg. If the swelling is indeed a saphena varix, he will feel a vibration.

Patients with ulcers are usually assessed initially in hospital. A Doppler machine uses sound to measure the blood flow and pressure in the veins around the ankle. Sometimes phlebography is performed, in which a dye is injected into the veins and an X-ray is then taken which will show their outlines.

# Orthodox Treatment

*Elastic Stockings*
Elastic stockings are used to prevent minor varicosities from getting worse and to prevent the development of varicose veins in pregnant women and people who have had a DVT. They are especially valuable for patients who, because of age or frailty, are unsuited to other forms of treatment, and for those who are on the waiting-list for treatment. NHS stockings used to be very hefty affairs but recently a completely new range has been introduced. They are no longer unsightly and are much easier to put on than the previous type. Unfortunately, tights are not available, although these can be bought privately.

People who have established varicose veins should put their

elastic stockings on before they get out of bed in the morning, thus preventing any back pressure on the valves, and they should take them off last thing at night. Patients are measured very carefully for their stockings but sometimes complain that they feel tight. This, however, is not due to poor fitting but to swelling of the leg under the stocking. It is an indication to the patient to do some gentle exercise (such as walking) in order to reduce the swelling. The only patients for whom elastic stockings are not suitable are those who have hardening of the arteries in the legs, resulting in inadequate amounts of blood reaching the lower legs and feet. In such a case, the compression produced by elastic stockings could make the problem worse.

_Drugs_
Some doctors prescribe oxerutins which may relieve the aching and swelling resulting from varicose veins. Stanozolol is some-times used for patients with lipodermatosclerosis. This is a steroid preparation which helps to break down the fibrin barrier that is thought to play an important role in the development of ulcers.

_Injection_
Patients with minor varices can be treated with injections, although these are not suitable if the varices are in the upper part of the thigh. The points at which the varicosites connect with the deep veins of the leg are determined and a sclerosing solution injected into them. This has the effect of closing off the vein at these points. Once the injections have been given, the leg is bandaged firmly with an elastic bandage and this is kept on for two weeks.

_Surgery_
For more advanced varicose veins, surgery is usually necessary. In the Trendelenburg procedure, the saphenous vein is discon-nected from the femoral vein (see diagram) and the individual branches of the saphenous vein are tied off. This may be combined with stripping (complete removal) of the vein. This is often done if there are large varicosities in the thigh. Between 60 and 70 per cent of patients have a good long-term result from operation.

*Treatment of Complications*

The treatment of haemorrhage is to lie the patient down, raise the leg that is bleeding and apply a pressure bandage over the bleeding point (a thick layer of folded handkerchiefs tied firmly in place with a scarf will do as a first-aid measure). It is most important that a pressure bandage is used and not a tourniquet, which would cut off all the blood supply to the leg. Bleeding will stop quite quickly with this treatment but the doctor should be called to inspect the injury and the patient will later need either injection or operative treatment for the varicose veins.

Phlebitis is treated with bed rest, the foot of the bed being raised. A bandage is applied to the leg which flattens out the superficial veins and increases blood flow through the deep veins. In severe cases, an anticoagulant (blood-thinning drug) may be necessary in order to relieve pain and prevent the thrombosis from spreading.

There are two main methods of treating varicose ulcers. The first is to put the patient to bed, with the foot of the bed raised, and keep the ulcer clean until it has healed. In severe cases, an elastic bandage may be needed in addition. Although this is an effective treatment, it may entail the patient remaining in bed for some weeks, which may be inconvenient for a younger patient and inadvisable for an older one. In such cases, the patient may be treated simply by tight elastic bandaging and regular dressing of the ulcer itself. Sometimes zinc-impregnated bandages are used since zinc helps to promote skin healing.

Over the past few years, some hospitals have been using dressings derived from seaweed in the treatment of ulcers. These have two great advantages over traditional gauze dressings. Firstly they form a gel which absorbs fluid from the ulcer, reducing the risk of infection. Secondly they are very easy to remove, as they can just be washed away. This means that not only is their removal painless but there is also no risk that delicate healing tissue will be damaged when the dressing is changed. Available over the counter under the name of Sorbsan, they are also suitable for treating other types of wound.

Some patients with varicose ulcers need skin grafting. This may be done by removing a slice of skin from another part of the

444

body (such as the thigh) or by a 'pinch graft' in which a number of tiny pieces of skin are used. Done under a local anaesthetic, pinch grafting can dramatically reduce the time needed to heal a bad ulcer.

Once an ulcer has healed, the patient must continue to wear elastic stockings in order to reduce the risk of a recurrence. Some patients with ulcers are not suitable for injection or operation but, in other cases, one of these may be necessary.

# Complementary Treatment

*Aromatherapy*
Cypress, lemon, lavender and rosemary are among the oils that may be recommended.

*Herbalism*
Various lotions such as marigold, witch hazel or horse chestnut may be prescribed for patients with varicose veins or ulcers. Marigold has a healing action on local tissues, both witch hazel and horse chestnut are astringent and help to prevent bleeding, and horse chestnut has additional anti-inflammatory properties. Lime blossom too, is anti-inflammatory, aids circulation and has a healing effect on the walls of the blood vessels.

*Homoeopathy*
Carbo veg. may be suitable for patients whose legs tend to be blue from poor circulation and whose feet and legs are always cold. For those whose legs are constantly painful and tired and who have purple blotches on the skin of the legs, hamamelis may be appropriate. Pulsatilla is useful for patients with painful inflamed veins whose symptoms are relieved by walking in cool air.

*Nutrition*
Rutin tablets help to strengthen the walls of blood vessels and may be recommended. In addition, supplements of vitamins C and E, which are essential for the health of the skin and blood vessels, may prevent varicose veins from getting any worse.

# Vertigo
## *and*
## Tinnitus

These two conditions commonly arise as the result of disorders affecting the ear and may occur together.

## Vertigo (Giddiness)

This word is often used by lay people to mean fear of heights. However, the medical term for fear of heights is acrophobia. Vertigo (pronounced vert-eye-go) is, in fact, a sensation of abnormal movement in which the patient feels that either he or his surroundings are going round and round or rocking to and fro. The sensation is often accompanied by vomiting, sweating and faintness. Frequently the patient will have other symptoms of ear disease, although vertigo can occur in someone with perfectly normal ears – after whirling round and round or after drinking a lot of alcohol, for example.

Although vertigo is usually the result of diseases of the ear (such as acute or chronic infections, injury, Ménière's disease or labryinthitis), it may also be due to conditions affecting the brain (such as stroke or migraine) or the blood supply to the ear (such as hardening of the arteries).

## LABYRINTHITIS

The labyrinth is the section of the inner ear which is concerned with the maintenance of balance. Acute labyrinthitis or vestibular neuronitis is sometimes known as viral labyrinthitis, although there is no firm evidence that it is caused by a virus. However, some experts think this is likely because the condition often occurs in little epidemics. It usually affects patients in the 30–50 age range and may follow a feverish illness. It often starts with severe vertigo which is made worse by movement or by putting the head in certain positions. Recovery is rapid over a period of two or three days and there are no after-effects. Some patients have repeated attacks but these become less frequent and less severe with time and have usually disappeared within 12–18 months. Occasionally, if labyrinthitis has followed an attack of mumps, the patient may be left with some degree of deafness.

Labyrinthitis may also occur as a complication of chronic suppurative otitis media (described fully in the section on ear infections). The patient may have had a discharging ear for many years but has not seen his doctor about it because he has not experienced any pain. Suddenly he develops severe vertigo and vomiting, which is made worse by moving his head and, sometimes, by pressing on the diseased ear. This is associated with headache and fever, and the patient feels very unwell.

## MÉNIÈRE'S DISEASE

This is a relatively uncommon condition which tends to affect middle-aged men and women. The cause is unknown, although it seems to be associated with an increased amount of fluid in the inner ear (the part housing the balance mechanisms and the nerve endings that transmit sound to the brain).

The first symptoms are usually deafness and tinnitus (a buzzing or ringing sound) in one ear. Then the patient starts to have attacks of severe vertigo, which may come on very suddenly but which are usually preceded by a worsening of the tinnitus. The giddiness is made worse by movement and is accompanied, often, by vomiting and, sometimes, by diarrhoea. The patient is pale and clammy and cannot hear with the affected ear. However, once the attack has subsided, after a period of between fifteen minutes and two hours, the hearing starts to return. If an attack is severe, it may be several hours or even days before the patient feels quite well again. But attacks may be quite mild and may consist simply of a slight degree of vertigo on waking in the morning, which gradually wears off after about an hour. Sometimes they are brought on by a sudden movement, coughing or sneezing, but this is the exception rather than the rule. Patients who are under stress seem more liable to frequent attacks but, as time goes on, most patients find that they become less frequent and less severe, although this improvement may be associated with gradually increasing deafness. If the inner ear is completely destroyed by the condition, the attacks will cease altogether but the patient will be profoundly deaf in that ear. Occasionally, in severe cases, both ears may become affected.

## TRAUMATIC VERTIGO
This may follow a head injury or an ear operation. Usually the patient recovers completely, although a fracture of the base of the skull may damage the labyrinth to such an extent that the problem becomes a long-term one.

## POSITIONAL VERTIGO
In this condition, the patient complains of fleeting episodes of vertigo which are brought on by moving the head or by bending down. What causes these attacks, which last only a few seconds, is unknown but most patients recover after a period of two or three months. In some cases, positional vertigo may be associated with arthritis of the spine, in which case the wearing of a cervical collar may considerably relieve the symptoms.

## INVESTIGATIONS
The doctor will first need to determine whether the patient is suffering from vertigo (due to a problem in the ears) or from another disorder of balance, which may be associated with eye problems or with an abnormality in the balance-sensing mechanism, which is made up of special nerve endings (proprioceptors) situated in the feet and legs and the major posture-maintaining muscles of the body. If the diagnosis seems to be one of vertigo,

then the ears will need to be investigated. Often such a diagnosis can be made from the history alone (such as in Ménière's disease) and investigations are necessary just to determine the cause.

The doctor will examine the patient's eyes and may test his sense of balance and coordination. Blood tests may be done, including one for blood sugar, since proprioceptor abnormalities may occur in diabetes.

The ears will be inspected through an auroscope and a hearing test performed. Sometimes, it may be necessary to X-ray the skull to determine whether there is any infection of the mastoids. A caloric test, in which cold water and then warm water is run into one ear helps the doctor to assess the normality of the balance mechanism in that ear. The test provokes nystagmus – a rhythmic movement of the eyes – which is due to irritation of the labyrinth. (Patients with labyrinthitis may develop nystagmus as part of their illness.) In a patient with Ménière's disease, where the labyrinth has been destroyed, the caloric test may fail to provoke nystagmus.

## ORTHODOX TREATMENT

The treatment of vertigo depends to a certain extent on its cause. Acute labyrinthitis needs nothing more than a few days' bed rest and, if necessary, a mild anti-vertigo drug. Labyrinthitis resulting from chronic suppurative otitis media, however, requires hospital admission, antibiotics and, as soon as possible, a radical mastoid operation (see the section on ear infections). Anti-vertigo drugs are also given, such as cinnarizine, cyclizine, dimenhydrinate, hyoscine, prochlorperazine, promethazine, thiethylperazine or betahistine hydrochloride.

Various treatments have been tried for Ménière's disease and, although none has proved outstanding, each is helpful in a number of cases. During the acute attack of vertigo, the patient needs bed rest and an anti-vertigo drug. Relief of stress, reducing salt intake and stopping smoking may result in fewer and less severe attacks. If the ear has become very deaf but vertigo continues, an operation to destroy the remaining labyrinth (which will also destroy any remaining hearing in that ear) will halt the attacks. Some specialists advocate the insertion of a grommet into the ear in cases where blockage of the Eustachian tube seems to be contributing to the problem. The Eustachian tube, running from the the ear to the throat, ensures that air pressure on both sides of the ear-drum are equal (see the section on ear infections). A grommet is a tiny plastic tube which is inserted through the ear-drum and thus provides the same service. This may produce a considerable improvement in the patient's condition. The grommet is removed after a period of at least three months.

# Tinnitus (Ringing in the Ears)

Tinnitus, or 'ringing in the ears', is a fairly common condition among elderly people. It affects about 15 per cent of the adult population and may be mild or severe. Usually the sound takes the form of a high-pitched hiss or a noise similar to that of running water. Rarely, tinnitus is caused by an abnormality in the blood flow to the ear and, in such cases, the noise may pulsate. The intensity of the sound may change from day to day but usually the patient is most aware of it when in quiet surroundings, especially when in bed at night.

Although tinnitus is usually associated with some degree of hearing loss, many patients have nothing else wrong with their ears. The sound is thought to be caused by damage to the nerve cells that transmit hearing to the brain, so that they send abnormal 'messages'. However, why the cells become damaged is unknown. Occasionally tinnitus may occur as the result of taking certain drugs such as quinine or aspirin. In such cases, the symptom usually disappears when the drug is stopped.

ORTHODOX TREATMENT
For some patients in whom tinnitus is combined with deafness, a hearing-aid may be useful since, by amplifying the background noise of their surroundings, it makes them less aware of the noise being generated in their ears. However, the standard treatment is to use a masker. This device, which is suitable for about two thirds of patients with tinnitus, is fitted into the ear in

the same way as a hearing-aid and produces a constant soothing noise. Unlike the sound of tinnitus, it doesn't fluctuate in any way and so is not distracting. Although it may take two or three months for a patient to adjust to a masker, in most cases it is very successful. It is not uncommon for patients to find that the effect lasts for some time after they have removed the masker and, in some cases, they may eventually be able to do without the device altogether.

Unfortunately, there is usually a wait of a year or so before a patient can obtain a masker on the NHS, but, for those who can afford it, they are available privately through hearing-aid firms.

RECENT ADVANCES

For patients in whom tinnitus occurs in a completely deaf ear, a new implant has been produced which although, only in the trial stage at the time of writing, seems to be proving extremely successful. Developed at University College Hospital, it consists of an electrical device which suppresses the abnormal activity of the nerve cells responsible for tinnitus. Unfortunately it is not suitable for implanting into ears with any degree of hearing because there is the risk that deafness may result.

# Complementary Treatment

*Acupuncture*

Vertigo is said to be due to over-active yang (the positive, masculine aspect of Chi) in the liver, retention of phlegm and damp within the body obstructing the flow of Chi, or a deficiency of Chi and of blood. Treatment consists of balancing the Chi of the liver, dispelling the phlegm and damp or stimulating the Chi and blood, and, in all cases, restoring the normal flow of Chi and of blood.

Tinnitus is said to be caused by a disturbance in the flow of Chi through the ear – there being either an excess or a deficiency. Points around the ear are used to restore the flow to normal.

Because the kidney is associated with the regulation of hearing in the Chinese theory of energy flow, points may also be chosen which will stimulate kidney function.

## Alexander Technique and Manipulation

Because vertigo may sometimes be caused by postural problems in the neck cutting off the blood supply to the ear, postural training by the Alexander system may be very effective in some cases. Similarly, osteopathic or chiropractic manipulation may be very beneficial by loosening the neck and restoring full movement.

## Aromatherapy

Onion may be recommended for tinnitus and a number of oils for vertigo, including caraway, aniseed, fennel and lavender.

## Herbalism

Balm, hawthorn, misteltoe and betony are among the herbs used to treat dizziness. Hawthorn and misteltoe are also used for patients with tinnitus. Balm has a relaxant effect on the nervous system as a whole, while betony, as well as acting as a relaxant, stimulates the blood supply to the brain and head.

## Homoeopathy

For patients who hear a roaring or humming sound when they are in bed at night, who are chronically giddy with a tendency to fall to one side and who have a chronic ear infection, sulphur may be effective. If the patient becomes dizzy when getting up after lying down, if this is associated with nausea and if he is very sensitive to noise of any kind, aconite may be prescribed. In cases of Ménière's disease when vertigo is brought on by sudden movement and the patient has a tendency to fall backwards, bryonia may be appropriate. Nux vomica is also used for patients who tend to fall backwards, when the dizziness comes on during or after a meal. Many other remedies are available to treat both tinnitus and vertigo.

## Hypnotherapy

This can be very effective in the treatment of tinnitus but the subject must be capable of going into a moderately deep trance. By using hypnosis, it is possible to make a patient have positive or negative hallucinations – that is, believe that something is there when it isn't or that it isn't there when it is. For patients with tinnitus, a negative hallucination is induced in which they are made to believe that they cannot hear the noise in their ears – after which it ceases to trouble them. Various techniques may be used, one of which is to suggest to the patient that he can see a dial that controls the tinnitus and that it is possible for him to use this to turn the sound off. The patient is taught self-hypnosis so that he can practise the technique at home and, after a while, he should find that he can 'turn off' his tinnitus for hours or days at a time.

## Self-help

Alcohol, smoking and strong tea or coffee may make tinnitus worse and should be avoided when this is found to be the case.

## Organizations

The British Tinnitus Association, c/o 105 Gower St, London, WC1E 6AH (tel. 071-387 8033) offers information about tinnitus and the treatment available.

# Warts

## Description and Cause

Warts are extremely common. They are caused by a virus, known as the human papilloma virus, or HPV, which causes localized excessive growth of the skin cells together with over-production of keratin, the substance that gives hardness to skin, nails and hair. They affect between 7 and 10 per cent of the population at any one time and are especially likely to affect children and young adults. No treatment has been discovered that can guarantee a cure; at the same time that some warts are being cured, others may appear on the neighbouring skin. About one fifth of all warts will disappear spontaneously within six months and two thirds within two years. However, some may take much longer.

## Types of Wart

The main sites for warts are the hands, face and neck, feet, genitalia and the skin around the anus. Those affecting the hands, face and neck usually fall into one of two categories – common warts or plane warts. The latter are fairly flat, often brownish and usually 2–3 mm in diameter. Common warts are raised, rough nodules which may appear in groups and which, most frequently, affect the fingers. Spread may be caused by injury – nail biters may get warts around their nails while thumb suckers may spread them from their hands to their mouths. A man may spread warts across his face while shaving. Apart from warts on the feet (plantar warts) and those around the nails, both of which may be painful, most warts remain painless unless they become infected by bacteria.

A plantar wart is often known as a verruca (although this is actually the medical term for any sort of wart). It may become painful because the pressure put on it when the patient stands or walks drives the wart into the flesh of the sole, pressing on nerve endings. Groups of warts (known as mosaic warts) may form, spread being encouraged by dampness.

Most warts are only slightly contagious but the exception is anal and genital warts which are easily spread by sexual contact. Growth in this area is encouraged by warmth and sweat and usually the warts are multiple, quite large, soft and fleshy, although those on the penis may be flat. Anal warts are commonest in male homosexuals although occurring in other people as well. In women, warts tend to occur around the vagina and certain strains of wart virus, when they affect the cervix, seem to be associated with the development of abnormal cells and, possibly, cancer. However, this has not yet been proved. Large fleshy warts may ulcerate or bleed and, if they become infected, may produce an unpleasant discharge.

## Investigations

Occasionally a wart on the foot may be difficult to differentiate from a corn or local hardening of the skin (callosity). In such a case, the doctor may take a scalpel and gently scrape away at the overlying layers. This is painless because there are no nerve endings in these layers of skin. In a wart, tiny blood vessels come quite close to the surface and these will be seen as tiny red or black points. Such points are not visible in a callosity.

# Orthodox Treatment

Most doctors recommend that, unless warts are particularly unsightly or uncomfortable, they should be left alone. The exceptions to this are anal and genital warts, which are very contagious, and plantar warts which can become very painful. The main reason for leaving warts untreated is that, eventually, they will resolve of their own accord without scarring whereas treatment can, occasionally, leave a scar which is more troublesome than the wart itself. The aim of all forms of treatment is to kill the wart virus, either directly or by changing the properties of the skin in which it is living, making its continued existence there difficult.

*Occlusion*
In some situations, an airtight plaster put over warts and changed weekly for six to eight weeks may destroy them by softening the underlying skin to such an extent that the virus can no longer live there. This is particularly useful when there is only a small group of warts situated on delicate skin, such as that around the nails or on the toes, which may react poorly to chemical treatment.

*Salicylic Acid*
This is available as a paint and is particularly suitable for treating multiple warts on the hands, head and neck. One of its actions is to soften the wart, making it less conspicuous. When treating a plantar wart, the patient has first to rub it with pumice stone or an emery board, to remove the top surface, before applying the paint. The wart is then covered with an airtight plaster. As the treatment starts to work, the wart turns white and the area becomes slightly tender.

*Formaline*
This method of treatment is suitable only for plantar warts. The patient smears Vaseline around the wart, to protect the surrounding skin, and then soaks the wart in a saucer of formaline solution for fifteen minutes every day. Treatment needs to be

continued for at least a month and, before each soak, the hard surface tissue must be scraped or rubbed away. Three dilutions of formaline are available. It is usual to start with the weakest and progress to a stronger solution if the treatment does not seem to be working.

*Podophyllin*
This is available as a paint or an ointment. Used two to three times a week, it may be effective for plantar warts when other treatments have failed and is the treatment of choice for anal or genital warts. It is also useful for warts around the nails or on the toes but should not be used on the face or neck. The surrounding skin must be protected with Vaseline and the podophyllin washed off after about six hours because, otherwise, there is a risk of burning. Treatment is usually effective within a few weeks. Like formaline, podophyllin comes in different dilutions and increasing strengths can be used if patients fail to respond. Because a small amount of podophyllin may be absorbed into the bloodstream and because it may cause foetal abnormalities, it should not be used by pregnant women.

*Cryotherapy*
Carbon dioxide snow or liquid nitrogen can be used to freeze warts but they are not suitable for treating large clusters. They may, however, be used for warts around the nails and for the toes and, if all else fails, for plantar warts. The treatment has about a 70 per cent success rate but, very occasionally, may leave a painful scar.

*Curettage and Cautery*
This is done under local anaesthetic. The wart is scooped out of the skin and the area is cauterized to stop bleeding and to kill any of the wart virus that may remain. It cannot be used on warts around the nails because it may damage the nail bed and result in nail deformities. It may be useful for genital and anal warts if these keep recurring or if there is no response to podophyllin. Like cryotherapy, it may, very occasionally, leave a painful scar.

_Other Treatments_
These include the use of preparations containing glutaraldehyde and silver nitrate. Lasers may also be used to burn out warts.

# Recent Advances

Interferons are proteins that occur naturally in the body and that are involved in the process of immunity, especially against viruses. In recent years it has become possible to make synthetic interferons and one of these (Intron A) has been used in a trial to treat genital warts. Injected into the warts three times a week for three weeks, it was found to produce good results. Up to 60 per cent of patients developed flu-like symptoms during treatment but these seemed to be the only side effects. Unfortunately, interferons are extremely expensive and so, for the time being, it seems likely that they will only be used for treating genital and anal warts that have not responded to any other form of treatment.

# Complementary Treatment

_Aromatherapy_
Lemon and tea tree are among the oils that may help to combat warts.

_Herbalism_
Various herbal remedies may be effective against warts. Patients may be advised to rub the wart each day with the sap from a fresh dandelion stalk, a slice of garlic, or the juice of a sour apple, a fresh pineapple or fresh green figs. Calendula juice, celandine juice and thuja (arbor-vitae) tincture may also be helpful.

_Homoeopathy_
Calc. carb. may be prescribed if the patient has large numbers of warts, especially on the sides of the fingers, the hands and arms. Thuja is useful if there are crops of warts on the backs of the hands and dulcamara if they are on the back of the fingers.

Fleshy warts may be treated with causticum or natrum mur. and flat, hard warts with antimony crud.

*Hypnotherapy*
Because 'mind over matter' may sometimes be effective in getting rid of warts, hypnotherapy may be useful if all else has failed.

# Orthodox Drugs *and* Their Trade Names

Some of the drugs mentioned in the text may be better known to patients by their trade names. A selection of these is given below.

Those drugs and groups of drugs about which specific information is given in the text will also be found in the main index.

**ACNE**

| | |
|---|---|
| Benzoyl peroxide | Acetoxyl, Acnegel, Benoxyl, Benzagel, Nericur, Panoxyl, Quinoderm, Theraderm |
| Sulphur | Dome-Acne, Eskamel |
| Tretinoin | Retin-A |
| Tetracycline | Achromycin, Economycin, Sustamycin, Tetrabid, Tetrachel, Tetrex, Deteclo, Mysteclin (with nystatin) |
| *chlortetracycline* | Aureomycin |
| *oxytetracycline* | Berkmycen, Imperacin, Oxymycin, Terramycin, Unimycin |
| Co-trimoxazole | Bactrim, Chemotrim, Comox, Fectrim, Laratrim, Septrin |
| Minocycline | Minocin |
| Doxycycline | Doxatet, Nordox, Vibramycin |
| Erythromycin | Arpimycin, Erycen, Erymax, Erythrocin, Erythrolar, Erythromid, Erythroped, Ilosone, Ilotycin, Retcin |

Cyproterone acetate      in Diane
Isotretinoin      Roaccutane

**ANXIETY AND PHOBIAS**

| | |
|---|---|
| Diazepam | Alupram, Atensine, Evacalm, Solis, Tensium, Valium |
| Chlordiazepoxide | Librium, Tropium |
| Nitrazepam | Mogadon, Nitrados, Noctesed, Remnos, Somnite, Surem, Unisomnia |
| Oxazepam | Oxanid |
| Temazepam | Normison |
| Lorazepam | Almazine, Ativan |
| Chlorpromazine | Chloractil, Largactil |
| Trifluoperazine | Stelazine |
| Clomipramine | Anafranil |

**ARTHRITIS**

| | |
|---|---|
| Ibuprofen | Apsifen, Brufen, Ebufac, Fenbid, Ibular, Ibumetin, Motrin, Paxofen |
| Indomethacin | Artracin, Imbrilon, Indocid, Indoflex, Indolar, Indomod, Mobilan, Rheumacin, Slo-Indo |
| Naproxen | Laraflex, Naprosyn |
| Aspirin | Aspergum, Claradin, Laboprin, Paynocil, Solprin |
| Sodium aurothiomalate | Myocrisin |
| Auranofin | Ridaura |
| Penicillamine | Distamine, Pendramine |
| Azathioprine | Azamune, Imuran |
| Methotrexate | Emtexate, Maxtrex |
| Steroids include: | |
| *betamethasone* | Betnelan, Betnesol |
| *cortisone* | Cortelan, Cortistab, Cortisyl |
| *dexamethasone* | Decadron, Oradexon |
| *hydrocortisone* | Hydrocortistab, Hydrocortone |
| *methylprednisolone* | Medrone |
| *prednisolone* | Delta-Phoricol, Deltacortril, Deltastab, Precortisyl, Prednesol, Sintisone |
| *prednisone* | Decortisyl |
| *triamcinolone* | Ledercort |
| Azapropazone dihydrate | Rheumox |

461

| | |
|---|---|
| Allopurinol | Aloral, Aluline, Caplenal, Cosuric, Hamarin, Zyloric |
| Probenecid | Benemid |

**ASTHMA**

| | |
|---|---|
| Sodium cromoglycate | Intal |
| Nedocromil sodium | Tilade |
| Theophylline | Biophylline, Nuelin |
| Aminophylline | Phyllocontin |
| Isoetharine | Numotac |
| Salbutamol | Asmaven, Cobutolin, Salbulin, Ventolin, Aerolin |
| Fenoterol | Berotec |
| Terbutaline | Bricanyl, Monovent |
| Steroids – see Arthritis | |
| Cetirizine | Zirtek |
| Methotrexate | Emtexate, Maxtrex |

**BACK PAIN**

| | |
|---|---|
| Indomethacin | Artracin, Imbrilon, Indocid, Indoflex, Indolar, Indomod, Mobilan, Rheumacin, Slo-Indo |
| Flurbiprofen | Froben |

**BED-WETTING**

| | |
|---|---|
| Imipramine | Praminil, Tofranil |
| Propantheline | Pro-Banthine |
| Desmopressin | Desmospray |

**BREAST LUMPS**

| | |
|---|---|
| Danazol | Danol |
| Bromocriptine | Parlodel |
| Tamoxifen | Noltam, Nolvadex, Tamofen |

**BRONCHITIS**

| | |
|---|---|
| Digoxin | Lanoxin |

**CONSTIPATION**

| | |
|---|---|
| Bran | Fybranta, Lejfibre, Proctofibe, Trifyba |
| Bulking agents include: | |
| *ispaghula husk* | Fybogel, Isogel, Metamucil, Regulan, Vi-Siblin |

462

| | |
|---|---|
| *methycellulose* | Celevac, Cellucon, Cologel |
| *sterculia* | Normacol |
| Lactulose | Dulphalac |
| Docusate sodium | Dioctyl |
| Senna | Agiolax, Senokot |
| Magnesium sulphate | Epsom salts |

**DEPRESSION**

| | |
|---|---|
| Imipramine | Praminil, Tofranil |
| Amitriptyline | Domical, Elavil, Lentizol, Tryptizol, and in Limbitrol and Triptafen |
| Nortriptyline | Allegron, Aventyl, and in Motipress and Motival |
| Doxepin | Sinequan |
| Mianserin | Bolvidon, Norval |
| Trazodone | Molipaxin |
| Viloxazine | Vivalan |

Monoamine oxidase inhibitors include:

| | |
|---|---|
| *phenelzine* | Nardil |
| *iproniazid* | Marsilid |
| *isocarboxazid* | Marplan |
| *tranylcypromine* | Parnate, and in Parstelin |
| Flupenthixol | Fluanxol |
| L-tryptophan | Optimax, Pacitron |
| Lithium carbonate | Camcolit, Liskonum, Phasal, Priadel |
| Carbamazepine | Tegretol |

**DIABETES**

| | |
|---|---|
| Tolbutamide | Glyconon, Rastinon |
| Glibenclamide | Daonil, Euglucon, Libanil, Malix |
| Acetohexamide | Dimelor |
| Chlorpropamide | Diabinese, Glymese |
| Tolazamide | Tolanase |
| Metformin | Glucophage, Orabet |
| Ponalrestat | Statil |
| Cyclosporin | Sandimmun |

**DIVERTICULAR DISEASE**

| | |
|---|---|
| Belladonna | Alka-Donna, Aluhyde, Bellocarb, Carbellon, Peptard |

| | |
|---|---|
| Dicyclomine hydrochloride | Kolanticon, Kolantyl, Merbentyl |
| Hyoscine | Buscopan |
| Propantheline bromide | Pro-Banthine |

**EPILEPSY**

| | |
|---|---|
| Sodium valproate | Epilim |
| Ethosuximide | Emeside, Zarontin |
| Phenytoin | Epanutin |
| Carbamazepine | Tegretol |
| Primidone | Mysoline |
| Phenobarbitone | Luminal |

**GALLBLADDER DISEASE**

| | |
|---|---|
| Chenodeoxycholic acid | Chendol, Chenocedon, Chenofalk |
| Ursodeoxycholic acid | Destolit, Ursofalk |

**HAIR LOSS**

| | |
|---|---|
| Minoxidil | Regaine |

**HERPES SIMPLEX**

| | |
|---|---|
| Povidone iodine | Betadine |
| Idoxuridine | Herpid, Idoxene, Iduridin, Kerecid, Ophthalmadine |
| Acyclovir | Zovirax |

**HIGH BLOOD PRESSURE**

| | |
|---|---|
| Digoxin | Lanoxin |
| Bendrofluazide | Aprinox, Berkozide, Centyl, Neo-NaClex |
| Chlorothiazide | Saluric |
| Cyclopenthiazide | Navidrex |
| Frusemide | Aluzine, Diuresal, Dryptal, Frusetic, Frusid, Lasix |
| Bumetanide | Burinex |
| Amiloride | Midamor |
| Triamterene | Dytac |
| Propranolol | Angilol, Apsolol, Berkolol, Inderal, Sloprolol |
| Oxprenolol | Apsolox, Slow-Pren, Trasicor |
| Metoprolol | Betaloc, Lopresor |

| | |
|---|---|
| Atenolol | Tenormin |
| Hydralazine | Apresoline |
| Minoxidil | Loniten |
| Prazosin | Hypovase |
| Labetalol | Labrocol, Trandate |
| Nifedipine | Adalat |
| Verapamil | Berkatens, Cordilox, Securon, Univer |
| Captopril | Acepril, Capoten; with hydrochlorthiazide – Acezide, Capozide |
| Enalapril | Innovace |
| Methyldopa | Aldomet, Dopamet |
| Clonidine | Catapres |

**IMPOTENCE**

| | |
|---|---|
| Bethanidine | Bendogen, Esbatal |
| Guanethidine | Ismelin |
| Metaraminol | Aramine |

**INCONTINENCE**

| | |
|---|---|
| Propantheline | Pro-Banthine |
| Terodiline | Terolin |
| Imipramine | Praminil, Tofranil |
| Bethanechol | Myotonine |

**INFERTILITY**

| | |
|---|---|
| Clomiphene citrate | Clomid, Serophene |
| Tamoxifen | Noltam, Nolvadex, Tamofen |
| Bromocriptine | Parlodel |
| Buserelin | Suprefact |

**INSOMNIA**

| | |
|---|---|
| Nitrazepam | Mogadon, Nitrados, Noctesed, Remnos, Somnite, Surem, Unisomnia |
| Flurazepam | Dalmane, Paxane |
| Flunitrazepam | Rohypnol |
| Loprazalam | Dormonoct |
| Temazepam | Normison |
| Triazolam | Halcion |
| Chloral hydrate | Noctec |

| | |
|---|---|
| Dichloralphenazone | Welldorm |
| Chlormethiazole | Heminevrin |
| Promethazine | Phenergan |
| Trimeprazine | Vallergan |
| Imipramine | Praminil, Tofranil |
| Trimipramine | Surmontil |

**IRRITABLE BOWEL SYNDROME**

| | |
|---|---|
| Mebeverine | Colofac, Colven |
| Propantheline | Pro-Banthine |
| Ispaghula husk | Fybogel, Isogel, Metamucil, Regulan, Vi-Siblin |
| Methylcellulose | Celevac, Cellucon, Cologel |
| Sterculia | Normacol |

**ISCHAEMIC HEART DISEASE**

| | |
|---|---|
| Glyceryl trinitrate | Coro-Nitro spray, GTN 300, Sustac, Nitrolingual spray, Nitrocontin, Suscard buccal |
| Isosorbide dinitrate | Cedocard, Isoket, Isordil, Sorbichew, Sorbitrate, Vascardin, Soni-Slo, Sorbid |
| Isosorbide mononitrate | Elantan, Imdur, Ismo, Monit, Mono-Cedocard |
| Propranolol | Angilol, Apsolol, Berkolol, Inderal, Sloprolol |
| Nifedipine | Adalat |
| Verapamil | Berkatens, Cordilox, Securon, Univer |
| Diltiazem | Calcicard, Tildiem |
| Labetalol | Labrocol, Trandate |
| Digoxin | Lanoxin |
| Clofibrate | Atromid-S |

**MENOPAUSE**

| | |
|---|---|
| Hormone replacement | Cyclo-progynova, Menophase, Prempack, Trisequens |
| Oestrogen cream | Hormofemin, Ortho Dienoestrol, Ovestin, Premarin |
| Clonidine | Dixarit |

**MENSTRUAL PROBLEMS**

| | |
|---|---|
| Flurbiprofen | Froben |
| Mefenamic acid | Ponstan |

| | |
|---|---|
| Naproxen | Laraflex, Naprosyn |
| Ibuprofen | Apsifen, Brufen, Ebufac, Fenbid, Ibular, Ibumetin, Motrin, Paxofen |
| Piroxicam | Feldene, Larapam |
| Norethisterone | Primolut N, Utovlan |
| Dydrogesterone | Duphaston |
| Ethamsylate | Dicynene |
| Tranexamic acid | Cyklokapron |
| Clomiphene | Clomid, Serophene |
| Danazol | Danol |

**MIGRAINE**

| | |
|---|---|
| Propranolol | Angilol, Apsolol, Berkolol, Inderal, Sloprolol |
| Metoprolol | Betaloc, Lopresor |
| Nadolol | Corgard |
| Timolol | Betim, Blocadren |
| Pizotifen | Sanomigran |
| Methysergide maleate | Deseril |
| Cyproheptadine | Periactin |
| Naproxen | Laraflex, Naprosyn |
| Clonidine | Dixarit |
| Metoclopramide | Maxolon, Metox, Metramid, Mygdalon, Parmid, Primperan |
| Ergotamine | Cafergot, Lingraine, Migril |

**MOUTH ULCERS**

| | |
|---|---|
| Carbenoxolone sodium | Bioplex |
| Benzocaine | Dequacaine, Medilave, Oral-B |
| Salicylates | Bonjela, Pyralvex, Teejel |
| Chlorhexidine | Corsodyl, Eludril |
| Steroids | Adcortyl, Corlan |

**NOSEBLEEDS**

| | |
|---|---|
| Tranexamic acid | Cyklokapron |
| Ethamsylate | Dicynene |

**OSTEOPOROSIS**
Hormone replacement – see Menopause

467

Etidronate disodium     Didronel
Calcitonin     Calcitare

**PEPTIC ULCER**
Cimetidine     Dyspamet, Tagamet
Ranitidine     Zantac
Famotidine     Pepcid
Nizatidine     Axid
Bismuth chelate     De-Nol
Sucralfate     Antepsin
Misoprostol     Cytotec

**PREMENSTRUAL SYNDROME**
Progesterone     Cyclogest, Gestone
Spironolactone     Aldactone, Diatensec, Laractone, Spiretic, Spiroctan, Spirolone
Bromocriptine     Parlodel

**PROSTATE PROBLEMS**
Prazosin     Hypovase
Cyproterone acetate     Androcur

**PSORIASIS**
Salicylic acid     Keralyt
Tar     Alphosyl, Carbo-Dome, Clinitar, Celcosal, Gelcotar, Meditar, Pragmatar, Psoriderm, PsoriGel, Polytar emollient, Tarcortin
Dithranol     Exolan
Methotrexate     Emtexate, Maxtrex
Etretinate     Tigason

**RHINITIS**
Astemizole     Hismanal
Terfenadine     Triludan
Xylometazoline     Otrivine
Oxymetazoline     Afrazine, Iliadin
Sodium cromoglycate     Intal
Ketotifen     Zaditen
Beclomethasone     Beconase

**RINGWORM**

| | |
|---|---|
| Griseofulvin | Fulcin, Grisovin |
| Clotrimazole | Canestan |
| Econazole | Ecostatin, Pevaryl |
| Miconazole | Daktarin, Monistat |
| Sulconazole | Exelderm |
| Salicylic acid | Phytex, Phytocil |

**SCHIZOPHRENIA**

| | |
|---|---|
| Chlorpromazine | Chloractil, Largactil |
| Thioridazine | Melleril |
| Trifluoperazine | Stelazine |
| Haloperidol | Dozic, Fortunan, Haldol, Serenace |
| Procyclidine | Arpicolin, Kemadrin |
| Benzhexol | Artane, Bentex, Broflex |
| Orphenadrine | Biorphen, Disipal |
| Fluphenazine | Moditen |

**SHINGLES**

| | |
|---|---|
| Idoxuridine | Herpid, Idoxene, Iduridin, Kerecid, Ophthalmadine |
| Acyclovir | Zovirax |
| Prednisolone | Codelsol, Delta-Phoricol, Deltacortril, Deltastab, Precortisyl, Prednesol, Sintisone |

**THRUSH**

| | |
|---|---|
| Nystatin | Nystan |
| Clotrimazole | Canestan |
| Ketoconazole | Nizoral |
| Econazole | Ecostatin, Pevaryl |
| Miconazole | Daktarin, Monistat |

**THYROID DISEASES**

| | |
|---|---|
| Thyroxine | Eltroxin |
| Tri-iodothyronine | Tertroxin |
| Carbimazole | Neo-Mercazole |

**URINARY TRACT INFECTIONS**

| | |
|---|---|
| Potassium citrate | Effercitrate |

## VAGINAL DISCHARGE

| | |
|---|---|
| Metronidazole | Elyzol, Flagyl, Metrolyl, Nidazol, Vaginyl, Zadstat |
| Tetracycline – see Acne | |
| Co-trimoxazole | Bactrim, Comox, Fectrim, Laratrim, Septrin |
| Erythromycin | Arpimycin, Erycen, Erymax, Erythrocin, Erythrolar, Erythromid, Erythroped, Ilosone, Ilotycin, Retcin |
| Tinidazole | Fasigyn |

## VARICOSE VEINS

| | |
|---|---|
| Oxerutins | Paroven |
| Stanozolol | Stromba |

## VERTIGO AND TINNITUS

| | |
|---|---|
| Cinnarizine | Stugeron |
| Cyclizine | Valoid |
| Dimenhydrinate | Dramamine |
| Prochlorperazine | Stemetil, Vertigon, Buccastem |
| Promethazine | Avomine |
| Thiethylperazine | Torecan |
| Betahistine | Serc |

## WARTS

| | |
|---|---|
| Formaldehyde (formaline) | Veracur |
| Podophyllin | Posalfilin |
| Glutaraldehyde | Glutarol |

## APPENDIX B

# Pronunciation Guide

**VOWELS**

| | |
|---|---|
| a | as in cap, mad, hat |
| ay | as in tape, date, male |
| ah | as in far, mark, jar |
| e | as in met, kept, wed |
| ee | as in meet, weak, seem |
| er | as in term, learn, perm |
| i | as in with, miss, list |
| ī | as in might, line, wide |
| o | as in soft, lost, dot |
| oh | as in spoke, boat, low |
| u | as in but, stud, shut |
| ū | as in put, wood, look |
| yoo | as in due, new, mute |
| aw | as in port, saw, naughty |
| oi | as in coin, annoy, void |
| oo | as in do, boot, fruit |
| ow | as in how, stout, loud |

There are some words in which, when one is speaking normally, one glosses over a vowel and this I have shown as 'eh' – for example, the word 'normally' would be shown as nawm-eh-lee rather than nawm-a-lee and 'ballerina' as bal-eh-ree-neh.

471

**CONSONANTS**

g       as in grand, grant, girl
j       as in jelly, just, giant
s       as in soft, speak, less
z       as in raising, was, exercise

The syllable on which emphasis is put is shown in capital letters

adenoma – a-den-OH-meh
adenomyosis – a-den-oh-mī-OH-sis
alkalosis – al-keh-LOH-sis
alopecia – a-loh-PEE-sheh
amenorrhoea – ay-men-eh-REE-eh
ampulla – am-PŪL-eh
anagen – AN-a-jen
androgens – AN-droh-jens
angiogram – AN-jee-oh-gram
ankylosing – AN-kil-oh-zing
aorta – ay-AW-teh
aortography – ay-aw-TOG-raf-ee
apnoea – AP-nee-eh
arthritides – ah-THRIT-id-eez
arthrodesis – ah-throh–DEE-sis

biguanide – bī-GWAN-īd
bronchi – BRON-kee
bronchioles – BRON-kee-ohls
bulimia – bul-IM-ee-eh

catagen – KAT-a-jen
cheilosis – kee-LOH-sis
chemonucleolysis – KEE-moh-nyoo-klee-O-li-sis
chenodeoxycholic – KEE-noh-dee-oks-ee-KOH-lik
chlamydia – kla-MID-ee-eh
cholangiogram – koh-LAN-jee-oh-gram
cholangitis – koh-lan-JĪ-tis
cholecystitis – KOH-lee-sis-TĪ-tis
cholecystokinin – KOH-lee-sis-toh-KĪ-nin

472

choledocholithiasis – koh-lee-DOH-koh-li-THĪ-eh-sis
cholesteatoma – koh-LES-tee-eh-TOH-meh
chymopapain – kī-moh-pa-PAYN
cilia – SI-lee-eh
cirrhosis – si-ROH-sis
coarctation – koh-ahk-TAY-shun
colporrhaphy – kol-PO-ra-fee
coronary – KO-ron-ree
cruris – KRAW-ris
curettage – KYAW-re-tazh
cystocoele – SIS-toh-seel

defaecation – de-feh-KAY-shun
*déjà vu* – DAY-zhah voo
diuretic – DĪ-yaw-re-tik
dysmenorrhoea – dis-men-oh-REE-eh
dysplasia – dis-PLAY-zee-eh
dysuria – dis-YAW-ree-eh

eicosapentaenoic – ī-KOH-seh-pen-teh-en-OH-ik
emphysema – em-fi-ZEE-meh
endometrium – en-doh-MEE-tree-um
enuresis – en-YAW-ree-sis
eosinophils – ee-oh-SIN-oh-filz
epidermis – e-pee-DER-mis
epididymitis – e-pee-di-dim-Ī-tis
erythrodermic – e-ri-throh-DER-mik
exogenous – eks-O-jeh-nus
exophthalmos – EKS-off-thal-mos

faecal – FEE-kal
fibroadenosis – FĪ-broh-a-de-NOH-sis
fluorescein – FLAW-re-seen

gingivitis – JIN-ji-VĪ-tis
glucagon – GLOO-ka-gon
glucosidase – gloo-koh-SĪ-dayz
goitre – GOI-ter

gynaecology – gī-neh-KO-leh-jee

haematoma – hee-meh-TOH-meh
haematuria – hee-meh-TYAW-ree-eh
haemorrhoids – HEM-eh-roids
herpes – HER-peez
hypertrophy – hī-PER-tro-fee
hypoglycaemia – hī-poh-glī-SEE-mee-eh

idiopathic – i-dee-oh-PA-thik
ileus – Ī-lee-us
intertriginous – in-ter-TRĪ-geh-nus
ischaemic – is-KEE-mik
interstitial – in-ter-STI-shal

keratolytics – ke-ra-toh-LI-tiks
ketoacidosis – kee-toh-a-si-DOH-sis

libido – li-BEE-doh
lipodermatosclerosis – li-poh-der-meh-toh-skleh-ROH-sis
luteinizing – LOO-ti-nī-zing

maceration – MA-ser-ray-shun
malleus – MA-lee-us
Meibomian – mī-BOH-mee-ehn
melaena – me-LEE-neh
menorrhagia – me-noh-RAY-jee-eh
methyl – mee-THĪL
myometrium – mī-oh-MEE-tree-um
myxoedema – miks-eh-DEE-meh

nephropathy – ne-FRO-pa-thee
neuropathy – nyaw-RO-pa-thee
nystagmus – ni-STAG-mus

oesophagus – ee-SO-fa-gus
onycholysis – on-ee-KO-li-sis
ophthalmoscope – off-THAL-mo-skohp

orchidectomy – aw-ki-DEK-to-mee
otitis – oh-TĪ-tis

paronychia – pa-roh-NI-kee-eh
pedis – PEE-dis
percutaneous – per-kyoo-TAY-nee-us
petit mal – PE-tee mal
phaeochromocytoma – fee-oh-KROH-moh-sī-TOH-meh
phlebography – fle-BO-graf-ee
phlegm – flem
photocoagulation – foh-toh-koh-ag-yoo-LAY-shun
phylloides – fi-LOI-deez
physiology – fi-zee-O-lo-jee
placebo – pla-SEE-boh
procidentia – pro-si-DEN-sheh
psoralens – SO-ra-lenz
psoriasis – so-RĪ-eh-sis
psoriatic – so-ree-A-tik
pulmonary – PUL-mehn-ree
pyelogram – PĪ-eh-loh-gram

rectocoele – REK-toh-seel
Reiter's – RĪ-terz
renal – REE-nal
retinopathy – re-ti-NO-pa-thee
rhinitis – rī-NĪ-tis

salicylic – sa-li-SI-lik
saphena – sa-FEE-neh
scintigraphy – sin-TI-gra-fee
sebaceous – seh-BAY-shus
seborrhoeic – se-beh-RAY-ik
sebum – SEE-behm
septicaemia – sep-ti-SEE-mee-eh
sphenoidal – sfee-NOI-dehl
sphincterotomy – sfink-ter-O-to-mee
sphygmomanometer – sfig-moh-ma-NO-mi-ter
spondylolisthesis – spon-di-loh-lis-THEE-sis
spondylosis – spon-di-LOH-sis

stapes – STAY-peez
sulphanylurea – sul-fa-nīl-yaw-REE-eh
suppurative – SUP-yaw-ray-tiv
systolic – sis-TO-lik

telogen – TEE-loh-jen
terbutylether – ter-byoo-tīl-EETH-er
testosterone – tes-TOS-ter-ohn
thyroxine – thī-ROKS-in
tinea – TI-nee-eh
tinnitus – TI-ni-tus
trachea – tra-KEE-eh
transhepatic – tranz-he-PA-tik
transurethral – tranz-yaw-REE-thral
trichomonas – trī-koh-MOH-nas
tri-iodothyronine – trī-ī-O-doh-THĪ-roh-neen
tumescence – tyoo-ME-sens
tympanic – tim-PA-nik

unguium – UN-gwee-ūm
urethra – yaw-REE-threh
urethrocoele – yaw-REE-throh-seel
uric – YAW-rik
ursodeoxycholic – ER-soh-dee-oks-ee-KOH-lik
uterine – YOO-ter-īn

varicella – va-ri-SE-leh
vasodilator – vay-zoh-dī-LAY-teh
ventricular – ven-TRI-kyoo-lah
vertigo – ver-TĪ-goh
vesico-ureteric – VEE-si-koh-yaw-ri-TE-rik
videocystourethrography – vi-dee-oh-sis-toh-yaw-ree-THRO-gra-fee

# How to Find a Qualified Complementary Practitioner

The following organizations hold registers of qualified practitioners. Not every practitioner is on every register covering his therapy (for example, some will appear only on that held by the school at which they qualified). So, if one organization is unable to give you the name of a practitioner near your home, try another.

The Institute for Complementary Medicine, 21 Portland Place, London, WIN 3AF (tel. 071-636 9543) has compiled the British Register of Complementary Practitioners and has public information points (PIPs) around the country which provide information about local therapists.

### ACUPUNCTURE

Register of Traditional Chinese Medicine, 19 Trinity Rd, London, N2 8JJ (081-883 8431)

Traditional Acupuncture Society, 1 The Ridgeway, Stratford-upon-Avon, Warwickshire, CV37 9JL (0789 298798)

International Register of Oriental Medicine, Green Hedges House, Green Hedges Ave., East Grinstead, Sussex, RHI9 IDZ (0342 313106)

### ALEXANDER TECHNIQUE

Alexander Teaching Associates, ATA Centre, 188 Old Street, London, ECIV 9BP (071-250 3038)

Society of Teachers of the Alexander Technique, 10 London House, 266 Fulham Rd, SWIO 9EL (071-351 0828)

## AROMATHERAPY

I am unaware of any register of aromatherapists, so would suggest asking the local Institute for Complementary Medicine PIP. Often a centre at which several complementary practitioners work together will have an aromatherapist.

## BACH FLOWER REMEDIES

Information, remedies and books are available from the Bach Centre, Mount Vernon, Sotwell, Wallingford, Oxon., OX10 0PZ

## CHIROPRACTIC

British Chiropractors' Association, Premier House, 10 Greycoat Place, London, SW1P 1SB (071–222 8866)

Institute of Pure Chiropractic, PO Box 126, Oxford, OX1 1UF (0865 246687)

## HEALING

The best way to find a healer is probably by word of mouth – people are always ready to recommend someone who has helped them, so ask around. The Institute for Complementary Medicine's PIPs may also be able to supply names.

There are many professional associations of healers including:
British Alliance of Healing Associations, 7 Clover Way, Thetford, Norfolk

Guild of Spiritualist Healers, 36 Newmarket, Otley, Yorks, LS21 3AE (0943 462708)

National Federation of Spiritual Healers, Old Manor Farm Studio, Church St, Sunbury-on-Thames, Middlesex, TW16 6RG (09327 83164)

Spiritualists' National Union, Britten House, Stansted Hall, Stansted Mountfitchet, Essex, CM24 8OD (0279 812705)

All the above organizations have a written code of practice.

## HERBALISM

National Institute of Medical Herbalists, 41 Hatherley Rd, Winchester, Hants., SO22 6RR (0962 68776)

School of Herbal Medicine, Bucksteep Manor, Bodle Street Green, Nr Hailsham, Sussex, BN27 4RJ

## HOMOEOPATHY

The Society of Homoeopaths, 2 Artizan Rd, Northampton, NN1 4HU (0604 21400)

## HYPNOTHERAPY

To see a medical hypnotherapist, one needs a referral from one's GP, who can obtain a list of practitioners in the area from: British Society of Medical and Dental Hypnosis, PO Box 6, 42 Links Rd, Ashtead, Surrey, KT21 2HT

## NATUROPATHY

British Naturopathic and Osteopathic Association, 6 Netherhall Gardens, London, NW3 5RR (071-435 8728)

British Register of Naturopaths, 1 Albemarle Rd, The Mount, York, YO2 IEN (0904 23693)

Natural Therapeutic and Osteopathic Society and Register, 63 Collingwood Rd, Witham, Essex, CM8 2AQ (0376 512188)

## NUTRITION THERAPY

Institute for Optimum Nutrition, 5 Jerdan Place, London, SW6 IBE (071-385 7984)

## OSTEOPATHY

British Naturopathic and Osteopathic Association, 6 Netherhall Gardens, London, NW3 5RR (071-435 8728)

General Council and Register of Osteopaths, 56 London St, Reading, Berks., RGI 4SQ (0734 576585)

Natural Therapeutic and Osteopathic Society and Register, 63 Collingwood Rd, Witham, Essex, CM8 2AQ (0376 512188)

Society of Osteopaths, 62 Bower Mount Rd, Maidstone, Kent, MEI6 8AT (0622 674656)

## RADIONICS

Radionics Register, Sycamore Farm, Chadlington, Oxon., OX7 3NZ

## REFLEXOLOGY

British School for Reflex Zone Therapy of the Feet, 15 Lichfield Grove, Finchley, London, N3 2SL (071-629 3481)

International Institute of Reflexology, 92 Sheering Rd, Old Harlow, Essex, CMI7 OLT (0279 29060)

# Glossary

**Achilles tendon:** the tendon lying at the back of the ankle joint

**Acute:** short-term, often having a sudden onset

**Adenoidectomy:** removal of the adenoids

**Adenoids:** lymphatic tissue lying at the back of the nose

**Allergen:** a substance capable of causing an allergic reaction

**Allergy:** overreaction to a substance which is normally harmless (such as grass pollen)

**Amenorrhoea:** absence of the monthly periods

**Amino acid:** one of the 'building blocks' out of which protein is made and into which protein food is broken down by the digestive system

**Anaemia:** a condition in which the number of red blood cells (which are responsible for carrying oxygen) is reduced

**Anterior:** at the front

**Antibiotic:** a drug which will kill bacteria; antibiotics have no action on viruses and therefore are not given to patients with viral infections

**Antibody:** a substance produced by the cells involved in the immune system to neutralize foreign invaders such as viruses

**Anticoagulant:** a drug which prevents the blood from clotting abnormally; sometimes known as a 'blood-thinning' drug

**Antihistamine:** a drug which prevents histamine being released from the cells that produce it

**Antispasmodic:** a drug which prevents spasm in the muscle layers of the intestines and airways and in other muscle which is not under voluntary control

**Anus:** the end of the digestive system, consisting of a ring of muscle which relaxes to allow the bowels to be opened

**Arrhythmia:** an abnormality of the heart's rhythm

**Arterial:** concerning the arteries (the blood vessels that take blood from the heart to the rest of the body)

**Arteriography:** an X-ray of arteries into which a radio-opaque substance has been injected

**Articulating surfaces:** the surfaces of two bones that move against each other at a joint

**Aspirate:** (verb) to draw off or suck out; (noun) that which is drawn off or sucked out

**Asymptomatic:** having no symptoms

**Atheroma:** a fatty substance which is laid down in plaques along the inside of arteries

**Atrophy:** wasting

**Auditory:** concerning the hearing

**Aura:** symptoms occurring before an attack of epilepsy or migraine by which the patient knows that an attack is imminent

**Auroscope:** an instrument for looking into the ears

**Auto-immune disease:** a disease in which the patient's immune system attacks his own body

**Bacteria:** tiny organisms which invade the body and can cause disease; germs

**Benign:** not malignant, relatively harmless

**Biliary:** concerning the bile and the organs that produce and transport it

**Biliary tract:** the bile ducts and gallbladder

**Biopsy:** the removal of a small piece of tissue in order to examine it under a microscope

**Bipolar depression:** depression which alternates with mania; manic depressive psychosis

**Bone marrow:** the central part of a bone in which the blood cells are manufactured

**Bronchi:** the larger airways of the lungs

**Bronchioles:** the smaller airways of the lungs

**Bronchodilator:** a drug which relaxes the muscles in the walls of the airways, allowing them to dilate

**Buccal:** concerning the cheek or mouth

**Calcified:** having calcium laid down in it

**Carbohydrate:** sugars and starches

**Carcinogen:** a substance capable of causing cancer

**Carcinoma:** one form of cancer

**Cardiac:** concerning the heart

**Cardiovascular:** concerning the heart and blood vessels

**Cartilage:** gristle; a firm substance of great strength and rigidity which is found on the articulating surfaces of bones and elsewhere

**Cataract:** an opacity in the lens of the eye which can cause blindness

**Catheter:** a tube

**Caucasian:** white races

**Cautery:** literally burning, but used to mean anything which will have the same effect of sterilizing the area and sealing off any bleeding vessels

**Cerebrovascular:** concerning the blood vessels of the brain

**Cervix:** neck (usually the neck of the womb); **cervical:** concerning the neck

**Chemotherapy:** literally treatment with chemicals, but usually applied to the drugs used in the treatment of cancer and related diseases

**Chromosomes:** the microscopic bodies within the nucleus of each cell which carry the hereditary factors; it is the chromosomes that are responsible for children inheriting the attributes of their parents, and it is abnormalities in the chromosomes that cause diseases such as Down's syndrome

**Chronic:** long term

**Compression fracture:** a fracture of an osteoporotic vertebra caused by the weight of the body pressing down on the thinned bone

**Congenital:** something that is present at or before birth

**Conjunctivitis:** inflammation of the conjunctiva, the membrane that covers the eyeball

**Contractile:** having the ability to contract

**Convulsion:** a fit

**Coronary:** to do with the heart

**Cranial nerves:** those nerves which arise directly from the brain and run to the head and parts of the neck and chest

**Curettage:** scraping material (e.g. pus) out of a cavity

**Cyst:** a sac containing liquid or semi-solid material

**Cystitis:** inflammation of the bladder

**Cystoscopy:** examination of the inside of the bladder with a small telescope, done under anaesthetic

**Cytotoxic:** cell killing; usually applied to drugs used to kill cancer cells

**Deep vein thrombosis:** clotting of blood in the deep system of veins in the leg

**Defaecation:** opening of the bowels

**Dehydrated:** lacking in fluid, dry

**Delusion:** a false unshakeable belief

**Dermatologist:** a specialist in skin diseases

**Desensitization:** treatment with a series of injections to try to reduce a patient's allergic state; starting with a very low concentration, increasingly larger doses of the allergen are given until the patient can tolerate large doses without reacting

**Detrusor:** the muscle in the wall of the bladder

**Dialysis:** a mechanism which acts as an artificial kidney

**Diaphragm:** the sheet of muscle that divides the chest from the abdomen

**Diffuse:** widespread

**Dilatation** (or **dilation**): stretching

**Dilate:** to stretch

**Diuretic:** a drug which makes the kidneys pass more water

**Double-blind trial:** a trial of a drug or other form of treatment in which neither the patients nor the doctors know until the end who has been given the real treatment and who has received a placebo

**Duct:** a canal or tube

**Duodenum:** the first part of the small intestine

**Dysmenorrhoea:** painful periods

**Dysplasia:** an abnormality of cells not necessarily signifying malignancy

**Dysuria:** pain on passing water

**Electrode:** a conductor of electricity

**Emollient:** a substance which softens and moisturizes the skin

**Emulsify:** to mix an oily substance in water, producing a uniform fluid

**Encephalitis:** inflammation of the brain

**Endometrium:** the lining of the womb

**Endoscope:** a flexible telescope used for inspecting the inside of the stomach and duodenum

**Enzyme:** a substance which speeds a chemical reaction within the body while remaining unchanged itself

**Eustachian tube:** the canal which links the middle ear and the throat

**Expectorant:** a medication which loosens phlegm on the chest, enabling it to be coughed up more easily

**Exudate:** fluid that oozes out through tiny blood vessels

**Faeces:** the waste matter expelled from the bowels; **faecal;** concerning the faeces

**Feedback mechanism:** a mechanism controlling the secretion of certain body chemicals and hormones. A lack of substance A causes gland B to secrete substance B; this stimulates gland A to secrete substance A. Once the level of substance A rises, this stops the secretion of substance B until the level drops again

**Fissure:** a split

**Fistula:** an abnormal hole between two body cavities, e.g. between the bowel and the bladder

**Flaccid:** limp, flabby

**Foetus:** an unborn child; **foetal:** concerning the foetus

**Follicle:** a small sac; **hair follicle:** the sac from which the hair grows

**Fracture:** a broken bone

**Frequency:** the need to pass water frequently

**Gait:** the way in which one walks

**Gangrene:** death of part of the body tissues, often due to an inadequate blood supply

**Gastric:** concerning the stomach

**Gastrointestinal:** concerning the stomach and intestines

**Genetically:** concerning heredity and inherited characteristics

**Genital:** concerning the genitalia

**Genitalia:** literally all the reproductive organs but, in a woman, usually used to mean the external genitalia – the vulva and vagina

**Goitre:** a swelling of the thyroid gland

**Gynaecology:** the science of diseases of women; **gynaecologist:** a specialist in women's diseases

**Haematuria:** blood in the urine

**Haemorrhage:** bleeding

**Hallucination:** a false perception – seeing, hearing, tasting, smelling or feeling something that is not there

**Hepatitis:** inflammation of the liver

**Histamine:** a chemical manufactured by the body which is involved in allergic reactions and also in the normal function of the nervous system

**Hormone:** a substance which is secreted by an endocrine gland (e.g. thyroid, ovaries) directly into the bloodstream and which has an effect on the function of other organs

**Hormone-like:** acting in a similar way to a hormone but not produced by an endocrine gland

**Hyperthyroid:** over-activity of the thyroid gland

**Hypertrophy:** overgrowth

**Hyperventilation:** overbreathing

**Hypoallergenic:** having a low capacity for causing allergic reactions

**Hypothermia:** a condition in which the body temperature drops below normal

**Hypothyroid:** underactivity of the thyroid gland

**Hysterectomy:** surgical removal of the womb, with or without the ovaries

**Idiopathic:** having an unknown origin

**Immune system:** the system which protects the body against invasion by bacteria and viruses and, probably, cancer, and which is made up of the lymphatic system and the white blood cells together with the substances that they produce (see also Antibody)

**Immunosuppressant:** a substance which suppresses the activity of the immune system

**Incision:** a cut

**Interstitial:** within the tissues

**Intertrigonous areas:** skin folds

**Intervertebral:** between the vertebrae

**Intra-abdominal:** within the abdomen

**Intraepithelial:** within or into the skin

**Intramural:** within the walls

**Intramuscular:** within or into the muscles

**Intrauterine:** within the uterus (womb)

**Intravenous:** within or into the veins

**Jaundice:** yellowing of the skin caused by bile in the blood

**Keratin:** a hard dead substance which forms the basis of hair and nails and which is found in the top layer of skin cells

**Keratolytic:** a substance that smooths the skin surface by encouraging the shedding of superficial scales

**Ketoacidosis:** a condition occurring in diabetics who have an excess of sugar in the blood; this is broken down into acidic compounds called ketones, which may cause vomiting, abdominal pain, kidney failure, coma and, if untreated, death

**Labyrinthitis:** inflammation of the inner ear

**Laryngeal:** concerning the larynx

**Larynx:** the voice-box

**Laser:** an extremely concentrated beam of light which is capable of cutting or burning tissue (see also Cautery)

**Lateral:** at the sides

**Ligament:** a strong fibrous band which supports an organ or holds bones together

**Lipodermatosclerosis:** a fan-shaped flare of blood-vessels over the ankle bone, associated with abnormal firmness and darkening of the skin, resulting from incompetent valves in the veins and pooling of blood

**Lobule:** a small, round section of an organ

**Low-grade:** subacute; usually used of an infection that is causing a minimum of symptoms

**Lymph glands:** patches of tissue which act as sieves, catching invaders (such as bacteria, viruses and cancer cells) in the lymphatic system in an attempt to prevent further spread

**Lymphatic system:** a system of vessels through which flows lymph, a colourless fluid containing white blood cells that are involved in the process of immunity

**Maceration:** waterlogging of skin which looks white and soggy

**Maintenance therapy:** treatment to keep a patient with a chronic disease in good health and to prevent a relapse into the disease state

**Malignant:** harmful; something which without treatment is likely to have a fatal outcome

**Mastectomy:** surgical removal of a breast

**Mastoid:** the section of the skull behind the ear which contains pockets of air and which communicates with the middle ear

**Membrane:** a thin layer of tissue, often acting as a lining to a body cavity

**Meningitis:** inflammation of the meninges, the membranes that cover the brain and spinal cord

**Menorrhagia:** excessively heavy, frequent or prolonged periods

**Menstrual:** concerning the periods

**Menstruation:** the monthly periods

**Micturition:** passing water

**Mucosa:** see Mucous membrane

**Mucous membrane:** a thin layer of tissue containing glands that secrete mucus

**Multinodular:** having many nodules

**Murmur:** an abnormal heart sound or sound heard over a large artery

**Musculoskeletal:** concerning the muscles and bones

**Myelogram:** an X-ray in which a radio-opaque substance is injected into the spinal canal to outline the spinal cord and show up any abnormalities of the intervertebral discs

**Myringotomy:** a cut made in the ear-drum to release fluid behind it

**Nail bed:** that part of the end of the finger from which the nail grows

**Neoplasia:** literally new growth, usually applied to cancer

**Neurological:** to do with the nerves and nervous system

**Neuropathy:** a disease affecting the nervous system

**Neurosis:** a mental condition in which the patient still retains touch with reality (c.f. Psychosis)

**Neurotransmitter:** a chemical that carries messages across the gap between two nerve cells and is essential to the normal functioning of the nervous system

**Nocturnal:** by night

**Nodule:** a swelling

**Nucleus:** the central part of each cell, containing all the equipment needed for the function of that cell, together with the chromosomes

**Oesophagus:** the gullet

**Oestrogen:** one of the female hormones secreted by the ovaries

**Ophthalmoscope:** an instrument for looking at the back of the eyes

**Optic disc:** the point at which the optic nerve enters the eyeball, seen at the back of the eye as a round, pale area

**Ossicles:** the tiny bones in the middle ear which transmit vibrations to the inner ear

**Ovulation:** the production of an egg by the ovary

**Pacemaker:** a device which, by means of an electrical stimulus, can keep the heart rhythm regular in a diseased or damaged heart

**Pancreas:** an organ in the upper part of the abdomen which secretes digestive juices into the intestines and insulin into the bloodstream

**Pancreatitis:** inflammation of the pancreas

**Paranoid:** having a fear of persecution

**Partial thyroidectomy:** removal of part (usually one half) of the thyroid

**Pedunculated:** on a stalk

**Pelvic cavity:** that part of the abdomen lying within the pelvis

**Pelvis:** the hip bones; **pelvic:** concerning the pelvis

**Percutaneous:** through the skin

**Perineum:** the area between the legs

**Peritonitis:** inflammation of the peritoneum, the membrane which lines the abdominal cavity and covers its contents

**Pessary:** something which is inserted into and retained within the vagina

**Phlebitis:** inflammation of the veins

**Phlebography:** an X-ray taken of veins into which a radio-opaque substance has been injected

**Phlegm:** mucus, catarrh, sputum

**Physiology:** the way in which the body works

**Pigment:** a coloured substance

**Pinna:** the ear flap

**Placebo:** a substance which has no medical action (e.g. a sugar pill)

**Placenta:** the structure which is joined to a growing foetus through its umbilical cord and by which it receives its blood supply; the afterbirth

**Plain X-ray:** an X-ray taken without any contrast medium being used (i.e. no radio-opaque substance is given beforehand)

**Polyp:** a tumour (usually benign) attached to the body by a stalk

**Posterior:** at the rear

**Post-partum:** after birth

**Precursor:** that which goes before; something from which another substance is derived

**Prodromal:** before the main illness

**Progestogen:** a substance having similar properties to progesterone

**Progesterone:** one of the hormones secreted by the ovaries

**Prognosis:** forecast of the likely outcome of a disease

**Prolapse:** dropping down

**Prophylactic:** preventive

**Psychogenic:** arising from the mental state

**Psychomotor:** the effect of the nervous system or the mind on movement

**Psychosis:** a mental condition in which the patient loses touch with reality

**Purulent:** involving pus

**Pyloroplasty:** cutting of the pylorus (the ring of muscle at the outlet of the stomach) to allow food to flow more freely into the duodenum

**Radio-opaque:** opaque to X-rays, showing up as white on an X-ray

**Rectum:** the back passage

**Referred pain:** irritation of a nerve which causes pain lower down the nerve as well as at the actual site of irritation

**Remission:** a state in which the symptoms and signs of a disease disappear, although they may return later

**Renal:** concerning the kidneys

**Renal colic:** pain caused by a kidney stone

**Reproductive organs:** the vagina, womb, tubes and ovaries in a woman, the penis, testes and the vas (tube) linking them in a man

**Resection:** cutting out

**Respiratory:** concerning the lungs and breathing

**Retina:** the light-sensitive cells at the back of the eye

**Retinopathy:** disease affecting the retina

**Retrograde:** backwards

**Retropubic:** behind the pubic bone which forms the anterior part of the hip bones

**Saline:** a salt solution, used as the basis for most intravenous drips

**Sciatica:** pain running from the back down the leg

**Sclerosing:** hardening

**Sebaceous cyst:** a cyst arising in the skin and containing a thick oily substance

**Second line:** not first choice (usually used of drugs); back-up where other treatments have failed

**Septicaemia:** infection of the bloodstream, blood poisoning

**Serum:** the fluid part which remains after blood has clotted

**Sign:** see Symptom

**Sphincter:** a ring of muscle which keeps an orifice (such as the anus) shut but which can relax to allow it to open

**Sphincterotomy:** cutting through a sphincter

**Spinal cord:** a continuation of the tissue of the brain, contained within the vertebral column and giving rise to the nerves that supply the body below the head

**Spleen:** an organ situated in the upper left side of the abdomen which, if ruptured, can bleed profusely, threatening life; it can safely be removed since it is not essential to the normal workings of the body

**Staphylococci:** a common type of bacteria

**Stenosis:** narrowing

**Stools:** the waste product eliminated from the bowels

**Streptococci:** a common type of bacteria

**Stress fracture:** a broken bone which is caused by continued stress being put upon it, often occurring in the foot

**Stress incontinence:** a condition in which anything that raises the intra-abdominal pressure (such as coughing) will cause a leakage of urine

**Subacute:** less dramatic than acute but usually not as long term as chronic

**Submucosal** (or **submucous**): below the lining (mucosa) of an organ

**Subserosal** (or **subserous**): below the outer covering (serosa) of an organ

**Suppository:** something which is inserted into and retained within the back passage

**Suppurative:** pus-forming

**Suspension:** a liquid in which something is evenly mixed although not dissolved

**Symptom:** what the patient feels; often used in a wider sense to include what the doctor sees (which, strictly speaking, is a sign); thus pain in the eye is a symptom but redness of the eye is a sign

**Syndrome:** a condition in which certain well-defined symptoms and signs appear together, although not all cases are necessarily due to the same cause – or the cause may be unknown

**Synovectomy:** removal of the synovial membrane within a joint

**Systemic:** generalized (e.g. systemic treatment is distributed to all the tissues by the bloodstream, a systemic illness affects the whole body)

**Tendon:** a fibrous band that attaches a muscle to a bone

**Testes:** the organs that produce sperm and are contained within the scrotum

**Thoracic:** concerning the chest

**Thyrotoxicosis:** over-activity of the thyroid gland

**Tinnitus:** ringing in the ears

**Tolerance:** when applied to drugs, means a state in which a higher dose is needed in order to achieve the same effect

**Topical:** applied to the skin

**Torsion:** twisting

**Tourniquet:** a very tight band that cuts off the blood supply to part of the body

**Trachea:** the windpipe

**Transhepatic:** through the liver

**Transurethral:** through the urethra

**Transvesical:** through the bladder

**Trauma:** injury

**Tumour:** a swelling, not necessarily malignant

**Ulna:** one of the bones of the forearm; **ulnar:** to the side of the ulna (the side of the little finger)

**Ultrasound:** the use of an instrument which sends an ultrasound beam through the body tissues and analyses the beam they reflect back; in some cases it can be used instead of X-ray

**Umbilicus:** the navel

**Unipolar depression:** depression in which the patient never has episodes of mania

**Urgency:** a condition of having to pass water immediately one feels the need or risk incontinence

**Urinary tract:** the kidneys, ureters, bladder and urethra

**Uterine:** concerning the womb

**Uterus:** the womb

**Vagina:** the female front passage, leading to the womb

**Vagotomy:** cutting of the vagus nerve to reduce acid secretion in the stomach

**Varices:** dilated veins (plural of varix)

**Vasectomy:** cutting of the vas or tube that leads from the testes to the penis, to prevent sperm from getting through

**Vertebra:** one of the individual bones making up the spine or backbone

**Vertigo:** giddiness

**Vesico-ureteric reflux:** a condition in which urine can flow backwards from the bladder up the ureter due to a faulty valve mechanism

**Virus:** a tiny organism, smaller than a bacterium, which causes disease by getting into the body cells; it is not affected by antibiotics

**Vulva:** the area surrounding the vagina

**Whitlow:** inflammation around a finger-nail

# Index

## OF COMPLEMENTARY REMEDIES MENTIONED IN THE TEXT

## HOMOEOPATHIC REMEDIES

# General Index

# FOR THE BEST IN PAPERBACKS, LOOK FOR THE 🐧

In every corner of the world, on every subject under the sun, Penguin represents quality and variety – the very best in publishing today.

For complete information about books available from Penguin – including Puffins, Penguin Classics and Arkana – and how to order them, write to us at the appropriate address below. Please note that for copyright reasons the selection of books varies from country to country.

**In the United Kingdom:** Please write to *Dept E.P., Penguin Books Ltd, Harmondsworth, Middlesex, UB7 0DA.*

If you have any difficulty in obtaining a title, please send your order with the correct money, plus ten per cent for postage and packaging, to *PO Box No 11, West Drayton, Middlesex*

**In the United States:** Please write to *Dept BA, Penguin, 299 Murray Hill Parkway, East Rutherford, New Jersey 07073*

**In Canada:** Please write to *Penguin Books Canada Ltd, 2801 John Street, Markham, Ontario L3R 1B4*

**In Australia:** Please write to the *Marketing Department, Penguin Books Australia Ltd, P.O. Box 257, Ringwood, Victoria 3134*

**In New Zealand:** Please write to the *Marketing Department, Penguin Books (NZ) Ltd, Private Bag, Takapuna, Auckland 9*

**In India:** Please write to *Penguin Overseas Ltd, 706 Eros Apartments, 56 Nehru Place, New Delhi, 110019*

**In the Netherlands:** Please write to *Penguin Books Netherlands B.V., Postbus 195, NL–1380AD Weesp*

**In West Germany:** Please write to *Penguin Books Ltd, Friedrichstrasse 10–12, D–6000 Frankfurt/Main 1*

**In Spain:** Please write to *Longman Penguin España, Calle San Nicolas 15, E–28013 Madrid*

**In Italy:** Please write to *Penguin Italia s.r.l., Via Como 4, I-20096 Pioltello (Milano)*

**In France:** Please write to *Penguin Books Ltd, 39 Rue de Montmorency, F-75003 Paris*

**In Japan:** Please write to *Longman Penguin Japan Co Ltd, Yamaguchi Building, 2–12–9 Kanda Jimbocho, Chiyoda-Ku, Tokyo 101*

## PENGUIN HEALTH

**Healing Nutrients**  Patrick Quillin

A guide to using the vitamins and minerals contained in everyday foods to fight off disease and promote well-being: to prevent common ailments, cure some of the more destructive diseases, reduce the intensity of others, augment conventional treatment and speed up healing.

**Total Relaxation in Five Steps**  Louis Proto

With Louis Proto's Alpha Plan you can counteract stress, completely relaxing both mind and body, in just 30 minutes a day. By reaching the Alpha state – letting the feelings, senses and imagination predominate – even the most harassed can feel totally rejuvenated.

**Aromatherapy for Everyone**  Robert Tisserand

The use of aromatic oils in massage can relieve many ailments and alleviate stress and related symptoms.

**Spiritual and Lay Healing**  Philippa Pullar

An invaluable new survey of the history of healing that sets out to separate the myths from the realities.

**Hypnotherapy for Everyone**  Dr Ruth Lever

This book demonstrates that hypnotherapy is a real alternative to conventional healing methods in many ailments.

## PENGUIN HEALTH

**Audrey Eyton's F-Plus**  Audrey Eyton

'Your short cut to the most sensational diet of the century' – *Daily Express*

**Baby and Child**  Penelope Leach

A beautifully illustrated and comprehensive handbook on the first five years of life. 'It stands head and shoulders above anything else available at the moment' – Mary Kenny in the *Spectator*

**Woman's Experience of Sex**  Sheila Kitzinger

Fully illustrated with photographs and line drawings, this book explores the riches of women's sexuality at every stage of life. 'A book which any mother could confidently pass on to her daughter – and her partner too' – *Sunday Times*

**Food Additives**  Erik Millstone

Eat, drink and be worried? Erik Millstone's hard-hitting book contains powerful evidence about the massive risks being taken with the health of the consumer. It takes the lid off food and the food industry.

**Living with Allergies**  Dr John McKenzie

At least 20% of the population suffer from an allergic disorder at some point in their lives and this invaluable book provides accurate and up-to-date information about the condition, where to go for help, diagnosis and cure – and what we can do to help ourselves.

**Living with Stress**  Cary L. Cooper, Rachel D. Cooper and Lynn H. Eaker

Stress leads to more stress, and the authors of this helpful book show why low levels of stress are desirable and how best we can achieve them in today's world. Looking at those most vulnerable, they demonstrate ways of breaking the vicious circle that can ruin lives.

# FOR THE BEST IN PAPERBACKS, LOOK FOR THE 🐧

## PENGUIN HEALTH

### Living with Asthma and Hay Fever   John Donaldson

For the first time, there are now medicines that can prevent asthma attacks from taking place. Based on up-to-date research, this book shows how the majority of sufferers can beat asthma and hay fever and lead full and active lives.

### Anorexia Nervosa   R. L. Palmer

Lucid and sympathetic guidance for those who suffer from this disturbing illness, and for their families and professional helpers, given with a clarity and compassion that will make anorexia more understandable and consequently less frightening for everyone involved.

### Medicines: A Guide for Everybody   Peter Parish

This sixth edition of a comprehensive survey of all the medicines available over the counter or on prescription offers clear guidance for the ordinary reader as well as invaluable information for those involved in health care.

### Pregnancy and Childbirth   Sheila Kitzinger

A complete and up-to-date guide to physical and emotional preparation for pregnancy – a must for all prospective parents.

### The Penguin Encyclopaedia of Nutrition   John Yudkin

This book cuts through all the myths about food and diets to present the real facts clearly and simply. 'Everyone should buy one' – *Nutrition News and Notes*

### The Parents' A to Z   Penelope Leach

For anyone with children of 6 months, 6 years or 16 years, this guide to all the little problems involved in their health, growth and happiness will prove reassuring and helpful.

End galley

# FOR THE BEST IN PAPERBACKS, LOOK FOR THE 🐧

## PENGUIN HEALTH

### Positive Smear  Susan Quilliam

A 'positive' cervical smear result is not only a medical event but an emotional event too: one which means facing up to issues surrounding your sexuality, fertility and mortality. Based on personal experiences, Susan Quilliam's practical guide will help every woman meet that challenge.

### Medicine  The Self-Help Guide
### Professor Michael Orme and Dr Susanna Grahame-Jones

A new kind of home doctor – with an entirely new approach. With a unique emphasis on self-management, *Medicine* takes an *active* approach to drugs, showing how to maximize their benefits, speed up recovery and minimize dosages through self-help and non-drug alternatives.

### Defeating Depression  Tony Lake

Counselling, medication and the support of friends can all provide invaluable help in relieving depression. But if we are to combat it once and for all we must face up to perhaps painful truths about our past and take the first steps forward that can eventually transform our lives. This lucid and sensitive book shows us how.

### Freedom and Choice in Childbirth  Sheila Kitzinger

Undogmatic, honest and compassionate, Sheila Kitzinger's book raises searching questions about the kind of care offered to the pregnant woman – and will help her make decisions and communicate effectively about the kind of birth experience she desires.

### Care of the Dying  Richard Lamerton

It is never true that 'nothing more can be done' for the dying. This book shows us how to face death without pain, with humanity, with dignity and in peace.

# THE RESEARCH-INFORMED TEACHING REVOLUTION
## NORTH AMERICA
### A HANDBOOK FOR THE 21ST-CENTURY TEACHER

EDITED BY CHRIS BROWN, JANE FLOOD
AND STEPHEN MACGREGOR

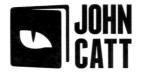

**First published 2021**
by John Catt Educational Ltd,
15 Riduna Park, Station Road,
Melton, Woodbridge IP12 1QT UK

Tel: +44 (0) 1394 389850

4600 140th Avenue North,
Suite 180,
Clearwater, FL 33762
United States

Email: enquiries@johncatt.com
Website: www.johncatt.com

**ISBN: 978 1 91362 286 2**

Set and designed by John Catt Educational Limited

*This book is dedicating to educators everywhere who kept our kids educated during the pandemic. We can't thank you enough.*

# CONTENTS

# ACKNOWLEDGEMENTS

This book would not have been possible without the help and support of Mark Combes at John Catt North America, who saw the value in this work and kept us on track. We would also like to thank the contributors for their fantastic efforts in helping us bring together this engaging and, vitally, practically useful text. We consider ourselves extremely fortunate to have been able to work with you all.

# ABOUT THE EDITORS

**Chris Brown:** Chris Brown is Professor in Education at Durham University's School of Education. With a longstanding interest in how evidence can aid education policy and practice, this is Chris's ninth book in this area (and his 16th overall). Chris has also presented and keynoted on the subject at a number of international conferences stretching the globe, from Africa to South America, and has extensive experience leading a range of funded projects, many of which seek to help teachers identify and scale up best practice. In 2018 Chris was awarded a Siftung Mercator Foundation Senior Fellowship. Each year Siftung Mercator identifies and invites just six people worldwide to apply each year for one of its fellowships. Potential Fellows are identified by a panel as "exceptionally talented and outstanding researchers and practitioners" from areas seen as relevant to the themes and fields of activity of Stiftung Mercator. The purpose of the Mercator Fellowship program is to offer selected fellows the space and freedom to also devote themselves to exploratory and unconventional research and practical projects (typically for six months). Previous fellows include advisors to former US President Barack Obama and current French President Emmanuel Macron.

**Jane Flood:** Jane has been an elementary school teacher for more than 20 years, working in a variety of schools in various roles. In 2018, she became a Founding Fellow of England's Chartered College of Teaching. Throughout her career, Jane has engaged in school-based research designed to raise pupil outcomes and involving the dissemination of this learning to colleagues. Jane is studying part time for a PhD at Durham University, focusing on ways to manage the competing priorities of teacher researchers and informal leaders in research learning networks. She has presented this work at national and international conferences.

She is currently head/principal at Netley Marsh CE Infant School in the south of England.

**Stephen MacGregor:** Stephen is an Ontario Certified Teacher and a PhD candidate at Queen's University, Canada. His doctoral research considers how multi-stakeholder networks, in education and other public service sectors, can mobilize research evidence to achieve societal impacts. A specific focus in his research is the role of higher education institutions and how they can build capacity in knowledge mobilization: a range of activities to connect research producers, users, and mediators. Stephen will soon begin a postdoctoral fellowship at the Ontario Institute for Studies in Education at the University of Toronto, where his research will explore knowledge brokering in research-intensive universities.

# INTRODUCTION

## THE IMPORTANCE OF TEACHERS ENGAGING WITH RESEARCH

Educators and education systems at large face countless decisions every day. Whether focused on meeting the learning needs of a diverse student population, cultivating stakeholder connections, or improving the mental health and well-being of students and school staff, optimal courses of action are rarely clear cut. Grounding educational decisions in research, we and others argue, can improve the likelihood of desirable teaching and learning outcomes and reduce the likelihood of unintended consequences (Brown et al., 2020; Nelson & Campbell, 2019). Empirical support for this claim is still nascent, but examples are emerging in areas such as teacher education and professional development (e.g., Cordingley, 2015; Mincu, 2015), research learning communities (e.g., Brown, 2017; Rose et al., 2017), and school- and district-level decision making (e.g., Penuel et al., 2017). At a more general level, Cain et al. (2019) argue that research evidence—"systematic inquiry *made public*" (Stenhouse, 1981, 104)—can have broad utility in informing bounded decision-making (i.e., connected to specific outcomes), teachers' reflection on their professional practice, and organizational learning.

At the same time, recent studies illustrate that acquiring, understanding, and using research evidence is a highly effortful process that takes place in complex social and political contexts (e.g., Farley-Ripple et al., 2018; Malin et al., 2020). Whereas discussions of research-informed teaching once invoked the language of *evidence-based* policy and practice, *evidence-informed* language has now become common parlance. This shift acknowledges that research is one among many types of evidence used in educational decision-making. Being "evidence informed" is therefore as much about engaging with research evidence as it is engaging with practice-based evidence (e.g., professional judgment) and data-based evidence (e.g., school performance data). By learning from examples and experts of integrating research with these other types of evidence, we can better understand how research can be embedded within everyday practice.

## WHAT THIS BOOK IS ABOUT

Much as we know about the benefits to teachers engaging with research and becoming evidence informed, we also know that such engagement doesn't always happen. So how might we remedy this situation? Our approach has been to reach out to those who are striving to realize the idea of research-informed practice and to see what they suggest. Specifically, we have brought together the best in the business—leading thinkers and doers in the field—and we've asked them to tell us what they have learned about connecting research and practice, as well as give us their general take on the subject. The result is 16 illuminating chapters that provide a wealth of advice and perspectives on the subject.

## SO, WHAT WE HAVE LEARNED?

In 2019, two of us (Chris Brown and Jane Flood) wrote a book for school leaders on how to maximize the benefits of engaging with professional learning networks (PLNs). The book was based on a small-scale research project looking at PLNs that were helping to promote teachers' engagement with research. However, we knew at the time that our conclusions had the potential to stretch beyond the case in hand. What we found with our study is that if school leaders are to lead change in a meaningful way, they needed to focus on three things:

1. Formalizing the change—that is, ensuring the change in question remains a key focus across the school and that its importance is recognized by all stakeholders

2. Prioritizing the change—ensuring appropriate support is available through the allocation of resources to enable the work associated with the change to be achieved.

3. Mobilizing the change—ensuring new knowledge and practice relating to, or emerging from, the change can be accessed and engaged with.

As we noted above, we have been privileged, along with our co-editor Stephen MacGregor, to be able to bring together a really talented group of practitioners, researchers, and other key players to express their views on how to make the research-informed revolution a reality. However, what has really struck us is how the themes from what people have written once again relate to these three core needs. Bringing together insights from across the book, therefore, we feel that a number of key lessons emerge for making research use a reality in schools. In terms of these ideas of formalizing, prioritizing, and mobilizing, these are:

**What we have learned about formalization.** It is vital that research-informed practice is formally linked to the policies and process of the school. Doing so signals the importance of the work. Also, that engaging in research is not "just another initiative" but something that is key to a school's culture and way of working. Approaches to formalizing research use encompass the inclusion of such activity in school improvement plans and teachers' performance management targets (making it clear, as intimated in the chapters by Victoria Parent, and Margaret Goldberg and Lani Mednick, that research use is part of teachers' roles). At the same time, such signals need to be meaningful. There is no point adding priorities to a school improvement plan if there are already so many that the notion of something being a "priority" no longer has currency. Other learning here includes the use of routines, such as learning sets; having in place the right supporting structures and tools; and showing that taking reasonable risks in the pursuit of innovation is okay.

**What we have learned about prioritization.** Ask any teacher in any education system around the world how they could best be supported to engage with a new initiative, and "more time" will always feature as part of their response. We know teachers are overburdened. We also know that if we want them to do more of something, we need to ensure that they can do less of something else (an idea nicely encapsulated in chapters by Matt Norris, Jeremy Hannay, and Lindsay Kemeny). This seems to be especially true for schools situated in areas of disadvantage where some of the teachers often admit they are struggling simply to stay afloat. Often, school leaders have the freedom to change structures within their school to free up time—for example, by reallocating meeting or teacher preparation time, or through smart approaches to timetabling. Affording time to teachers will go a long way to helping them engage in research effectively, but time also needs to be allocated to help teachers engage with their colleagues to ensure the mobilization of research can occur. This also means that processes within the school should be used to facilitate research-related collaboration (something nicely touched upon in Kyair Butts's chapter). For instance, timetables should reflect that the need for collaboration between particular groups of teachers. Under the heading Prioritization we also have suggestions from Kyair Butts and Elizabeth Farley-Ripple for building the capacity of teachers to engage effectively and critically with research.

**What we have learned about mobilization.** Mobilization is complex and teachers and school leaders still have much to learn in this area. The work here has provided some vital clues as to how mobilization can be improved. In particular, as well as enforcing the notion that passive dissemination is ineffectual (e.g., see the chapters by Sofia Malik, Elizabeth Farley-Ripple, and Jeremey Hannay), it has shown that the most impactful forms of mobilization involve school staff 1) actually engaging with innovations, 2) collaboratively testing out how new practices can be used to improve teaching and learning, and 3) continuing to use and refine new practices in an ongoing way (thus achieving what one of our authors, Eleftherios Soleas, describes as "pedagogic alchemy"). This is because supporting staff to actively engage and experiment with new practices helps them to develop as experts. In turn this means that the use of research-informed innovations and practices will be both refined and sustained over time, allowing students to benefit from their ongoing improvement. In addition, who is doing the mobilizing matters. If teachers are to be the types of change agent envisaged in Kyair Butts's chapter, they need, as Elizabeth Farley-Ripple notes, to hold prominent enough positions within their school (either in a formal or in an informal capacity) so that they can influence whether and how innovations are adopted by others. Also key is ready access to research, but also to accessible research findings, or tools or proformas, which transform research into something usable (areas that are explored by Joshua Pigeon, Sofia Malik, Heather Braund, Elizabeth Farley-Ripple, and Bill Langley). However, as Andrew Lyman-Butler does well to suggest, you can also share your research-informed practices openly and freely so that others can benefit from them too.

In addition to understanding more about formalizing, prioritizing and mobilizing, as we have read through the chapters in the book, the following key learnings have emerged:

**Reflection:** In her chapter, Heather Braund reminds us of the powerful importance of reflection (something also discussed by Eleftherios Soleas, and Derek Tangredi and colleagues). Of course, the notion of reflection is not new. Writing almost 90 years ago, John Dewey considered reflection as a key part of any teacher's toolkit: describing it as a process of "active, persistent and careful consideration of any belief [or knowledge] in the light of the grounds that support it and ... the conclusions to which it tends" (1933, 9). However, reflection continues to matter because when done well, it leads to teachers actively and collectively questioning ineffective teaching routines while finding ways to respond to them. We also now know more about how to facilitate the process of reflection; for example, through utilizing approaches such as "reflective dialogue"— conversations about serious practice-related problems that involve the application of new knowledge in a sustained manner; the "deprivatization of practice"—the frequent examining of practice through collaborative observation and joint planning and development; teachers seeking new knowledge; and teachers applying new ideas and information to problem solving and solutions that address the needs of students. So, if we can get it right, ongoing reflection, centered on educational research, should result in a cadre of expert teachers who work to continually ensure their understanding and practice is as effective as possible (see Brown et al., 2021, and Brown & Rogers, 2015, for more).

**Networks and collaboration:** Chapters by Elizabeth Farley-Ripple, Heather Braund, Joel Knudson, and Michael Fairbrother and Jacqueline Specht also serve to reinforce the importance of utilizing networks and working collaboratively. With humans being an ultra-social species, networks have always mattered because they serve to provide us with access to a multitude of resources: from aid and assistance to knowledge and norms (i.e., knowing how to behave appropriately). In terms of education, networks can be used to foster knowledge sharing and practice development across schools (what Matt Norris refers to in his chapter as "capital"). However, leveraging educational networks requires effective collaboration, which isn't always easy. In fact, it's worth thinking about the types of collaboration that are present within your school or institution and how these can be improved. We argue that, when it comes to engaging with research, collaboration must involve the inducement of mutual obligation, foster interdependence, expose the practice of teachers to the scrutiny of others, and encourage initiative in terms of developing new approaches to teaching and learning. Yet, as Judith Warren-Little (1990) posits, many types of collaboration exist, and these differ vastly in terms of the extent to which they trigger these key factors. In Warren-Little's case, prominent types of collaboration include storytelling and scanning, aid and assistance, sharing, and joint work. Further detail on each is provided in Box 1, below, with *joint work* emerging as the preferred option. Warren-Little also argues that teachers will also be more motivated to collaborate with one another when the success of their efforts depends on it. Furthermore, as a result of this interdependence, over time schools are likely to establish new norms based on the thoughtful, explicit examination of practices and their consequences. Such new ways of working should ultimately result in the sustained learning of teachers.

## BOX 1: FOUR TYPES OF COLLABORATION

1. *Storytelling* represents the occasional and opportunistic forays undertaken by teachers as they seek out specific ideas, information, solutions, or reassurances. At the same time, teachers remain autonomous and free to choose which of these stories they engage with or act upon. Within this mode of collaboration, independent trial and error acts as the principal route to developing competence.

2. *Aid and assistance* reflects the idea that teachers offer help and support when asked, but only when asked. This is because, in schools where this mode of collaboration is prevalent, discussions about teaching practice become associated with judgments on the competence of teachers: both judgments about those seeking support and judgments relating to the competency of those supplying support.

3. *Sharing* spotlights the routine exchange of materials and methods as well as the open interchange of ideas and opinions. Acting in this way provides teachers with an opportunity to learn about others' practices and to compare this with their own. Even so, sharing can be variable in nature: Different teachers may engage with more or fewer teachers; their engagement may be fully or only partially reciprocated; and teachers may reveal much or little of their thinking, ideas, practice, or materials.

4. Finally, the term *joint work* represents encounters among teachers that are grounded in "shared responsibility for the work of teaching (interdependence), collective conceptions of autonomy, support for teachers' initiative and leadership with regard to professional practice, and group affiliations grounded in professional work." This fourth type is generally preferred because of the collegial norms that result.

**Trust:** Effective collaboration centered on the use of research will also be grounded in trust existing between participants and across hierarchies (e.g., see the chapter by Derek Tangredi and colleagues), where trust relates to our beliefs regarding the competence, the benevolence, and the integrity of others (Ehren, 2018). In particular, high levels of trust are associated with a variety of reciprocal efforts, including where learning, complex information sharing, problem solving, shared decision making, and coordinated action are required. This is because in high-trust situations, individuals feel supported and "safe" to engage in risk taking and the innovative behavior associated with efforts at sharing, developing or trialing new research-informed teaching practices. In particular, a trusting work environment is instrumental to the type of "double-loop" learning that is a prerequisite if teachers are to both 1) openly and collegiately challenge and question their foundational assumptions and 2) engage in ongoing and open disclosure about problems and challenges, with both 1) and 2) occurring as part of a process of seeking to continually improve teaching and learning through an engagement with research (see Argris & Schön, 1996; Brown, 2020).

No doubt there are many more lessons to be learned from engaging with our 16 chapters, and we would love to hear what you think. Also, let us know whether you feel we have not covered a key facilitator of research use that you believe to be vital. Before you can tell us that, however, you need to reflectively engage—either alone or, preferably, with colleagues—with what each of our authors have to say. So, we'll leave you here to start this process and to begin treading the path of your own research-informed teaching journey. Happy reading and viva la research-informed teaching revolución!

*Chris, Jane, and Stephen.*
*August 2021*

## REFERENCES

Argris, C., & Schön, D. (1996). *Organisational learning II: Theory, method, practice, increasing professional effectiveness.* Jossey Bass.

Brown, C. (2017). Research learning communities: How the RLC approach enables teachers to use research to improve their practice and the benefits for students that occur as a result. *Research for All, 1*(2), 387–405.

Brown, C. (2020). *The networked school leader: How to improve teaching and student outcomes using learning networks.* Emerald.

Brown, C., & Flood, J. (2019). *Formalise, prioritise and mobilise: How school leaders secure the benefits of Professional Learning Networks.* Emerald.

Brown, C., MacGregor, S., & Flood, J. (2020). Can models of distributed leadership be used to mobilise networked generated innovation in schools? A case study from England. *Teaching and Teacher Education, 94,* 1–11.

Brown, C., Poortman, C., Gray, H., Groß-Ophoff, J., & Wharf, M. (2021). Facilitating collaborative reflective inquiry amongst teachers: What do we currently know? *International Journal of Educational Research, 105.* Advance online publication.

Brown, C., & Rogers, S. (2015). Knowledge creation as an approach to facilitating evidence-informed practice: Examining ways to measure the success of using this method with early years practitioners in Camden (London). *Journal of Educational Change, 16*(1), 79–99.

Cain, T., Brindley, S., Brown, C., Jones, G., & Riga, F. (2019). Bounded decision-making, teachers' reflection and organisational learning: How research can inform teachers and teaching. *British Educational Research Journal, 45*(5), 1072–1087.

Cordingley, P. (2015). The contribution of research to teachers' professional learning and development. *Oxford Review of Education, 41*(2), 234–252.

Dewey, J. (1933). *How we think: A restatement of the relation of reflective thinking to the educative process.* Houghton Mifflin.

Ehren, M. (2018, December 12). *Accountability and trust: Two sides of the same coin?* [Invited talk]. University of Oxford's Intelligent Accountability Symposium II, Oxford, UK.

Farley-Ripple, E., May, H., Karpyn, A., Tilley, K., & McDonough, K. (2018). Rethinking connections between research and practice in education: A conceptual framework. *Educational Researcher, 47*(4), 235–245.

Malin, J. R., Brown, C., Ion, G., van Ackeren, I., Bremm, N., Luzmore, R., Flood, J., & Rind, G. M. (2020). World-wide barriers and enablers to achieving evidence-informed practice in education: What can be learnt from Spain, England, the United States, and Germany? *Humanities and Social Sciences Communications, 7*(1), 1–14.

Mincu, M. E. (2015). Teacher Quality and School Improvement: What is the role of research? *Oxford Review of Education, 41*(2), 253–269.

Nelson, J., & Campbell, C. (2019). Using evidence in education. In A. Boaz, H. Davies, A. Fraser, & S. Nutley (Eds.), *What works now? Evidence-informed policy and practice* (pp. 131–145). Policy Press.

Penuel, W. R., Briggs, D. C., Davidson, K. L., Herlihy, C., Sherer, D., Hill, H. C., Farrell, C., & Allen, A.-R. (2017). How school and district leaders access, perceive, and use research. *AERA Open, 3*(2).

Rose, J., Thomas, S., Zhang, L., Edwards, A., Augero, A., & Roney, P. (2017). *Research learning communities: Evaluation report and executive summary.* Education Endowment Foundation.

Stenhouse, L. (1981) What counts as research. *British Journal of Educational Studies, 29*(2), 103–114.

Warren-Little, J. (1990). The persistence of privacy: Autonomy and initiative in teachers' professional relations. *Teachers College Record, 91*(4), 509–535.

# NOT ANOTHER REFLECTION!

## LEARNING HOW TO REFLECT DEEPLY AND INTEGRATE RESEARCH

**HEATHER BRAUND**

**Heather Braund recently completed her PhD at Queen's Faculty of Education focused on assessment and self-regulation in kindergarten classrooms. She has taught a variety of courses at Queen's Faculty of Education including Self as Professional, Numeracy, and Elementary Mathematics. She also is a guest lecturer in topics including the development of self-regulation and metacognition, research methods, and mobilizing evidence-based practices for teachers, students, researchers, and health professionals.**

Close your eyes and think back to teacher's college. Imagine sitting in one of your classes, likely in a building with few windows (we wouldn't want to distract your learning!). You are sitting in class and likely wondering how you will apply what you are learning in your teaching training. Now the instructor asks you to complete a reflection detailing what you have learned in the course and how you will apply it in your future teaching practice. You think silently, "Not another reflection!" but you wouldn't dare say a thing, as reflection is a buzzword in all of your classes. This experience was probably not unique to you and might be something that many of us teachers have in common.

One of the concepts that I have studied tirelessly in my graduate work is that of reflection. I have delivered many guest lectures, workshops, and lessons that incorporated reflective thinking. When I teach, there is *always* an assignment where my students have to reflect. When I guest lecture, one of my favorite questions is to ask everyone who is tired of hearing the word "reflection" to raise their hand. It likely comes as no surprise that all students raise their hand. Our students are clearly tired of reflecting, yet we continue to bombard them with reflection assignments. With the number of reflections that students are asked to write, do you really think that they are engaging in deep reflection? They might be, but I would argue that the reflection is probably shallow in nature.

I am going to challenge you to think about how you encourage reflective thinking in your teaching. What is working well? What isn't working well? What can you learn from me? I hope that this chapter will describe some ways in which I have learned from being a student myself and how I have worked to integrate research into my teaching practice.

## GOING THROUGH THE MOTIONS IS NOT REFLECTING

Despite having been a pre-service teacher myself, I continued to incorporate reflection assignments in my first few courses that I taught. I remember the first few times I integrated reflection in my teaching, thinking that it was going to result in a deep classroom dialogue, and I would be thrilled to read the reflection responses. Unfortunately, that was not the case. Many of the reflections read the same way and had very similar content. Ironically, I was reflecting myself as to why this activity was a flop. Why didn't it work? I had studied reflective thinking in great detail and had figured that would result in clear translation into practice. After some deep reflective thinking on my part, I realized that I was just having my students go through the motions. They answered generic reflection prompts and wrote what they thought I wanted to hear. As with many students, mine wanted to achieve high grades and their writing followed the prompts but suggested that they may not have told me what they were really thinking. Hence, their assignments suggested that they were engaging in reflective thinking at a more surface level rather than at a deep level.

I decided that I didn't want to have students going through the motions of reflective thinking without having them engage in deep reflective thinking. I realized that the focus needed to be on *why* teachers should reflect and *how* they can reflect. I found myself guilty of not taking the time to explain the importance of reflective thinking. By not highlighting the importance, students may not understand why reflective thinking is necessary and how it can benefit them in their practice. To be honest, I can relate. I remember doing what felt like hundreds of reflections, but no one actually took the time to explain why we should care about reflective thinking. Teachers may not fully understand the importance of reflective thinking until they are out in independent practice. However, we can help increase buy-in and encourage students to be authentic and deep in their reflective thinking by discussing the importance early on in their educational journeys.

In order to revamp my reflection assignments, I went back to the research on reflective thinking and highlighted the importance as articulated in the literature. Before I could teach my students about the importance of reflective thinking, I had to find accessible and meaningful research to share with them. Once I shared what reflection entailed and why it was important, I had students find their own research related to reflection. This helped them to learn how to access research and how to sift through the hundreds of results that populated when they searched *reflection*. I was trying to teach them to be critical not only of themselves as educators and learners but also of the available research.

A key component of reflective thinking is to learn from the experience that you are reflecting on. We need to be clear that reflection is not just thinking about what happened. Reflective thinking is far more encompassing and includes the systematic thinking about one's performance, actions, emotions, and reactions (Boud et al., 1985). However, the act of reflecting also needs to result in learning (Boud et al., 1985) and the development of new understanding (Moon, 2004). Further, reflective thinking should be challenging and used to identify any biases that an individual has within a given context (Jasper & Rolfe, 2011). These were some of the key components of reflective thinking I discuss with my students, guided by evidence. I recognize that I had focused too much on the theoretical literature and not enough on the practical application of reflection. A one-size-fits-all mentality never works with anything in the classroom, and it certainly doesn't with reflection. I had tried to integrate standardized reflection questions despite research suggesting that it might be more worthwhile for students to identify their own reflection prompts. I decided to make my teaching practices more student centered by encouraging my students to generate their own reflection prompts rather than aiming for standardization across students.

## LEARNING FROM OUR SUCCESSES AND FAILURES

I hope the story that I shared above about my experiences highlights the importance of constantly reflecting as a teacher. One of the worst things that we can do as teachers is to let our teaching practices become stagnant. It is more natural to engage in reflective thinking when a lesson flops or something does not go as planned. However, we need to reflect following positive experiences as well. In fact, we can learn just as much reflecting on a positive teaching experience as on a more negative experience. Thus, it is equally important to learn from your successes and your failures. However, remember that you only fail if you don't reflect and try again!

It is also important that we learn from the successes and failures of our students. It might seem cliché for me to say that I aim to learn as much from my students as they hopefully learn from me. But, it is true. When we reflect as teachers, it is about far more than just the material we were trying to teach or the level of engagement. When you reflect, make sure that you think about the experience from the perspective of your students. Yet again, research can provide you with the opportunity to learn from others and try something new. We likely encourage our students to think outside of the box, but we may be hesitant to do the same with our teaching practices. This is your time to step outside of the box and use research to identify new strategies and practices that you want to try with your students. Delving into the research on a consistent basis will help to ensure that your teaching practices don't become stagnant, because you will be staying informed with current evidence-based practices.

## MOBILIZING RESEARCH INTO PRACTICE

You likely hear the phrase "evidence-based practices" regularly as people encourage you to integrate them into your teaching. What if I were to tell you that it also makes your teaching more efficient by using instructional strategies and activities that are grounded in the research? Why spend time trying different strategies when there are teachers and scholars that recommend the use of certain strategies? This isn't to say that you can always find the answers in research, but starting with the research can be useful. Having the mindset that research will make your life easier as a teacher and may lead to greater efficiency will help you to prioritize delving into the research rather than thinking of it as an add on and something that you have to do above and beyond your daily work.

Teachers are busy and likely don't have a lot of extra time to wade through piles of research. There are many resources and a lot of research but not enough time! This is a main barrier impacting the mobilization of research into practice. Another barrier includes being inundated with research from around the world. It can be difficult to identify what is relevant for you and your students. If you are having trouble finding research that is relevant, try different key words, try a different database (e.g., Google Scholar), and befriend a librarian who might be able to direct you to more relevant research. The other challenge with integrating research into practice is that research is typically context specific and it might not fit within your context. However, this is an opportunity for you to modify the empirically based practice to fit within your classroom context as necessary.

There are numerous facilitators that can help you and other teachers to integrate research into practice. One facilitator is sharing resources with others. Remember that there isn't a need to reinvent the wheel; if you find research that is helpful, share it with your colleagues. This will help you to develop a network of research-oriented teachers. Another avenue that can be helpful is to stay up to date with current research. Find one or two teacher-oriented conferences (e.g., Canadian Society for Studies in Education, Ontario Association of Math Educators, Science Teacher's Association of Ontario, International Study Association on Teachers and Teaching, American Educational Research Association, Utah Early Childhood Conference, The American Associated for Teaching and Curriculum Conference) that would be high yield for you to attend. Use the opportunity to network and hear about recent research. Shorter versions of research studies can also be found in newsletters (e.g., *Canadian Teacher, Research in a Nutshell, Education Week*) and practitioner-oriented journals (e.g., *Professional Speaking, Journal of Teacher Action Research, Education Forum*). Find those sources that are highest yield and check them regularly for new research.

## CONCLUSION

The best teachers try new things in order to meet the needs of their students. They may know what works from years of experience and they might have a repertoire of strategies ranging from instructional to classroom management to engagement. They definitely have a repertoire of resources that they consult when they are puzzled or needing to seek additional information. Consider research as one of your resources that provides you with recommendations, strategies, and activities from around the world. I am going to leave you with my top three recommendations for mobilizing research into your practice: 1) Create a research network, share with colleagues, and encourage them to share with you; 2) Stay informed, things change rapidly; and 3) Find accessible content without too much theoretical jargon.

## REFERENCES

Boud, D., Keogh, R., & Walker, D. (Eds.). (1985). *Reflection: Turning experience into learning*. Kogan Page.

Jasper, M., & Rolfe, G. (2011). Critical reflection and emergence of professional knowledge. In G. Rolfe, M. Jasper, & D. Freshwater (Eds.), *Critical reflection in practice. Generating knowledge for care* (pp. 1–10). Palgrave Macmillan.

Moon, J. (2004). *A handbook of reflective and experiential learning. Theory and practice*. Routledge.

# A SERIES OF DECREASINGLY FREQUENT FAILURES

## INTEGRATING RESEARCH INTO YOUR TEACHING PRACTICE

### ELEFTHERIOS SOLEAS

**Eleftherios Soleas is a biology, history, and math teacher who had a few research questions and then left the classroom to figure them out. He left to figure out how to help teachers better capitalize on opportunities to make their teaching inclusive, and stayed out to figure out how to help teachers motivate innovation. That last one will take him a while beyond his recently completed PhD, so the education system will have to do its level best to soldier on without him.**

Translating research into practice was always an interest of mine; it was the process by which I would intake, contemplate, and enact the latest research to which I was exposed. In my classroom, I often found myself trying new things based on what I had read in the latest paper on my pile, making me something of a pedagogical alchemist (Rooke & Torbert, 2005). I would try something, see if it worked, and then if and only if it worked, it became part of my standard practice—not an add-on but part of who I was as a teacher.

Some things worked for me and my students (e.g., Universal Design for Learning, Bloom's Revised Taxonomy, and formative assessment activities), and some things certainly did not work for me (e.g., Tribes [Benard, 2005; Phillips, 2011] and Prezi). I readily added graphic organizers into my practice based on reading a paper and attending a workshop; they worked for me, and I still ask questions on my tests, assignments, and projects that require the expression of processes and complex ideas beyond expository words. I saw them work for my students and their thinking, and they and enabled me to make my assessments multimodal. It became a permanent part of who I would be as a teacher. SMART Boards, however, did not work for me (I am sure they work for lots of other folks, though). I decided early on that they simply did not suit my conversational and discussion-based style of teaching. They were neat; I appreciated them and the work that went into teaching me how to use them, but that SMART Board might as well have been an overhead projector based on how often I used it. Therein lies the salient point: I was doing what worked for me rather than what evidence was pushing us toward. I rejected what did not immediately work in my classroom and actively channeled what did. I gave up on ideas too soon. I did not give them a real chance. Taking a "what works for me right now" mindset was making me stagnant. I needed to look for new tricks to stay fresh and up to date.

I use the metaphor of a baseball pitcher. I had one or two pitches that I was good at, but I taught myself many more by reading the latest and greatest in journals and experimenting. It took reflection and many failures, but I learned how to experiment with new ideas successfully. Over time, the duds (by my perception of their utility; none of these ideas were bad in and of themselves) became fewer, and I grew in my ability to integrate new things successfully, especially the ideas I was initially uncomfortable with. I stopped seeing what did not work for me and started noticing how to make something work—a subtle shift with tremendous implications for my teaching.

## THE COURAGE TO TRY NEW THINGS

As a new teacher, by virtue of fear and by the pragmatism and busyness inculcated into us by our well-meaning teacher education institutions, it is easy to have a "what works" mindset. However, who is this what works mindset programmed to serve? Stagnation is as easy as deciding not to try new or uncomfortable things in the classroom (Darling-Hammond, 2010; Darling-Hammond et al., 2020). I was driven to try new things to fight the obsolescence that I could see seeping into my teaching. I could see that I could become set in my ways, teaching precisely the way I was taught, something that I had told myself as a teacher candidate was a teaching fate worse than death. The source of renewal was innovation (Dewey, 1938; Glassman, 2001) as inspired by my reading and idea exchange with peers in my school and around my classroom. If I paid attention and was willing to be deliberative, there was an unrelenting conveyer belt of ideas from my peers that I could enact and have readily available as collaborators in my implementation.

I realized early on in my teaching that I would teach as I was taught without the push of reflecting on my practice. Every teacher needs the benefit of hindsight to improve their teaching, and mine came through critically self-appraising my assignments and teaching. I could also seek out the perspectives of my students by asking them for their thinking and preferences. I told my students that my classroom was a "benevolent dictatorship" wherein I depended on an iterative feedback cycle with my students and consistent inputs of new evidence like articles, presentations, trends, and patterns to help me decide. I quickly concluded that relying on instinct without evidence was a stopgap and that, at best, it was getting me from point A to point B. I needed to critically appraise my teaching and seek out the evidence-based practices that would patch holes in my teaching game and open up all sorts of new potential integrations of strategies, approaches, and activities. I had never lost my connection to research given that I was working on my master's degree and reading voraciously, which helped me identify good ideas and made utter hokum easier to detect. The easiest way to learn to detect hokum was to understand the anatomy of misinformation. For me, this was seeing unsubstantiated claims, something being too good to be true, and it not having been scrutinized by peer review. If it had not experienced the joy of being challenged by reviewer 2, I was not interested.

## THE RESOLVE TO IMPLEMENT AND THE AFTERMATH

Reading and consuming research and ideas is the easy part; the harder part is enacting them in your practice. That is why we have a whole field of research on knowledge translation and implementation science. The chasm between "this is a good idea" and it happening in my classroom was a wasteland of good intentions that I promised would never get larger. It is quite easy to fall into a mentality of quickly deciding that something does not work for me and going back to what I thought worked before, but what really should go into that decision? What if what worked for you did not work for your students? Sorry to be the bearer of bad news, but it is not all about you. If teachers stuck to what worked for them without a bit of a push for the new, we would still be assessing mostly through summative assessment (Black & Wiliam, 2003; Egan, 2011). Formative assessment is more work for teachers, but it has impressive benefits for students (Gofton et al., 2017; Hudesman et al., 2013). What drove me to implement the things that I read?

The answer was convincing evidence. When I saw it, I felt personally responsible for making changes happen in my classroom. I would do the mental math—either I was going to do this or I was going to short-change my students out of an opportunity. I read the early work on formative assessment (e.g., Black & Wiliam, 2009) and quickly identified it as a solid option for enhancing the quality of work that I was going to be marking and, more importantly, as setting students on a footing for being reflective, resilient thinkers (CAST, 2011). To say that it worked overnight is an understatement. Students lined up to tell me that the formative feedback strategy that I used first—establishing shared success criteria—worked. I knew that it worked because more students were getting to our negotiated goals (understanding how DNA replication works, if anyone is interested), and there were fewer confused looks on the way there.

The first sign I had whether an idea was working was tangible student engagement. I was well aware, even before my PhD, that motivation and a great deal of engagement are latent and extremely difficult to measure (Blau & Shamir-Inbal, 2018; Maehr & Meyer, 1997; Soleas, 2020). For the tangible engagement, I could see if students were immersed in the learning activity, or if they were participating vigorously in their workgroups, or if the assignment had initially captured their imagination. The best notion I had of whether an idea was working was my students' response. I obtained this honest feedback in a few ways. I would ask openly, and the bravest and most outspoken would tell me their immediate thoughts. The rest I would have to ask in a safe way, often using a mixture of exit cards and anonymous surveys. It is not enough to gather evidence or even a lot of evidence; it has to be the right kind of evidence. Is the evidence definitive, holistic, trustworthy, context specific, delimited, and methodologically sound? I told myself that I was making decisions on what I would do to connect students with their chosen future; the evidence had better be good.

## EXAMPLES OF INTEGRATING RESEARCH INTO MY PRACTICE

### Universal Design for Learning

The Universal Design for Learning (UDL) guidelines (CAST, 2011) changed my teaching life because it finally gave me an inventory of what good teaching should look like. They were easy to read and think about because they were modular and generalizable, had easily accessible and verifiable evidence, and best of all were designed with teachers in mind. I felt assured that I was making the right move for my students and that they would benefit. The UDL guidelines were easy to follow, and I had a resource that I could carry with me anywhere. I could view any lesson I would give and see if it was meeting the guidelines; if not, I had delineated options for doing so. It was a hit; I could see the efficacy of aligning my teaching with the guidelines and the tangible benefits for student learning. The outcomes were the combination of immediate and long-vesting that made me commit early and stay committed to using the UDL guidelines. Truly, it was a resource made for being implemented.

### Bloom's Taxonomy and Authentic Assessment

I had learned about Bloom's Taxonomy and had heard the term "authentic assessment" in my teacher education courses, but I quickly concluded that they were buzzwords and were doing little to enhance my teaching. I was bitter about how my teacher education courses were not practicing what they were preaching. I outright laughed in class when our special education and differentiated instruction class was evaluated solely by multiple-choice exams. I initially did not give these crucial concepts the time they needed. However, after reading more, and having started to integrate UDL, I saw how Bloom's Revised Taxonomy (Krathwohl, 2002) was a spur for integrating more possibilities and options for my teaching. I combined the two ideas (as many others did) to make sure that my teaching and assessments were striking at different types of thinking. This led me to ask different and what some would call "off-beat" questions on my assignments and design projects that approached learning from new angles. For example, one of my history tests asked learners to explain the French Revolution as a food fight. People wrote about how Robespierre was a sous-chef who got out of control and started having people get "marinara-ed" and how a deficit of biscuits led to the Tennis Court Oath. Students were demonstrating enduring learning by applying their knowledge in a new situation. The facts were all there, and it was not a simple regurgitation of memory; students had to do something with it, and the increased engagement to create a story or parable made for better answers and increased confidence from me that they had enduring learning. Other examples included asking folks to design a zoo for the Diversity of Living Things unit or to make their own organism for the evolution unit in Biology.

## Practice Points

Evidence-based teaching practice is an iterative process of reading, planning, implementing, conversing, and reflecting that keeps you current. It is a commitment to being the best teacher that you can be. I want to conclude this story of my decreasingly frequent failures with a few points for practice.

1. Teaching, as you were taught, is effectively staying in the Stone Age until you run out of rocks.
2. Transition yourself from "knowing what works" to "knowing how to make something work for me."
3. Develop the skill to detect or suspect misinformation by asking questions of veracity and rigor for claims in education and beyond.

## REFERENCES

Benard, B. (2005). *What is it about Tribes? The research-based components of the developmental process of Tribes learning communities.* CenterSource Systems.

Black, P., & Wiliam, D. (2003). "In praise of educational research": Formative assessment. *British Educational Research Journal, 29*(5), 623–637. https://doi.org/10.1080/0141192032000133721

Black, P., & Wiliam, D. (2009). Developing the theory of formative assessment. *Educational Assessment, Evaluation and Accountability, 21*(1), 5–31. https://doi.org/10.1007/s11092-008-9068-5

Blau, I., & Shamir-Inbal, T. (2018). Digital technologies for promoting "student voice" and co-creating learning experience in an academic course. *Instructional Science, 46*(2), 315–336. http://10.0.3.239/s11251-017-9436-y

CAST. (2011). *Universal Design for Learning guidelines–Version 2.0.* http://www.cast.org/library/UDLguidelines/

Darling-Hammond, L. (2010). Teacher education and the American future. *Journal of Teacher Education, 61*(1–2), 35–47.

Darling-Hammond, L., Flook, L., Cook-Harvey, C., Barron, B., & Osher, D. (2020). Implications for educational practice of the science of learning and development. *Applied Developmental Science, 24*(2), 97–140. https://doi.org/10.1080/10888691.2018.1537791

Dewey, J. (1938). Education and experience. In *The Educational Forum* (Vol. 50, Issue 3). Simon & Schuster.

Egan, R. (2011). Adjusting curricular design to "CREATE" a culture of self-regulation. *Canadian Journal for the Scholarship of Teaching and Learning, 2*(2). https://doi.org/10.5206/cjsotl-rcacea.2011.2.6

Glassman, M. (2001). Dewey and Vygotsky: Society, experience, and inquiry in educational practice. *Educational Researcher, 30*(4), 3–14.

Gofton, W., Dudek, N., Barton, G., & Bhanji, F. (2017). *Work based assessment implementation guide: Formative tips for medical teaching practice* (pp. 1–12). The Royal College of Physicians and Surgeons of Canada. http://www.royalcollege.ca/rcsite/documents/cbd/wba-implementation-guide-tips-medical-teaching-practice-e.pdf

Hudesman, B. J., Crosby, S., Flugman, B., Issac, S., Everson, H., & Clay, D. B. (2013). Using formative assessment and metacognition to improve student achievement. *Journal of Developmental Education, 37*, 2–13.

Krathwohl, D. R. R. (2002). A revision of Bloom's taxonomy: An overview. *Theory Into Practice, 41*(4), 212–218. https://doi.org/10.1207/s15430421tip4104_2

Maehr, M. L., & Meyer, H. A. (1997). Understanding motivation and schooling: Where we've been, where we are, and where we need to go. *Educational Psychology Review, 9*(4), 371–409. https://doi.org/http://dx.doi.org.library.capella.edu/10.1023/A:1024750807365

Phillips, G. A. (2011). The effect of Tribes training in a beginning-teacher-education program (Publication number XXXX) [Doctoral dissertation, University of Toronto]. *ProQuest Dissertations and Theses*, 246. http://hdl.handle.net/20.500.12424/786209

Rooke, D., & Torbert, W. R. (2005, April). Seven transformations of leadership. *Harvard Business Review*, 1–12.

Soleas, E. K. (2020). Expectancies, values, and costs of innovating identified by Canadian innovators : A motivational basis for supporting innovation talent development. *Journal of Advanced Academics*, 1–25. https://doi.org/10.1177/1932202X20904772

# CAPITAL DEVELOPMENT

**MATT NORRIS**

Matt Norris currently teaches Grade 6 in a First Nation community in Northern Canada. He has taught in nine different school settings (primary, high school, and university level, internationally and in Canada). He continues to reflect on and inform the processes in both his professional and personal life using the best available evidence, and does his best to model that for his students.

In this chapter, I intend to provide the most practical advice for research in practice that I can. My recommendation comes from my teaching and research experience, and being identified by my peers, family, and colleagues as being pragmatic, sometimes to a fault. Some examples of my pragmatic fault would be always considering cost-efficiency and time-efficiency: like eating at a restaurant versus making the same dish at home, being content stocking up at a warehouse store and not having to leave the house to buy almost anything for months if desired, preferring the place with the largest and cheapest schooners of basic beer for a night on the town, or insisting on using only one square of toilet paper for each trip to the bathroom during the COVID-19 crisis. (The last example was a joke.) I was also raised in an entrepreneurial family, and I did my undergraduate degree in business law with a minor in business. I am currently a grade 6 teacher in a First Nation community in Northern Canada.

## CAPITAL DEVELOPMENT IN SCHOOL

As educators, we individually provide value to our school and school board. To improve our value, sometimes we take it upon ourselves to improve independently (such as attending graduate school), or our employers invest in us to attend professional development. In my experience, these are the two typical situations where educators can engage in informing practices with research. The additional value gained from professional development is then expected to be captured and reflected in the improved growth of our students. This investment into and expected return of surplus value are the elements of capital in a capitalist society (Lin, 1999).

There are three important areas of capital related to professional development: human, social, and decisional. First, *human capital* is "the economic value of a worker's experience and skills. This includes assets like education, training, intelligence, skills, health, and other things employers value such as loyalty and punctuality" (Kenton, 2020, para. 1). As such, to improve individual employability from improving competencies, "the delivery of more holistic 'coping and enabling' services" (Lindsay, 2007, 539) can be used as a more human development aligned approach: by supporting and accommodating the employee to develop capacity for developing competencies.

Second, *social capital* is the "success that can be attributed to personal relationships and networks, both within the organization and outside of it" (Kenton, 2021, para. 1). The strength of social capital and relationships can be determined in the success of situations: success in a job search, or getting help to move homes, or having the opportunity to write a chapter in a book. Having stronger relationships with relatedness provides an increased opportunity in preserving or maintaining access to resources (Lin, 1999) such as human capital, other people's time and effort, or very basically, commodities such as food or shelter. As such, the impact of social capital is instrumental regarding access to "information, influence, social credentials and reinforcement" (Lin, 1999, 31). A popular saying captures the benefit of social capital in accessing information and accessing research: "It is not what you know but who you know. What you know extends from who you know."

Third, *decisional capital* is the "capital that professionals acquire and accumulate through structured and unstructured experience, practice and reflection- capital that enables them to make wise judgements" (Hargreaves & Fullan, 2015, 114). Like with the development of human capital, making connections can help individuals develop how to make judgments and decisions. Having a teaching mentor (like during a teaching practicum) can help guide reflection on practice and decisions and improve future outcomes: "Get the reflection *on* action right and it enables you to start reflecting *in* action more effectively too" (Hargreaves & Fullan, 2015, 119).

Social capital, human capital, and decisional capital can be viewed similarly in that if an investment is made into capital or value generation, there is an expected beneficial return to the individual: "a product of a process" (Lin, 1999, 29), but the process itself may sometimes be unclear.

## PRACTICAL FRAMEWORK

From my experiences, the way I can relate to the two areas of human capital and social capital is through self-determination theory (SDT; Deci & Ryan, 1985) because it makes it practical. SDT hypothesizes that individuals are motivated and experience positive effects to well-being (Niemiec et al., 2014) when psychological needs are satisfied: competence, relatedness, and autonomy. In understanding human capital and social capital, I interpret human capital development as being related to the psychological need of competence, and social capital development as being related to the psychological need of relatedness.

Competence, like human capital, includes your knowledge, skills, etc. If someone is competent at playing hockey, they would likely say, "I'm a hockey player." Because we are competent at teaching (after all, we went to school for it), we say, "I'm a teacher." Therefore, to be a teacher, we must be competent. If we do not feel competent, then we are likely not motivated and we do not experience positive effects to well-being. This is likely relatable for most teachers experiencing the recent transition to online teaching during the COVID-19 pandemic: Teacher-perceived competence or self-efficacy may not have been satisfied without proper capacity or competence development to effectively develop and manage a completely online learning experience.

Relatedness includes the feeling of connection. Relatedness, like social capital, can include the connections, networks, relationships, and so forth a person can have. With more and stronger relationships, and increased communication, it is possible to maintain or increase access to resources (i.e., information, research). The relationships and connections developed through hobbies, sporting activities, exercise, education, employment, and so forth are able to satisfy the psychological need of relatedness—often because of going through, and communicating about, shared experiences.

Autonomy is the freedom an individual feels when making a choice, considering perceived controlling forces in the situation. A person is more autonomously motivated when the decision is their own choice without extrinsic control. Control can be anything that forces you to decide to act in a certain way. This could include a salary; a superior like a parent, a coach, or a boss; or the ability to exercise professional discretion (decisional capital), time, or actual physical control (like being in prison). With less controlling factors, a person can be autonomous and may decide to take a vacation just because they can, or they may decide to try to satisfy other psychological needs.

SDT is a framework I used to complete my master's thesis in education, because it is holistic and helps to "permeate the motivational landscape" (Keegan et al., 2014, 561). By understanding the psychological needs that are able to capture why someone may be motivated, and by understanding how these psychological needs relate to capital development, it is possible to create opportunities that should both satisfy the individual teacher as a person and employee, and the organization as employer and service provider. After all, autonomy and competence are the psychological needs that affect burnout of the teacher the most. Research shows that "over the school year, changes in teachers' perceptions of the school environment (demands and resources) are likely to predict changes in burnout components (emotional exhaustion, depersonalization, and personal accomplishment) through motivational factors (autonomous motivation and self-efficacy)" (Fernet et al., 2012, 522). This means teachers experience burnout because of issues related to feeling controlled/not autonomously motivated, or negatively perceived competence/self-efficacy issues. These two issues are both captured by SDT.

## APPLYING THE PRACTICAL FRAMEWORK
Pursuing the psychological needs of competence and relatedness can provide the opportunities needed to access research/information through the development of our own human capital and social capital.

## Research Club

Applying the framework, the first idea emerges from my experience at graduate school: the on-campus opportunities. This includes being a teaching assistant, research assistant, and language instructor while completing my course requirements and thesis, but even more enjoyably being able to meet and learn directly from colleagues and professors (occasionally at the campus pub over a cider). At meetings, we talked about research, statistics, philosophies, methods, methodology, the latest thing we read and how it related to our interests, new research ideas, and so on. These meetings satisfied my three psychological needs and, by association, increased my human and social capital.

In an attempt to mimic my capital development experiences in graduate school, I recommend a voluntary "research club": educators of a school meeting throughout the school year to share, explore, and consider research and how the research can be used in practice. For the research club, an educator would be responsible to find a research article they are interested in or one that is related to an issue they or others may be having in the school, or what teachers use to guide their practice or interventions, and so forth. Then, the educator creates a half-page point form summary with important and practical information with citation. The educator would then be responsible to provide the half-pager to the other teachers at the research club and present it for a short time (e.g., 5 minutes) followed by conversation/discussion if needed. With all educators divided over many meetings over the year, the number of presentations per meeting may vary. In the initiation of a research club, one research article per educator per year is a good starting point to build capacity. Over time, teachers will access a lot of research, all while increasing their capital.

This club is conceptualized as an enabling and coping service to accommodate already stretched-thin educators by supporting self-efficacy, communication, and the sharing of expertise in a school. First, it is enabling because it minimally infringes on teacher autonomy because of the distributed investment of time and effort among colleagues to access and share research. Second, this research club would ideally occur during time provided (invested) by employers to enable employees to develop their capital; otherwise, the investment of time and effort is required outside the workplace by employees, and this can interfere with work/life balance. For example, this can be done by designating 20–30 minutes of time after monthly meetings in order to accommodate and provide time for the research club. Luckily, in my current school board, there are professional development opportunities throughout the school year during school time, in addition to a week-long conference in the city (employer investment) with capital development in mind. Investment like this by employers supports the movement of research into practice, and it also ensures that research use is treated as an integral part of the role. It also can function as a coping service. Some educators may struggle with capacity or competence development and would benefit from the available support and communication with colleagues at the research club to cope with difficulties or to help identify who has what expertise. Teachers would likely feel more comfortable doing this in a high-trust, supportive culture (Brown et al., 2016). Therefore, the research club attempts to overcome what I see as one of the biggest barriers for teachers to inform their practices with research: infringements on autonomy and/or not supporting competence/capacity development. It is also supported by research. If a professional development is designed with a motivational framework, it should enhance teacher engagement (Qian et al., 2018). Also, active learning opportunities can increase "the effect of the professional development on teacher's instruction" (Desimone et al., 2002, 81).

Overall, educational leaders can create and contribute to capital development by investing organization time to work on developing competence and relatedness; for example, half a day of bowling, and half a day exchanging premade half-pagers like a research club. People are self-determined when psychological needs are satisfied. If leaders aren't supporting it, teachers can advocate for it because it improves teacher employability and skills, and ultimately it is in everybody's best interest, especially the students. Although, even with a defined process, the execution relies on the context in which it is being used.

## CONTEXTS

I have taught in nine different school settings (primary, high school, and university level, internationally and in Canada), and I have learned that each context can be facilitating or limiting because of different factors. Each context needs its own approach because of different considerations.

I am currently enjoying teaching grade 6 in a First Nation community in Northern Canada. As I teach, I must consider historical, cultural, and systemic factors that exist in this context. Historically, First Nation people have had to endure residential schools, the Sixties Scoop (a period in which policies were enacted in Canada that enabled child welfare authorities to forcibly remove thousands of Indigenous children from their homes in an attempt to assimilate them into mainstream culture by placing them with non-Indigenous families), and fighting for their own land, among other things, and this has affected generations of First Nation families. With trauma and broken trust, it is understandable why some may have a difficult relationship with school generally. Culturally, students often participate in seasonal hunting and land-based learning, and these critically important activities must be considered in tandem with school-based teaching and learning. Systemically, the geographic location of the community sometimes means there are muddy or icy roads; extremely cold days (no buses for -35°C/-31°F or lower, no students at school for -40°C/-40°F or lower); days with no water, power, and/or internet; forest fire risk; repairs for buses, which cannot be done instantly; and so forth. Considering the context, teachers in my school need to be responsive to First Nation needs, considerations, and traditions while incorporating research-informed practices. To navigate these considerations and to incorporate research, I believe educators benefit from sharing expertise and insight relating to the same workplace context. After all, peers are the strongest source of innovation (Mourshed et al., 2010).

## OVERCOMING BARRIERS

Ideally, after receiving systemic and organizational support of autonomy by educational leaders for capital development, educators would have more freedom to invest their time and energy to pursue satisfying their competence and relatedness needs. Educators would also have to overcome their own competence barriers by taking steps to become more comfortable interacting with research. In graduate school, I learned an effective way to explore research: read abstracts first, and then read the conclusion if necessary. If it does not meet your needs, move on. If an article is useful, it is then worth the time and effort to read about the study population, data collection methods, context, takeaways, and so forth. With increased exposure to research, and an investment of time and effort, competence can be developed and educator practices can become informed by research. If it is still difficult, support can be found by pursuing elements of the SDT framework, such as making a connection with someone (even outside the workplace) who may have the research knowledge or experience in that area.

## SUCCESSES

In my opinion, research in practice doesn't have to be a rigid thing. With exposure to research, it is possible to understand a takeaway from a study and use it if it applies. This could include proven strategies/interventions, such as Jolly Phonics (Ariati et al., 2018), or recommended teacher behaviors or approaches, and so forth. A success is knowing I am relying on research in my practice based on the experiential and student-led learning-focused classroom structures I use and by having SDT and other actionable research in my mind. When a situation jolts it, as when interacting with someone who may have experienced trauma, research suggests I should do what I can to avoid triggers that remind the person of their traumatic experience, or a fight, flight, or freeze response may occur (Guarino & Chagnon, 2018). Research can have an impact simply through the ways it informs our thinking, and it is often underplayed in comparison to instrumental/tangible change.

## THREE BULLETED TOP TIPS/SUGGESTIONS/RECOMMENDATIONS

- Systemic accommodation provides time for collaboration, communication, innovation, and growth with minimal infringement on autonomy and well-being, while improving competencies.
- Share research responsibilities to be practical with time, and increase relatedness and contextual application.
- Reading abstracts and conclusions is the quickest way to find an appropriate article, and looking through the references helps locate related articles.

# REFERENCE

Ariati, N. P. P., Padmadewi, N. N., & Suarnajaya, I. W. (2018). Jolly Phonics: Effective strategy for enhancing children English literacy. *SHS Web of Conferences, 42*, 1–7.

Brown, C., Daly, A., & Liou, Y.-H. (2016). Improving trust, improving schools. *Journal of Professional Capital and Community, 1*(1), 69–91. https://doi.org/10.1108/JPCC-09-2015-0004

Deci, E. L., & Ryan, R. M. (1985). The general causality orientations scale: Self-determination in personality. *Journal of Research in Personality, 19*, 109–134.

Desimone, L. M., Porter, A. C., Garet, M. S., Yoon, K. S., & Birman, B. F. (2002). Effects of professional development on teachers' instruction: Results from a three-year longitudinal study. *Educational Evaluation and Policy Analysis, 24*(2), 81–112.

Fernet, C., Guay, F., Senécal, C., & Austin, S. (2012). Predicting intraindividual changes in teacher burnout: The role of perceived school environment and motivational factors. *Teaching and Teacher Education, 28*(4), 514–525.

Guarino, K., & Chagnon, E. (2018). *Leading trauma-sensitive schools action guide. Trauma-sensitive schools training package.* National Center on Safe Supportive Learning Environments.

Hargreaves, A., & Fullan, M. (2015). *Professional capital: Transforming teaching in every school.* Teachers College Press.

Keegan, R. J., Spray, C. M., Harwood, C. G., & Lavallee, D. E. (2014). A qualitative synthesis of research into social motivational influences across the athletic career span. *Qualitative Research in Sport, Exercise and Health, 6*, 537–567.

Kenton, W. (2020, September 4). *Human capital.* Investopedia. https://www.investopedia.com/terms/h/humancapital.asp

Kenton, W. (2021, July 24). *Social capital.* Investopedia. https://www.investopedia.com/terms/s/socialcapital.asp

Lin, N. (1999). Building a network theory of social capital. *Connections, 22*(1), 28–51.

Lindsay, C., McQuaid, R., & Dutton, M. (2007). New approaches to employability in the UK: Combining 'human capital development' and 'Work First' strategies? *Journal of Social Policy, 36*(4), 539–560.

Mourshed, M., Chijioke, C., & Barber, M. (2010). *How the world's most improved school systems keep getting better.* McKinsey & Co.

Niemiec, C. P., Soenens, B., & Vansteenkiste, M. (2014). Is relatedness enough? On the importance of need support in different types of social experiences. In N. Weinstein (Ed.), *Human motivation and interpersonal relationships* (pp. 77–96). Springer Netherlands.

Qian, Y., Hambrusch, S., Yadav, A., & Gretter, S. (2018, February). Who needs what: Recommendations for designing effective online professional development for computer science teachers. *Journal of Research on Technology in Education, 50*(1), 1–18. DOI: 10.1080/15391523.2018.1433565

# CLASSROOM TEACHERS AS SCHOLARS
BRINGING PRACTITIONER RESEARCH INTO CONVERSATION
WITH THE LITERATURE TO INFORM PROFESSIONAL PRACTICE

**DEREK TANGREDI, MARY OTT, KELLY HOLBROUGH AND KATHY HIBBERT**

Derek Tangredi is an award-winning mathematics and science instructor from Western University. He has received an Award of Excellence from Western for his work in relation to research and assessment with teacher candidates. He is an award-winning educator with Thames Valley District School Board and currently a mathematics consultant with the board. Finally, Derek is a speaker, a consultant, and the Director of Education with Inksmith.

Mary Ott believes that relationships and research mindsets are the heart and soul of our work as teachers. She coordinates and researches an innovative course for Western University's teacher education candidates, led by mentors in small communities of practice to develop habits of professional and collaborative inquiry.

Kelly Holbrough is an academic superintendent with the London District Catholic School Board. In her 33 years in education as a teacher and administrator, she has been leading school and board improvement planning looking for next best moves based on evidence-based data and how it improves student learning.

Kathy Hibbert is an Associate Dean of Teacher Education at Western University in Ontario, Canada. After nearly two decades

**in professional practice, she returned to academia. Her experiences as a former classroom teacher and consultant have informed the subsequent 20 years as a teacher educator and administrator— especially her thinking about classroom teachers as scholars.**

Famed Brazilian educator and activist Paulo Freire (2000) gave educators a gift when he wrote *Pedagogy of the Oppressed* in 1968. He offered clear assertions: 1) Teachers, like all humans, seek to grow and develop. 2) Oppression in any form interferes with this growth and development. 3) Change requires revolution. Oppression, he explained, is only successful insofar as its legitimacy is internalized and upheld by both the oppressed and the oppressors.

Yet, since the publication of Friere's clarion call to action, two competing trends can be seen in education in Canada and much of North America. On one hand, we see external mechanisms introduced to "professionalize" teaching. By the mid-1970s, teachers were required to have a university degree and a teaching degree; in the mid-1990s, professional bodies (such as the Ontario College of Teachers) were formed to regulate, set standards for, and govern their members. Coincidental to these professionalization efforts was the introduction of a mandatory standardized curriculum, standardized provincial testing, and standardized reporting. Cuts to professional development (PD) budgets within boards of education and centralized control over priorities (e.g., literacy and numeracy) repositioned teachers again as passive receivers of knowledge.

Many scholars have written about this contradiction as a shift toward deprofessionalizing teachers. This shift was reflected in the language such as "teacher training," "covering content," and "delivering curriculum." The market was quick to respond with "purchased solutions that both supplant active decision-making on the part of the teacher and neglect the child as informant" (Hibbert & Iannacci, 2005, 717).

At the same time, societies have been subject to a digital transformation that has altered our relationship to knowledge. In the early phase, most of us were passive receivers or consumers of information. As technology advanced, so did our skills and our expectations. We became capable of engaging, collaborating, interacting, and producing information and new knowledge through the internet. The semantic web has elevated our individual capacity to personalize experiences and interactions that will continue to grow. How we engage with knowledge today is at odds with the way teachers are positioned in a system clinging to antiquated managerial practices from a time gone by, while expecting educators to engage students in 21st-century competencies. This chapter joins the call for a revolution in North American education for 21st-century teachers so that they may well serve the students they teach.

## THE CLASSROOM TEACHER AS SCHOLAR

In *Shifting Minds: A 21st Century Vision of Public Education for Canada* (C21 Canada, 2012), there is an explicit call to modernize and innovate and support teachers in their efforts to "ensure learners attain 21st [C] learning competencies" that comes about through "fostering creative and innovative minds" (5). Susan Kidd Villaume (2000) has long argued that "progress in teaching comes from an ongoing search for discrepancies between our beliefs and our practices (Hibbert, 2013, 27). Teachers are routinely confronted by unexpected or surprising incidents and outcomes that they are called upon to respond to, make sense of and try to plan for. This "grappling" with our craft is in part what makes it so intellectually appealing. Most teachers welcome

> ...the opportunity to articulate what it means to be a teacher; to tangle with social issues beyond the technicalities of teaching; and having some agency within which to question and challenge the wider structures surrounding teaching and learning; and in the process gaining some ownership of the determination of one's own pedagogical work (Spivak, 1988).

To do this, we need to break free of outdated managerial practices imposed on highly educated professionals and instead give them the agency, space, and tools to grow and thrive as scholars of their professional practice. Because this handbook is specifically interested in how we ensure that research makes its way into practice, we see "classroom teachers as scholars" as an opportunity for teachers to engage in the necessary immersion, reflection, and capacity to respond that are critical to the deep learning necessary to transform practice.

To be considered scholarship, Shulman (1993) argued that it must meet certain threshold criteria:

i. the creation of some kind of artifact or product (lesson);

ii. the public sharing of the work;

iii. inviting peer review and critique (in alignment with accepted standards);

iv. opportunity to reproduce, build on and improve the work by others.

To embody the ideas we are discussing here, we engaged in a scholarship activity as a group of authors for the writing of this chapter. We purposefully engaged as a group of authors uniquely positioned to bring different perspectives.

## PROCESS

Using the guiding questions provided by the editors, each of the chapter's authors wrote an independent response. In addition, we considered a series of analytic questions, adapted from Smyth's (1998) "passionate plea for discontent" (191):

1. How do our responses imagine schools as learning communities?

2. What are the structured spaces within schools' and teachers' work where pedagogical knowledge and understandings can be systematically challenged, shared, and reconstituted?

3. What internal processes are feasible and manageable for schools as they invent for themselves ways of initiating, sustaining, and maintaining professional pedagogical dialogue?

4. How can a notion of "classroom teachers as scholars" support teachers' ability to develop the agency needed to resist narrow technicist constructions of their work and their professional identities? (192)

Our independent responses to these questions were shared with each other using collaborative technology. We later met and recorded an analysis session exploring where our perspectives converged and where they diverged. Our intent was that by both drawing on the expertise of our diverse group in ways that make our own learning and scholarly practice visible, we would invite you, the reader, to engage with these ideas. We seek to bring all voices, including those that may be viewed as "disruptive" into a conversation among teachers seeking to move fully into their professional roles.

## FINDINGS

Guided by our analytic questions, all responses emphasized the value of "making space" (Kathy) for teachers to act as scholars. For example, Kelly reflected on "creating a culture for learning" (Kelly); Mary about "how we are moved by research ... to the point that it embodies practice" and the time and space constituents of "effectively embedding research in practice" (Derek). Our divergence centered on how we expanded these space-making ideas further.

Kathy, Kelly, and Derek focused on space as an external, shaping force. Kathy's concerns as a university administrator were about how the organic nature of culture work was too often co-opted by mandatory structures and processes that shifted the experience from one of growth and discovery as professionals, to one that was part of a broader accountability system. Similarly, as a superintendent, Kelly focused on the logistics of finding time for teachers to learn together in a context where Ministry of Education mandates determined the focus of all PD sessions, and teacher unions restricted when and how leaders could bring their staff into PD sessions. Derek also noted the competing pressures of time at work and outside of work, where the expectation for PD has crept into the "outside-of-work" hours. While acknowledging the financial costs to bringing PD into the work day, he cautioned that when recent research and PD are not readily available, "teachers continue to teach the way they were taught, demonstrating a generational perpetuation of practice in curriculum, instruction, and assessment" (Gallavan & Webster-Smith, 2012, 53).

On the other hand, Mary's focus on space was on the inside out, concerning the formation of professional identity. She viewed the site of the struggle to be located in that identity shift from student to professional pedagogue and the need to disrupt the "habits of being" from one, in order to transform into the space of the other. In Mary's view, this shift requires us to think about the context of our teaching as a formative "inquiry space."

We all agreed, however, that strong systems and leaders have roles to play in the space for teacher scholarship. As senior administrators,

Kathy and Kelly noted the importance of support "from the top": from the Ministry of Education, the Ontario College of Teachers, boards of education, principals, and internal champions. We also noted how important it is to have some alignment with school improvement plans and board initiatives, although Kathy articulated the need to create conditions for teachers to engage as independent scholars of the "problems of practice" unique to their context. Mary and Derek focused on the need for leadership in "actively modeling" research practices through "pedagogical documentation and collaborative inquiry" (Mary) or through the establishment of "collaborative networks" where teachers voices are central to the inquiry and the problem-solving process (Derek). As we were grappling with our ideas, our discussion echoed the space Spivak described previously in this chapter. Mary posed, "We have to think about where the structured spaces and times are within schools where teachers' pedagogical knowledge and understandings can be systematically challenged, shared, and reconstituted."

## DISCUSSION

Our dialogues about co-creating knowledge led us to acknowledge the role of using system data to inform our practice, but also to leverage the affordances of collaborative inquiry for seeing differently – to extend, enrich, or contend with standard forms of data collection and "baked-in assumptions about system prioritiesIt is this ability to grapple that moves research. In an agentic, professional vision of teachers moving research into practice, "Teachers need to know, not only, how to use research evidence critically but also how to actively engage in research with their pupils as co-researchers as an integral part of their everyday teaching and learning practice" (Evans et al., 2017, 405). Valuing perspectives, challenging assumptions, making space for difference—these actions foster a community where the expectation is that teachers engage as scholars; autonomous professionals who are accountable of course, but provided the respect and freedom to grown and learn with their students as co-creators of knowledge.

We must stop positioning teachers as receivers of knowledge, regulated by narrow visions of what it means to "implement" curriculum. This process leads to an embodiment of identity where teachers are "performing" to standardized criteria. However, "procedural display"—

where we learn to "echo," "mirror," and "comply" (Hibbert, 2013)—is the antithesis of the critical inquiry and design-based innovation needed in 21st century curriculum making (Latta et al., 2017; Ott & Hibbert, 2020).

## CONCLUSION

We cannot hope for teachers to become what we do not enable them to be. Space for teaching as scholarship and teachers as researchers must be created and supported where individual teachers are able to set and develop their own unique learning goals (Ott & Hibbert, 2021). Too often, professional learning goals have been universally set by a government or school board or school leader. In a context where we are aiming for differentiating the teaching of students, we ought to be honouring the diverse knowledge, experience, and professionalism of our teachers.

Priestley and colleagues (2021) argue that teachers preparing students in the 21st century are not passively "implementing – or ... delivering – somebody else's curriculum product," but rather, they are engaging in a process of meaning making that demands the time for grappling, reflecting, and engaging "in their own contexts alongside a number of other social actors, including their students" (1–2). In the past year, we have learned through the context of a global pandemic, that innovation emerges when greater flexibility and autonomy is extended. The pandemic forced us to extend that flexibility, and a world of possibilities opened up. How might we bring that flexibility into the professional lives of teachers to honor their capacity for growth?

## RECOMMENDATIONS

- Respect teachers' autonomy as professionals, holding them accountable to their professionalism.
- Teacher professionalism as scholarship is marked by "grappling": creative, iterative, and sometimes disruptive acts of inquiry into learning as co-learners with students, colleagues, and school communities.
- What makes space to move research into practice is context dependent and requires interrogation and active exploration between teachers and leaders acting in systems. However, the space to grapple requires a commitment of time.

# REFERENCES

Evans, C., Waring, M., & Christodoulou, A. (2017). Building teachers' research literacy: Integrating practice and research. *Research Papers in Education, 32*(4), 403–423. https://doi.org/10.1080/02671522.2017.1322357

Freire, P. (2000). *Pedagogy of the oppressed* (30th anniversary ed.). Continuum.

Glassick, C. E. (2000). Boyer's expanded definition of scholarship, the standards for assessing scholarship, and the elusiveness of a scholarship of teaching. *Academic Medicine, 75*(9), 877–880.

Hibbert, K. (2013). Finding wisdom in practice: The genesis of the salty chip, a Canadian multiliteracies collaborative. *Language and Literacy, 15*(1), 23–38. https://doi.org/10.20360/G23G6H

Hibbert, K., & Iannacci, L. (2005). From dissemination to discernment: The commodification of literacy instruction and the fostering of "good teacher consumerism." *Reading Teacher, 58*(8), 716–727.

Latta, M. M., Hanson, K., Ragoonaden, K., Briggs, W., & Middleton, T. (2017). Accessing the curricular play of critical and creative thinking. *Canadian Journal of Education Toronto, 40*(3), 191–218.

Ott, M., & Hibbert, K. (2020). Assessment in 21st century learning: Improvisation and inquiry. In C. Martin, D. Polly, & R. Lambert (Eds.), *Handbook of research on formative assessment in pre-K through elementary classrooms* (pp. 346–367). IGI Global. doi:10.4018/978-1-7998-0323-2.ch017

Ott, M., & Hibbert, K. (2021). Designing assessment for professional agency. In J. Nickle & M. Jacobsen (Eds.), *Preparing teachers as curriculum designers*. Canadian Association of Teacher Education (CATE) Polygraph. https://cate-acfe.ca/wp-content/uploads/2021/01/Preparing-Teachers-as-Curriculum-Designers_ebook_FINAL.pdf

Shulman, L. S. (1993). Teaching as community property: Putting an end to pedagogical solitude. *Change, 25*(6), 6–7.

Smyth, J. (1998). Finding the 'enunciative space' for teacher leadership and teacher learning in schools. *Asia-Pacific Journal of Teacher Education, 26*(3), 191–202. DOI: 10.1080/1359866980260303

Spivak, G. (1988). Can the subaltern speak? In C. Nelson & L. Grossberg (Eds.), *Marxism and the interpretation of culture* (pp. 271–313). University of Illinois Press.

# BECOMING AN EDUCATOR
## EMBRACING RESEARCH-INFORMED PRACTICES

### KYAIR BUTTS

Kyair has worked in education for eight years having graduated from Drake University and completing graduate studies with Lesley University where he earned a double M.Ed. in Elementary & Special Education. He currently serves students in Baltimore City Public Schools as a sixth-grade literacy educator. He won Teacher of the Year for Baltimore City in 2019 in addition to facilitating professional development with *Wit & Wisdom* (Great Minds, n.d.).

Becoming a teacher is something that not many people have at the forefront of their minds. The current globalization of work and pace of humanity and technology has people racing to become engineers, software developers, and business wunderkinds. Where are the teachers? In teaching, we have a profession that relies on cutting-edge technology and innovative ways of thinking. In teaching, we bring creative minds together to solve persistent problems of equity, funding, access, and opportunity. Teaching is for the doer, the maker, the believer, and the change agent-in-waiting.

The path to becoming a highly effective teacher is fraught with highs and lows. Much study and application have to be considered and executed before being the teacher of record and making life-altering decisions for your students. There are those who come into the profession by way of having studied education in college. There are those (like me) who decided after undergrad that teaching was the route we wanted to take and thus we turned to alternative certification programs. These are programs that offer the opportunity to be a classroom teacher while taking graduate classes and helping with various benchmarks toward licensure (certification) to become an official teacher of record. (In this sense, think Teach for America. I was a member of a different program, Urban Teachers. While these programs, and there are many, have their nuances, they serve a similar purpose for people like me.)

In becoming an educator, we are tasked with understanding the prevailing literature/research around education to make informed decisions, adapt practices, and embed/imbue our pedagogy with the best that is available. Becoming an educator means that necessary and sufficient means need to be exacted in order to become highly effective. This is likely why higher education and alternative certification programs place such an emphasis (more could be done, however) on research-informed practices to boost student achievement both in academics and in social-emotional learning/wholeness (SEL or student wholeness).

In this chapter, I argue as much for teachers to see their jobs as change agents as I will argue for better access and learning to position teachers to accelerate learning for students. Research-informed practices and their application/implementation in the classroom can change someone's life. I see this as a chance for teachers to see themselves as true agents of change and advocates for advancement in the profession. As the years have rolled by, the respect for teaching has seemingly eroded, leaving behind the caricature of the weathered teacher longing for summer vacation. Teaching is a testament to the selfless, an ode to the resilient, and a call to the transformative and innovative.

## CELEBRATING RESEARCH | MOVING TOWARD BETTER

Research informs much of our daily lives, leading to new technology and various methods that not only make our lives safe but, it could be reasonably argued, have made our lives better. Research should not be limited to the latest medical advancements, but rather, research in education should be celebrated, reviewed, and widely discussed among teachers, teacher-leaders, and school/district leaders. Research maintains a standard of excellence that is acceptable within an industry and the standard in teaching is life or death. Now, I know this sounds hyperbolic but in some districts like mine (Baltimore City), excellent teaching can put students on a path toward academic success, whereas mediocre teaching or worse can severely derail a student's progress. If that student is already behind various benchmarks (let's say a sixth-grade student reading at a second-grade level), then the trajectory looks bleak. It is imperative that teachers, teacher-leaders, and school/district leaders not only understand the research and what it says but also discuss the research then implement the research using cycles of professional development to refine teaching practices and understand problems of practice.

Several years ago, the Baltimore City Public Schools CEO (superintendent) produced a plan that valued research, placed an emphasis on equity, and valued student wholeness. This intentional design is called our Blueprint for Success (Literacy, Leadership, and Student Wholeness make up the core pillars of the Blueprint for Success). Like any blueprint, its purpose is not just prescriptive, but it becomes predictive when teachers, leaders, and the district intentionally focus on research-based practices in those three core areas. Let's take literacy as a first example.

You might have to be a true literacy wonk and of a certain age to understand this idea of "Reading Wars," which were a real thing (more so arguments and discourse and less so librarians waging war against overdue library books or battles with alphabet soup spilling into the streets). The Reading Wars were very real (and intense) approaches to literacy (especially phonics) and the research therein during the 1990s and to some extent persist today. Phonics, phonological awareness, understanding of high-frequency words, access to vocabulary, and comprehension of fiction and nonfiction are big drivers in the literacy field. Add to that a growing tidal wave of research on knowledge building supporting those domains, and all of a sudden, the bottom line is that teachers need to be aware of the research—and not just aware but equipped to apply research-based practices in their classrooms.

Meredith and David Liben (2019) wrote a book, *Know Better, Do Better*, that talks specifically about the research, what it says, and why it is important. As a literacy teacher, it's crucial to understand what the experts are saying so I can do better by knowing better. Further, writing research has also changed over the years. I am only in my eighth year in education, but in these eight years the pendulum has swung again. As such, The Vermont Writing Collaborative produced an amazing look at writing research, and it is a "must-have" book for educators (all educators, it can be argued, support writing). Their book, *Writing for Understanding: Using Backward Design to Help All Students Write Effectively* (Vermont Writing Collaborative, 2008), has taken my writing practice to new heights, and as such, reluctant writers are producing amazing works within my classes because I listened to the research, discussed it with colleagues, and have a district leader who sees the value of having research at the foundation of our Blueprint for Success.

## REIMAGINE, RETHINK, RESIST | WHY RESEARCH MATTERS

Chalkboard, eraser, projector, transparencies, and students in a column/row desk orientation in terms of seating. Something tells me that at some point the research was compelling enough that teacher-centered classrooms were less effective than student-centered classrooms. The research is also clear about print-rich classrooms and what that can do for students. Common classroom set-ups now involve groupings for student desks/chairs, softer/warmer colors, less fluorescent lighting, opportunities for dialogue, and student check-ins with each other and with their teacher. Research has forced (too strong a verb?) teachers to reimagine teaching as a more interpersonal and interactive exchange than the "Matilda" approach (*I am right, you are wrong. I am big, you are small. I am the adult; you are the child*). In reimagining teaching, students are at the forefront of learning and equal partners in the process. Great teachers stop, rethink, and adjust their practices given the plethora of research for us to consume, digest, and implement. In doing this, we should resist the urge to carry on "business as usual," knowing full well this does not work and is not working for every student. At the point it does not work for every student, that's a complicit admission that it's holding students back, and I refuse to be complicit in a process that harms students. I am not only compelled by research, but I am motivated by research. I'll show you what I mean.

When I first started teaching in Baltimore City Public Schools, lessons seemingly operated in vacuums. I recall being in a math classroom where lessons were taught one skill a day, and we drilled those skills (likely killing any enthusiasm for math with the "drill-and-kill" approach). The next year, I was moved to a new content area: reading. The curriculum Baltimore City Public Schools had at the time was not a research-informed curriculum. In fact, it emphasized an isolated approach wherein I used different texts to teach different skills. My students were often lost trying to track the various texts and make connections to the various skills, and it seemed as if more harm than good was done. Did the isolated approach really work? All of my anecdotal evidence seemed to say "no."

At present, Baltimore City Public Schools is in its third year for a majority of its K–8 schools using the *Wit & Wisdom* curriculum produced by Great Minds. This literacy (English Language Arts) curriculum is the opposite of what I had my first through fifth years of teaching (isolated approach). *Wit & Wisdom* emphasizes the integrated approach and a depth of knowledge. Now, my students are reading about the Great Depression and making connections to their lives about resilience, transformation, and hardship, all using the core texts (the main books we read for the module/unit). Our writing lessons also are based in and around the content of the module using those core texts (integrating content across skill areas). Now, yes, I admit this is convenient for me as a teacher, but the research is astounding. Take, for instance, the research that comes out of The New Teacher Project (TNTP) and their findings in *The Opportunity Myth* (2018). Curricula that offer deep engagement, productive struggle opportunities, grade-level assignments, and a belief that students can do the work increase academic performance by some two months of additional learning at minimum and even six or more months of additional learning. That research should halt you in your place.

Teachers have reimagined education; we have had to rethink our practices and approaches, but we must resist the urge to not want to use research-based practices. Sometimes, I'll admit, there's an ease or convenience to reusing and recycling lessons, but this is not best practice. I learned early on that it did not benefit students to reuse my lessons. Each crop of students is different year-to-year even if the content is the same for you. This to me is especially true for those of us who teach Black and Brown kids. I make this point because some (not all; I will not overly generalize) Black and Brown students need extra supports, but maintaining an "it has worked for years" mentality or an "it is them" mindset serves your interests and does not equitably serve the children in our charge.

One of the best ways that I became invested in the research was by becoming invested in the curriculum that Baltimore City Public Schools chose (*Wit & Wisdom*). I wanted to become an expert in the curriculum, which led to applying for and being awarded a fellowship opportunity. Investing in the curriculum was and continues to be an investment in myself and my students. As simple as this sounds, I pay attention in professional development, I stay behind and ask questions, I seek out other educators who are doing this well, and I follow teacher leaders and district leaders on social media (specifically Twitter). I participate in education chats on Twitter and open up my practice for those who want to collaborate and/or observe. This makes me better because I am an active participant in my own success and in the acceleration of my students' academic success. Teachers, in my opinion, are similar to cars that need routine oil changes to continue running well. Teachers need regular and robust professional development where they can engage with each other and discuss the prevailing research with colleagues in empowering spaces.

In short, I am asking you as a colleague and as someone who is deeply invested in students and their success (just as I am) to not just value the research but believe the research and apply the research to your practice. Here are a few tricks I have used:

- Follow the experts on social media
- Invest time to research the research
- Invest in the curriculum (it's an investment in yourself)
- Participate in education chats on social media
- Give yourself credit, and finally
- Understand that research-based practices are meant to make your job easier and, in turn, make you better

The shift doesn't happen overnight, but the results for students are long term and long lasting.

## SUCCESS STORIES AND STRUCTURES | RIDING RESEARCH

I am in awe of where I am now considering how my first year of teaching went. I am from Des Moines, Iowa (it's a city… not a farm, so hold the chicken). When I moved to Baltimore, I was the outsider trying to become a teacher. I was worried about fitting in (all of a sudden, my school dances are darting across my memories) to a city and culture different from those of my youth. I am a Black man, but teaching in a city whose student population is majority Black and Brown didn't mean I would fit in or be respected automatically. I needed to research how best to become a teacher especially as an outsider. I was honestly worried about being Black enough to teach in Baltimore. That worry plagued me for my entire first year, with academic challenges for my students and classroom management issues for me. Flash forward to 2019, and I am the first Black man to win Teacher of the Year for Baltimore City Public Schools. The honor was presented to me at age 29, and now I am a teacher leader in the district and even nationally with the curriculum company Great Minds (*Wit & Wisdom*). I lay this groundwork to explain that research informed how I could better build rapport with students to establish mutual respect. Research informed my practice and my presence in the classroom to make me better and, in turn, students excelled.

## CONCLUSION | REINVEST IN RESEARCH-BASED PRACTICES

Baltimore City Public Schools, like many districts around the nation and certainly globally, still have room to grow, but the structures, shifts, and mindsets that are practiced by our CEO (Dr. Sonja Santelises) help sustain research-based practices within the district. Our Blueprint for Success has research at its roots. As a teacher, I respect that research informs what my district is doing and how much students will grow. Teachers need leaders to believe in the research, to give space for teachers to adequately process the implications of the research, to ensure that coaches can work with teachers, and to engage teachers in cycles of professional learning where problems of practice are analyzed and discussed, with action plans being created. Teachers also need to see what is being asked of them, so we know that research-informed practices are being modeled by expert teachers at the top of their game.

- Time and space for professional development centered on research
- District leaders establishing a culture of research-based practices
- Teachers engaging in cycles of professional learning and analysis of best practices

## REFERENCES

Great Minds. (n.d.). *Wit & Wisdom.* https://greatminds.org/english

Liben, M., & Liben, D. (2019). *Know better, do better: Teaching the foundations so every child can read.* Learning Sciences International.

The New Teacher Project. (2018). *The opportunity myth.* https://tntp.org/publications/view/student-experiences/the-opportunity-myth

The Vermont Writing Collaborative. (2008). *Writing for understanding: Using backward design to help all students write effectively.* Author.

# A CONFESSION

## JOSHUA PIGEON

After graduating from the Queen's University teacher education program, Joshua Pigeon started his career as an occasional teacher in Ottawa, Ontario. He had placements throughout the city and was given the opportunity to experience several schools. He fell in love with the culture in one of those schools and ended up pursuing several long-term occasional teaching contracts ranging from grades 7 to 12 there. He found himself immersed in the teaching and learning of grade 7/8 students and transitioned into his first permanent teaching position at the grade 7/8 level. His primary focus was to help bridge the gap between the intermediate and secondary panels, which later supported his move into a permanent position teaching grades 9–12. When the COVID-19 pandemic struck, he chose to try teaching in the virtual environment. It was a taxing and revolutionary journey where he realized something beautiful: the fundamental ideologies that drove practice and supported student learning in person still held —even through a screen.

For me, the first few years of teaching were filled with doubt. I remember being surrounded by veteran teachers who outwardly contradicted most of the practices taught to me throughout my teacher education. It didn't make sense. The literature suggested that students were more successful when teachers did (insert your favorite practice here) over traditional approaches, but only a handful of teachers listened. I tried these practices. I made pods. I used randomized groups. I had an evolving, flexible seating plan. Yet my students' success paled in comparison to that of my colleagues. I was stressed. I was tired. I questioned my career. And I quickly realized that if I wanted to survive in this profession, I needed to learn from the veterans who possessed a wealth of knowledge grounded in years of practical experience. After taking their advice, I started to think that theory and practice might be mutually distinct. I was missing something. It is not that the pedagogical practices that I learned in theory were ineffective, it was that I didn't implement them correctly.

*Teaching* is the implementation of instructional technique, assessment practice, and classroom management strategy in conjunction with determining classroom layout and fostering classroom culture. *Effective teaching*, on the other hand, utilizes pedagogical practices grounded in theory and practice that simultaneously influence each of the aforementioned parts. The challenge for practitioners is that the literature generally focuses on one practice and its impact on student learning. Determining how to use that practice to teach effectively is left to the classroom teacher. And that's hard. It was only when I viewed the classroom as a multifaceted, living entity with a network of interconnected moving parts that my students met with success.

Regardless of the pedagogical practice implemented, there are three fundamental tools that I use in every class:

1. **The lesson and goal page:** a template that students use to document and reflect on learning from the lesson.
2. **Bell work:** a question that students engage with when they enter the classroom.
3. **The "4 things" (which are modified based on grade and stream):** structured study materials comprising a review page, a documentation page, a definition page, and a set of cue cards.

The development of these tools, all of which morphed over the course of several years, is the focus for this chapter. Their co-evolution happened with constant interplay between my classroom experience and professional learning. These tools are not mutually exclusive; they depend on each other and provide a smooth transition through every component of a lesson. Throughout this chapter, I will reference these tools regularly because they drove each other to their most recent form.

## THE LESSON AND GOAL PAGE

My first long-term occasional contract was baptism by fire. In an attempt to gain control of my classroom, I drew on the concept of learning goals from my teacher education. Teachers were posting learning goals in their classroom and not changing them for months. These goals became dusty, unreferenced objects invisible to students. I wanted students to engage with the learning goal in every class. My idea was that when students walked into my classroom, they would pull out their lesson and goal page (figure 6.1) and write the date. This would signify to me that they were ready to learn.

### WHAT HAVE I LEARNED?

| DATE | LESSON | GOAL |
|------|--------|------|
|      |        |      |
|      |        |      |
|      |        |      |

Figure 6.1. A snapshot of the table that would be distributed to students (paper or digitally).

The lesson and goal for the class would then be written (by me) in a corner of a white board (figure 6.2), and the students would copy it down.

Writing the date was supposed to engage my students as they walked into my classroom. Instead, a handful of students wrote the date and started talking, a few pulled out their goal sheet and started talking, and the rest … started talking. This was not their fault—it was mine. I realized that the first second of class is the most important moment, and writing the date didn't create enough academic pressure. A question would have been (and was) more effective. Bell work kept students engaged and provided a transition into the lesson and goal.

I started my class with bell work and the lesson and goal page, as seen in figure 6.1, for a year and a half. Around that same time, I introduced the 4 things to help my students study. To hold students accountable, I had them record when they studied—and which concepts they studied—on their documentation page. One of my students added a rating system, of their own accord, assessing how much they understood from each study session. It was brilliant. After that day, I required all of my students to self-assess their understanding on the documentation page. My student's rating system consisted of 10 dots, which later became integrated into the goal sheet as seen in figure 6.3.

With bell work, the lesson and goal page, and the 4 things, I could keep my students learning until just a few minutes before the bell. But 2 minutes at the end of class, for 180 classes in the school year, was 360 minutes (or 6 hours) of wasted instructional time. I needed a way to keep them learning until the bell, and I wanted to dismiss them in the same way that I greeted them—individually.

In the next school year, I was excited to implement my new structures from day 1. They worked, but I still filled the last minutes before the dismissal bell by talking to my class about what we learned that day. One day, my timing was off and the bell rang while my students were filling out their documentation page. I feared that my students would stand up and leave without my dismissal. Then a student said, "Sir, do you need to check this?" and it hit me: I could dismiss students by checking the 10 dots on the documentation page. After a week of this, we decided that we should add the 10 dots to the lesson and goal page, and the reflection should be based on understanding of the entire lesson.

Over that same year and a half, I remember sitting in several professional development sessions and discussing the use of exit cards. Teachers raved about how they could now get immediate, formative feedback from students after every class. What everyone failed to mention was how they would collect the 30 pieces of paper at the end of class, how long they would spend reading them, how they would distribute them, and how they would document the learning, and they also never discussed what constituted a good exit card question. What worked was embedding a daily, metacognitive exit card—in the form of 10 dots—into the lesson and goal page (figure 6.3). At the end of class, students would flip over to their lesson and goal page (with the same consistent verbal cue) and fill out their 10 dots based on how much they felt they learned/understood from the lesson. I would then come around and check. Upon checking, I would dismiss the students from class—individually.

## WHAT HAVE I LEARNED?

| DATE | LESSON | GOAL | UNDERSTANDING (1-10) |
|------|--------|------|----------------------|
|      |        |      | ○○○○○ ○○○○○ |
|      |        |      | ○○○○○ ○○○○○ |

Figure 6.3. The addition of the 10 dots to the lesson and goal page.

The lesson and goal page from figure 6.3 leveraged instruction through its direct interplay with bell work and the learning goal. It leveraged assessment through daily metacognition and through consistent feedback based on individual students reporting. It leveraged classroom management as it started and ended the class. It leveraged classroom culture as I was able to connect with each student individually and appropriately respond to their needs. But it failed to interact with the classroom space. At the time, I had a whiteboard where, in between the action and consolidation of the lesson, I would write down the concepts that students told me they learned from the class. Students constantly referenced this wall to populate their 4 things. When I moved to teaching senior grades, the number of concepts grew much faster, and when I went to erase it, my grade 11 students suggested that we add a component for concepts to the lesson and goal page. This suggestion gave rise to the new structure of the lesson and goal page as seen in figure 6.4.

## WHAT HAVE I LEARNED?

| DATE | LESSON | GOAL | CONCEPT LIST | UNDERSTANDING (1-10) |
|------|--------|------|--------------|----------------------|
| Sept. 18, 2020 | The Natural Numbers | To use both representation | N={0, 1, 2, 3, ...} Number Line Blocks | ●●●○○ ●●●○○ |
| | | | | ○○○○○ ○○○○○ |

Figure 6.4. The most recent lesson and goal page with the first row completed as an example.

The final pieces had been added to the lesson and goal page: a transitional component through all major landmarks of a lesson and consistent interplay with the classroom space via the concept wall. At the same time, the lesson and goal page heavily relies on an introductory task to interact with, which is bell work.

## BELL WORK

The only thing that teachers can control is time, and the first second of class is the most important.

Prior to using bell work, the expectation in the first second of class was to fill in the date on the lesson and goal page. It didn't work. Students wouldn't do it. When I reached out to the veteran teachers, they would say something along the lines of, "Step one, get control of your class: structure, routine, consistency. They are going to eat you alive; classroom management is everything." But, more often than not, these phrases were said in the absence of implementation. Believe it or not, I did manage to get those grade 7 students to sit down quietly and write down the date on the goal sheet. I remember, during that one short-lived moment, thinking to myself, "They are actually expecting me to teach them now." The thought that they were—in all seriousness—going to listen to me was novel. And so, I began "teaching." That class went well. The next one didn't. The key piece was that my students needed (and wanted, although they wouldn't admit it) something educational to do. Bell work—and the expectation to engage with it—worked.

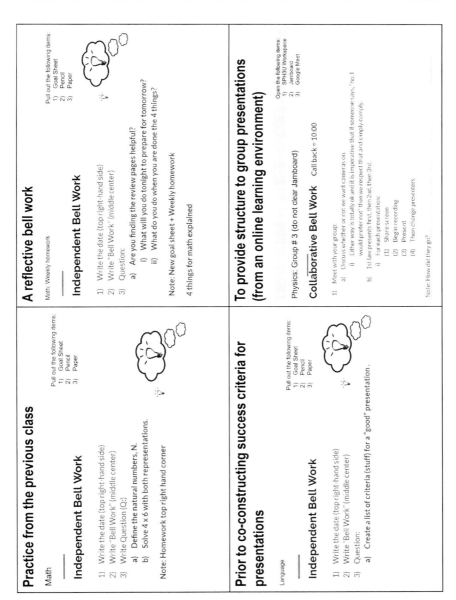

**Practice from the previous class**

Math

Pull out the following items:
1) Goal Sheet
2) Pencil
3) Paper

**Independent Bell Work**

1) Write the date (top right-hand side)
2) Write "Bell Work" (middle center)
3) Write Question (Q):
   a) Define the natural numbers, N.
   b) Solve 4 x 6 with both representations.

Note: Homework top right hand corner

**Prior to co-constructing success criteria for presentations**

Language

Pull out the following items:
1) Goal Sheet
2) Pencil
3) Paper

**Independent Bell Work**

1) Write the date (top right-hand side)
2) Write "Bell Work" (middle center)
3) Question:
   a) Create a list of criteria (stuff) for a "good" presentation.

**A reflective bell work**

Math; Weekly homework

Pull out the following items:
1) Goal Sheet
2) Pencil
3) Paper

**Independent Bell Work**

1) Write the date (top right-hand side)
2) Write "Bell Work" (middle center)
3) Question:
   a) Are you finding the review pages helpful?
      i) What will you do tonight to prepare for tomorrow?
      ii) What do you do when you are done the 4 things?

Note: New goal sheet + Weekly homework

4 things for math explained

**To provide structure to group presentations (from an online learning environment)**

Open the following items:
1) SPH3U Workspace
2) Jamboard
3) Google Meet

Physics: Group # 3 (do not clear Jamboard)

**Collaborative Bell Work**   Call back = 10:00

1) Meet with your group:
   a) Discuss whether or not we want cameras on.
      i) Either way is totally ok and it is imperative that if someone says, "no, I would prefer not" then we respect that and simply comply.
   b) 1st law presents first, then 2nd, then 3rd.
      i) For each presentation:
         (1) Share screen
         (2) Begin recording
         (3) Present
         (4) Then change presenters

Note: How did they go?

Figure 6.5. Some examples of bell work questions.[1]

---

1. I have always had access to a projector. However, in the absence of technology, bell work can be modified for the classroom space and the students' exceptionalities.

Bell work can be anything (figure 6.5). For example, it could be

1. grounded in curriculum (e.g., answer this question),
2. grounded in metacognition (e.g., list 3 things describing how yesterday's task went),
3. grounded in events in the school (e.g., Do you know someone affected by cancer?).

Further, a careful construction of bell work can leverage the instructional practice implemented in a class. If used as a review question based on the previous class, the teacher can discuss that question and transition into the next lesson. Alternatively, if bell work is used as an open-ended, minds-on question with multiple entry points, it can easily morph into a collaborative task.

Bell work cannot be implemented by displaying a question and then taking it up. Students need anchor charts to support their learning by modeling for them what they should write down. Students need you to check in on them frequently and keep them on task. Students need you to collect data on their thoughts by looking at their work and providing them feedback. Students need you to believe in bell work and ensure they are successful at it—even if that means something as simple as checking that they underlined their work.

Bell work leveraged instructional technique as I could build it into whatever I wanted. It leveraged classroom management via the presence of structure, routine, and consistency. It fostered classroom culture by the one-to-one interactions and the expectation to complete it. And it influenced classroom layout by its sheer presence—you could direct attention simply by the choice of where to project it (my personal favorite is to place it directly opposite of the classroom door). After professional learning on a triangulated approach for assessment (Ontario Ministry of Education, 2010), the formative data that I collected from observing my students' bell work—daily—finally held quantifiable weight.

With the assessment piece in mind, I found that bell work, in tandem with the lesson and goal page, changed the way I viewed teaching. Students who originally demonstrated distaste for the expectation of "instant work," learned to love it and crave it. The consistent transitions provided the structure and routine that students, including those with exceptionalities, needed to be successful, and with the principles of the

Universal Design for Learning, the entire class benefited. It worked, but I had no idea why.

At the 2019 Ontario Association for Mathematics Education mathematics conference, I learned about cognitive load theory (Penfound, 2010) and it suddenly made sense. The inherent structure/routine of the bell work in tandem with the lesson and goal page decreases the load on the student's working memory, leaving space available to use for learning. I like to think of this approach as a proactive discipline—preventive—executed prior to the progressive discipline. However, the bell work and the lesson and goal page only create the backbone of the classroom lesson by supporting transitions. What students do in between those transitions is equally important.

## THE 4 THINGS

During my first long-term occasional teaching contract, I was teaching grades 7/8 in a rotary-based system. (A rotary-based system is where students move throughout the school, teacher to teacher, for 50-minute class blocks through six periods a day.) I taught five different subjects (math, language, science, social studies, and religion) and had one prep period. I remember gratefully taking work from fellow teachers and trying my best to ... well ... teach. One of the teachers advised me to hand out a list of questions, spend one period working on those questions with the students (as a test preparation), and then give those same questions the next day as a test. Interestingly, all of my students failed. This was when I realized that my students lacked the learning skills they needed to study. In conjunction with trying to bring my students success and trying to survive, I developed the 4 things seen in table 6.1. The 4 things were used to explicitly instruct study strategies, and then once finished, they were used to study collaboratively in class.

| "THING" | PURPOSE |
|---------|---------|
| Yellow page | This was a yellow piece of paper that every student had that was their review page. It was meant to house a summary of all concepts learned in the course. |

| Green page | The documentation page seen below is the most recent version. For each concept, students would write down how much (out of 10 dots) they felt they understood. |
| --- | --- |

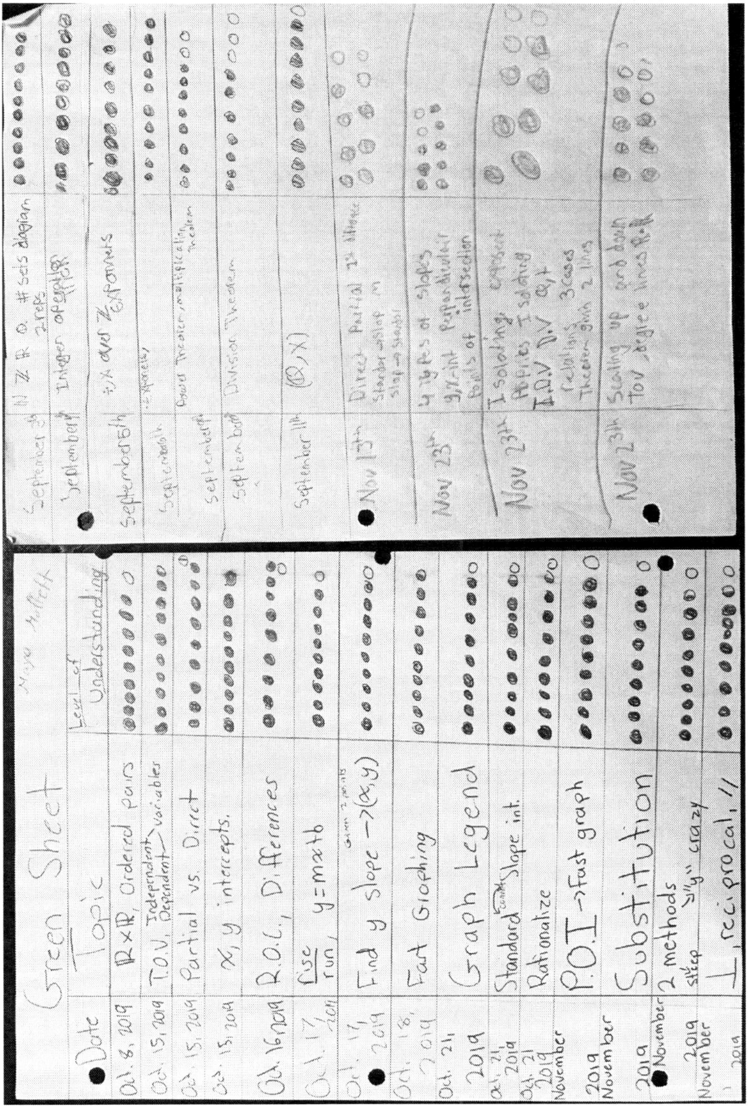

| Cue cards | Each concept in the course would be added to a cue card. |
|-----------|----------------------------------------------------------|

| Definition page | Each definition in the course would be written. |
| --- | --- |

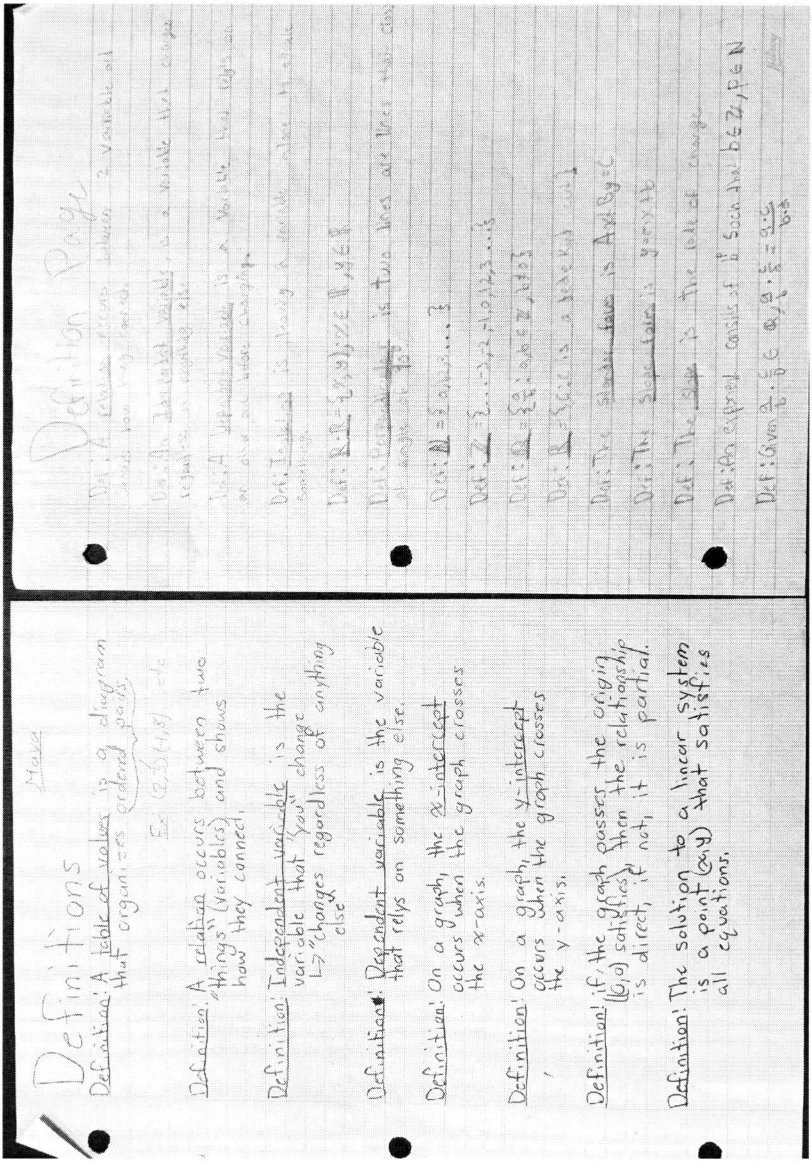

Definitions

Definition: A table of values is a diagram that organizes ordered pairs.

Ex (2,3),(4,8) etc

Definition: A relation occurs between two "things" (variables) and shows how they connect.

Definition: Independent variable is the variable that "you" change → "changes regardless of anything else"

Definition: Dependent variable is the variable that relys on something else.

Definition: On a graph, the x-intercept occurs when the graph crosses the x-axis.

Definition: On a graph, the y-intercept occurs when the graph crosses the y-axis.

Definition: if the graph passes the origin (0,0) satisfies, then the relationship is direct, if not, it is partial.

Definition: The solution to a linear system is a point (x,y) that satisfies all equations.

A digital example:

| Topic: Indicative Sample Set | Topic: Bias |
|---|---|
| Definition: | Definition: |
| | if a sample set refers to inaccurate representation of the population |
| An indicative sample set reflects the population in question | |
| Example: Some students from each grade of a school | |
| | Example: Only Males in one T.O.V And only females in the second T.O.V |

Table 6.1. The 4 things. The students would get the concept list from the 4-things wall/concept wall mentioned in the previous sections.

I worked the 4 things into the routine of my class and required it as part of student learning. For students to be able to engage with the 4 things, it required dedicated class time and explicit instruction on how to complete them. On the day of a formal assessment, the 4 things would be due. Originally, I gave a "bonus" for its completion and "removed" marks for its incompletion. However, a much more effective approach came to me when teaching high school: Integrate it into a portfolio/ end-of-semester rich summative task. Regardless of how I utilized the 4 things, students from grades 7 to 12 all benefited from the strategy. Of course, the approach was differentiated based on the grade and the stream. Nonetheless, the 4 things allowed me to have an additional routine consolidation at any point in time. If students finished their work, whatever it was, they could use the rest of the class time to study with the 4 things strategy. Many students continued using the 4 things as they grew up, but as they figured out their own style for learning, the 4 things turned into 3, then 2, then maybe 1. Regardless of whether or not students used the 4 things in the future, many told me that it gave them a foundation for creating their own study strategy. It was the explicit instruction of studying (with the support to do it) that brought my students success.

The 4 things directly link to instruction, assessment, and classroom management. In a similar way that bell work invokes expectation, the 4 things foster that same supportive pressure and bring safety and success to classroom culture. The problem was that students lost their work. With an idea posed to me by a colleague and some reading on *design thinking*, I realized that I should have a place for all of my students' work to be kept. I labeled some file folders in a filing cabinet with each student's name. Each student now had their own space in my classroom to keep whatever they needed (primarily the 4 things). This idea was extended into portfolios and keeping all students' completed assessments in class for reflection. At the end of the school year, prior to exams/final tasks, students would be given all of their 4 things and assessments back. They would then have the opportunity to create a portfolio and reflect on their progress throughout their learning. Hearing a grade 8 student say, "Sir, I am not proud of this work—look at how much better I am now" is remarkable. The 4 things, in conjunction with all other tools mentioned in this chapter, provided that student the structure he needed to be successful. That same student entered my grade 8 class modified to the grade 5 level and pursued academic classes in grade 9 where he met with success.

## FINAL THOUGHTS

When I left my teacher's education, I wanted the same thing every teacher wants: to help students be successful. In the absence of proper implementation, my passion was meaningless. Bell work, the lesson and goal page, and the 4 things provided a tangible transition piece for my students, allowing me to implement any pedagogical practice I wanted. As long as I used these tools as landmarks throughout the lesson, I could teach.

Figure 6.6 illustrates how my classroom would function daily.

---

What I do in each class:

1. Welcome students in and expect them to engage with bell work right away.
2. Walk around and connect with each student as they are doing bell work.
   a. Provide feedback on bell work (individually) and collect data on student thoughts (based on the bell work question).
3. Take up bell work (as a class or morph into a collaborative task).
4. Everyone would write down the lesson and goal (this may come after if the students are discovering the lesson/goal after the instructional component).
5. The "main action" (walking around, giving feedback, coaching … teaching)
6. Transition
   a. …by having students head back to their desks (if collaborating) with a verbal cue along the lines of, "…head back to your/a seat and write down 3 things that you learned today underneath your bell work from today's class."
      i. Then discuss what we learned and then transition to step 7.
   b. … if students are at their desks, move to step 7.
7. Go to the concept wall (4-things wall) and have students tell me what they learned (these concepts will be added to the 4 things later as a study tool)—students add this to their lesson and goal page.
8. Consolidation (when students finish the planned consolidation, they do their 4 things)
9. 10 dots
   a. Use the information from the 10 dots to inform future teaching, implement the proper intervention, and/or engage in conversations.
10. Dismissal

---

Figure 6.6. The order of "things."

Recently I transitioned into teaching in a virtual environment, and I run my classroom in the exact same way. However, with an asynchronous component, I have the ability to include a daily metacognitive reflection after the 10 dots (with an explanation of next steps and a reflection on engagement), rounding out the entire experience (figure 6.7).

| Date | Write the date of the class. | |
|---|---|---|
| **Session** | AM/PM | |
| **Lesson** | **Goal** | **Concept List** |
| Write the lesson for this session. | Write the goal of this session. | Write down the concepts covered on this day. |
| **Understanding /10** | **What next:**<br><br>How well do you think you understand the concepts from today's class? What are your next steps to take to encourage your learning? | |
| **Engagement /10** | **Why:**<br><br>How well did you engage with your classmates/individually today? Give real examples of what you are proud of and/or where you can improve for the next day. An honest and genuine reflection is what counts | |

Figure 6.7. The virtual lesson/goal page with an asynchronous reflection.

When teaching, I think we need to

1. Accept that students want to learn—despite any resistance—and give them educational tasks to do the moment they enter the classroom space.
2. Show students that they can learn—some don't believe they can—by believing in them and bringing them moments of success.
3. Realize that all students will get lost in transitions. They need us to ground them at each one.
4. Know that the only thing that we control is our timing. Use class time for student learning.

Our classrooms are ever evolving, but if we lack structure in our day-to-day lessons, students cannot learn.

## REFERENCES

Ontario Ministry of Education. (2010). *Growing success: Assessment, evaluation and reporting in Ontario's schools: Covering grades 1 to 12.* Ministry of Education.

Penfound, B. (2019, October 1). *Cognitive load theory* [Conference presentation]. Ontario Association for Mathematics Education.

# RECONCILING PEDAGOGY AND PRACTICE
## ACTION RESEARCH FOR THE EVERYDAY EDUCATOR

**VICTORIA PARENT**

**Victoria Parent is a 10th-grade English teacher in Richmond, Virginia. She holds a BA in English Literature and an MEd in Secondary English from the University of Mary Washington. Victoria is committed to her role as a teacher-researcher and is energized by studying the experiences of marginalized students in public schools, fostering young adult literacy, and revolutionizing writing instruction to empower students beyond the classroom.**

Action research, defined as a "disciplined process of inquiry conducted by and for those taking the action" has been a best practice in education for years, and it is increasingly important today (Sagor, 2000, page 1). Our classrooms are becoming more diverse, emerging best practices for literacy and instruction have improved, and our canonical curriculum is overdue for an overhaul. Systemic change in education rarely occurs from the policy makers and leaders at the top; change occurs when coalitions of experienced classroom teachers and school communities challenge outdated pedagogies through real interventions and collect the evidence to support these changes. Action research, then, becomes not only possible for busy teachers, but also it becomes our professional responsibility.

## PEDAGOGY AT ODDS WITH PRACTICE
During my first few years of teaching, I found myself in one philosophical dilemma after another. The realities of being a classroom teacher were far

more demanding, and at times restrictive, than I had experienced in student teaching. The particular concern that I had was about the curriculum and the subsequent effects it could have on students. I was perplexed over the continued use of antiquated, canonical texts as anchors for our literacy instruction and especially concerned that the stories we were expected to teach were not representative of the lives and experiences of our racially, ethnically, and socioeconomically diverse students. I was troubled by the implications and effects that these curricular decisions could have on our students' sense of identity and belonging in our classrooms.

When there is conflict between what you know is pedagogically best practice and the actual practice that is being implemented, action research can be the avenue to enact an intervention, collect data, and then present your findings to the appropriate individuals in your school and division in order to achieve lasting and meaningful change.

## INQUIRY-DRIVEN RESEARCH

My concerns over the quality of our curriculum and the accessibility of our resources were the beginning of my most recent inquiry-based action research project. I knew that our curriculum was not responsive to or representative of the students in our classes, and I was curious about what effect this would have. I also knew that I was not the first educator or researcher to have this concern, so I dove into the literature.

In my undergraduate and graduate programs, we learned about a pedagogy for teaching and learning called *culturally responsive teaching* (CRT). One of the leading scholars in the field of education and culturally responsive practices, Dr. Gloria Ladson-Billings, was one of our educators in residence and it was a gift to learn from her. CRT "is a pedagogy that recognizes the importance of including students' cultural references in all aspects of learning" (Ladson-Billings, 1994, page 29). Dr. Ladson-Billings defines some of the characteristics of CRT as "positive perspectives on parents and families; communication of high expectations; learning within the context of culture; student-centered instruction; culturally mediated instruction; reshaping the curriculum; and teacher as facilitator" (1994, page 30). As an Asian American woman who has had varying experiences with belonging and alienation as a student, CRT's pedagogy was particularly compelling. I wanted to become an educator who was culturally responsive and helped create meaningful and positive learning experiences for *all* of my students, with consideration for those who have been historically marginalized.

In lieu of a formal literature review, I chose to read several books and articles about CRT to deepen my understanding of the framework and to learn more about the practices and positive effects of implementing this pedagogy. I started with *The Dreamkeepers: Successful Teachers of African American Children* by Gloria Ladson-Billings (2009); I eventually read excerpts from *Culturally Responsive Teaching and the Brain: Promoting Authentic Engagement and Rigor Among Culturally and Linguistically Diverse Students* by Zaretta Hammond (2015) with the research team I began working with; and I was influenced by the article published by Learning for Justice called "A Crooked Seat at the Table: Black and Alone in an Honors Class" by Kiara Lee-Heart (2019).

When getting started with your own action research, reflect on what you've observed in your classroom and determine what you're curious to learn more about. Educators are constantly observing and absorbing the intertwined social and academic tones within their classroom and school communities. We strategically develop seating charts to create safe and focused learning environments, we analyze formative assessments to guide instruction, and we differentiate to meet the social and academic needs of all of our students. All of these seemingly small, everyday observations already drive our decision making. Action research builds on what educators already do in their classrooms to transform our natural observation-based inquiries into accessible research that directly improves our effectiveness.

## WHERE TO BEGIN

Finding a place to start when you have an inquiry can be a major barrier to engaging in the action research process. It's not necessary to conduct a formal literature review prior to each research project, but it is important to take some time to evaluate what's already out there. Evaluating the current research in the field can help you redefine your research question, give you strategies to immediately implement with your students, and even give you a model of a research project that you could duplicate or adapt for your classroom.

When getting started, the following resources can be a great place to start:

## 1) PRACTITIONER BLOGS, PUBLICATIONS, AND ORGANIZATIONS SUCH AS:

- Learning for Justice (formerly Teaching Tolerance)
- Understood.org
- NEA Today
- The National Council for Teachers of English (there's one for each content area!)
- Teach Thought
- ASCD Education Leadership and Educator Update
- Cult of Pedagogy

Since the beginning of my teaching career, I have been inspired, motivated, and informed by reading articles from these resources. Many of these resources are available at no cost, but for some of the professional publications that require subscriptions, such as Education Leadership or NCTE, inquire as to what support your school or district will provide in purchasing these subscriptions for your department or professional learning community (PLC) to share.

Another way to work through the plethora of articles and resources is to create a routine with your department or PLC to read one article a month from a relevant education publisher. There could be months where everyone reads the same article, and others where each colleague reads a different article about a related theme or topic and shares their findings with the group.

## 2) START WITH A BOOK THAT IS RELATED TO YOUR ACTION RESEARCH INTEREST.

- Interested in studying equity-based practices? Try *We Got This: Equity, Access, and the Quest to Be Who Our Students Need Us to Be* by Cornelius Minor (2019).
- Interested in studying classroom conversations about race? Try *Not Light, but Fire: How to Lead Meaningful Race Conversations in the Classroom* by Matthew R. Kay (2018).
- Interested in studying the workshop models, independent reading, and daily routines by master teachers? Try *180 Days: Two Teachers*

*and the Quest to Engage and Empower Adolescents* by Kelly Gallagher and Penny Kittle (2018).

- Interested in studying mindfulness? Try *Mindfulness for Teachers: Simple Skills for Peace and Productivity in the Classroom* by Patricia Jennings and Daniel J. Siegel (2015).

The topics and recommended texts above are just a few of the hot topics within education action research, but there are many more. One of my favorite publishers for high-quality and accessible professional texts is Heinemann. Talk with your PLC at your school and see if your colleagues are interested in starting a book study, or maybe divide up a book into chapters or read excerpts.

## 3) JOIN THE BEST AND MOST ACCESSIBLE PROFESSIONAL DEVELOPMENT NETWORK: TWITTER

Teacher-Twitter is one of my favorite corners of the internet. It is the home to the most accessible and exciting conversations about education, policy, curriculum, and action research. It can provide you with professional connections outside of your school and district; introduce you to books, articles, and podcasts; and help you crowdsource information and think aloud with like-minded individuals when you're stuck with your research and don't know how to move forward.

## ENGAGING IN THE ACTION RESEARCH PROCESS WITH A COMMUNITY

After a year of researching independently, I had the opportunity to join a team of action researchers at my school who were working with an organization called the Metropolitan Education Research Consortium (MERC). MERC is based out of a local university, Virginia Commonwealth University (VCU), and received a grant to study CRT practices and at the larger scale was studying action research teams as a form of professional development.

Through MERC, I connected with teacher-researchers at my school and throughout our region across different schools, grade levels, and content areas. We had monthly meetings and virtual workshops where we would read, discuss, plan, and reflect on topics related to our research goals all under the umbrella of CRT. Having this community was integral to my experience as a teacher-researcher because it deepened my understanding of CRT, provided me with evidence-based research in which to root my practices and my own research, and gave me a professional and supportive community to tackle systemic challenges in our school system.

I narrowed down the topic of my CRT action research to focus on the experiences of students of color in honors classes. My research focus was informed first by what I was observing in my classroom: Students of color were distinct racial minorities in honors-level classes. Were these students aware of the racial differences between themselves and their majority-white classmates? Did this impact how they spoke, acted, and participated in the class? If so, what were the potential effects on their adolescent ethnic-racial identities? Second, the article I read in Learning for Justice informed me of the complicated, and often painful, experiences of racially marginalized students in these elite honors classes. I hypothesized that the students of color in my honors classes would report similar conflicted feelings but would respond positively to a series of CRT interventions, including culturally responsive literature, equitable classroom discussions, and self-selected affinity groups.

Over the course of my research, I primarily relied upon qualitative data collection to gather in-depth testimonies of my students' experiences, perceptions, and feelings of belonging in school. As an English teacher, qualitative data speak to me because these data points contain the nuanced and unique stories of our students, schools, and teachers. I conducted interviews with my students, distributed and analyzed surveys, transcribed and coded classroom discussions looking for trends, and took risks when making my curriculum changes.

Our research group aimed to complete four research cycles over the course of the school year. In my first cycle, I learned that the students of color whom I interviewed had some negative emotions with regard to feelings of belonging in the honors classroom. They were grossly aware of racial dynamics, particularly racial tension, in the classroom; they had experienced racial microaggressions as minority students in their classes; and they would code-switch and were overly cognizant of their behaviors to avoid slipping into negative stereotypes in these spaces. Curriculum-wise, they *noticed* and *appreciated* when the curriculum was representative of speakers, scholars, poets, and authors who were racially diverse. Many reported growing tired of always reading and learning about one demographic, white people, in their English classes. I was thrilled to hear the positive feedback about the culturally responsive texts, but I was also saddened and frustrated. These results confirmed what I suspected: Our curriculum and classroom environments were not holistically evolving to meet the needs of our diverse students, and the majority of our students of color did not wholeheartedly feel a sense of belonging in our program. As teachers and leaders in our school, when this suspected information is confirmed, we have an obligation and responsibility to address it.

In my second cycle, I tackled creating equitable classroom discussions where all students were engaged and felt valued in the discourse. I hypothesized that if students were given the option to prepare for a formal discussion in small groups, minority students may self-select racial affinity groups, which would be indicative of an increased level of comfort and sense of belonging in those spaces. As I hypothesized, students self-selected racial affinity groups and had productive conversations in their small groups, which led to increased levels of participation in the formal whole-class discussion that was later conducted. This cycle taught me the significance of allowing our students to have self-selected safe spaces, which can sometimes be determined over ethnic and racial identities. When students had the opportunity to practice for a formal discussion in a safe space, they were more engaged in discussion and there was increased equity in the participation from students. One of the most compelling emergent findings from this cycle was that students of color were more likely to make real-world connections when discussing race, inequity, and injustice, whereas other students kept the discussion and analysis closer to the events from the book they were discussing.

In my third and final research cycle, I culminated my action research study by assessing how my students had grown from the beginning of the school year. I went back to journal entries from the beginning of the school year and coded them to measure their level of critical consciousness, which is "the ability to recognize and analyze systems of inequality and the commitment to take action against these systems" (El-Amin et al., 2020, para. 1). Through coding, which is essentially annotating for themes, their writing from the beginning of the year, I had a baseline to compare to their final reflection assignments after studying systemic and social injustices within literature and in modern society over the year. I was pleased to see that the majority of my students demonstrated growth by the end of the school year. The collective growth in critical consciousness could also potentially strengthen community ties and feelings of safety within our classroom of diverse students, which was a byproduct I had hoped for.

At times, it felt ambitious to complete this many research cycles, especially as we juggled our primary teaching duties. When conducting your classroom research, you can adapt the research process to meet your needs. It is more important to participate in the recursive process of asking questions, implementing an intervention, collecting data, and reflecting on that data than it is to rigidly follow a cookie-cutter plan for research. Just as we differentiate delivery instruction and assessments for our students, you can differentiate the action research process for yourself.

## THE RIPPLE EFFECTS OF ACTION RESEARCH

The findings from my previous research cycles provided me with school-based evidence to share with colleagues within and outside of my department, and with our administrators. Also, because of the team of action researchers at my school collecting data from their projects, we have a wealth of evidence to support a schoolwide effort to implement CRT. Now, CRT has become an ongoing topic for our school-based professional development, largely thanks to the work of the MERC team at our school advocating for its positive impact on students.

Our school's renewed commitment to CRT and ensuring positive experiences for *all* of our students is incredible, but the most worthwhile effect of this research has been the relationships that I've cultivated with my students along the way. When I interviewed some of my kids to inquire about their experiences in school thus far, several of them shared that no teacher had ever asked them to reflect and articulate their experiences as racial-ethnic minorities before.

My students reported feeling safe and that they felt like they belonged in my classroom, not solely because of the CRT practices I was implementing but because of the educator and person CRT had helped me become. My research allowed me to understand and see my students holistically and as individuals, which should be every teacher's goal.

## CONCLUSION

Action research is the gateway to change in our education system. It empowers educators, students, and communities; it is worth every bit of time, energy, and effort. To help you get started, remember the following:

- Create a culture of action research within your community: It is necessary to cultivate a professional culture in your workplace that is committed to learning about relevant research and evidence-based practices. When possible, create a team of action researchers at your school to study some of the pertinent education topics in your classrooms, or work within your department and PLC to establish routines for regularly reading newly published research in the field.

- Evaluate your existing action research practices: Learning the process for action research and practicing it over time is imperative to growing into a confident and effective teacher-researcher. Most teachers already use action research practices in their classrooms! Learning the structure and terminology provides a common language and understanding for sharing your research and findings with other professionals.

- Finally, embrace this work as a professional responsibility: Redefine yourself as a *teacher-researcher*. The teacher-researcher identity affirms our roles as professionals who navigate, grow, and lead within our connected webs of schools and society; it reinforces the notion that our work in the classroom can have larger implications that shift and redefine pedagogies, practices, and student outcomes. Embracing the teacher-researcher identity has revived my passion for education and sustained my belief in the professional nature of teaching.

## REFERENCES

El-Amin, A., Seider, S., Graves, D., Tamerat, J., Clark, S., Soutter, M., Johannsen, J., & Malhotra, S. (2020, December 10). Critical consciousness: A key to student achievement. *Kappanonline.org.* https://kappanonline.org/critical-consciousness-key-student-achievement/

Gallagher, K., & Kittle, P. (2018). *180 days: Two teachers and the quest to engage and empower adolescents.* Heinemann.

Hammond, Z. (2015). *Culturally responsive teaching and the brain: Promoting authentic engagement and rigor among culturally and linguistically diverse students.* Corwin.

Jennings, P. A., & Siegel, D. J. (2015). *Mindfulness for teachers: Simple skills for peace and productivity in the classroom.* W.W. Norton.

Kay, M. R. (2018). *Not light, but fire: How to lead meaningful race conversations in the classroom.* Stenhouse.

Ladson-Billings, G. (1994). The dreamkeepers: Successful teachers of African American children (1st ed.). Jossey-Bass.

Ladson-Billings, G. (2009). *The dreamkeepers: Successful teachers of African American children* (2nd ed.). John Wiley & Sons.

Lee-Heart, K. (2019, October 1). *A crooked seat at the table: Black and alone in an honors class.* www.learningforjustice.org/magazine/a-crooked-seat-at-the-table-black-and-alone-in-an-honors-class

Minor, C. (2019). *We got this: Equity, access, and the quest to be who our students need us to be.* Heinemann.

Sagor, R. (2000). *Guiding school improvement with action research.* Association for Supervision and Curriculum Development.

# LESSONS FROM THE FIELD
## MOBILIZING RESEARCH IN ONTARIO EDUCATION

**SOFYA MALIK**

Dr. Sofya Malik began her career as a public-school teacher at the second largest school board in Canada, where she later served as Chief Research Officer. Over the course of her career, Sofya has collaborated with educational leaders, educators, community groups, school boards, universities, government, and nonprofit organizations to build capacity for the improved use of research to effectively inform strategy, evaluation, and impact. Sofya earned a PhD in Educational Leadership and Policy at the Ontario Institute for Studies in Education (OISE), where she is an Assistant Professor, Teaching Stream. She holds a BA Honours from the University of Toronto, a Bachelor of Education from Queen's University, and Master of Education from the University of Ottawa.

This chapter describes insights and approaches to using research evidence in applied research settings. Included is a framework for understanding knowledge mobilization (KMb) and lessons learned from research conducted in Ontario education organizations. Using evidence from the field, I define KMb as the active and dynamic process whereby stakeholders such as researchers, practitioners, policy makers, and educators share, create, and use research evidence to inform programming, policy, decision making, and practice.

## BACKGROUND AND INTEREST

My interest in KMb began early in my career as an education researcher. As Research and Community Coordinator for the federally funded

Understanding the Early Years Malton (UEY Malton) project, I designed and implemented a KMb plan in a socioeconomically vulnerable community in the Malton neighborhood of Mississauga, Ontario. As the project sponsor, the Peel District School Board (PDSB) was one of 16 communities across Canada in its cohort managing the project's activities. The main goals of the project were to transfer knowledge and insights from research to the Malton community, to facilitate the use of evidence for decision making at the community level, and to build community capacity with the overall aim of developing sustainable neighborhood supports for children and families (Favaro & Malik, 2010; Malik, 2009). In collaboration with the PDSB team, local service providers, and a community coalition, I developed research-based products (e.g., parent toolkits), organized events (e.g., community forums), developed networks with service providers and community agencies (e.g., informal and formal partnerships), and provided capacity-building opportunities (e.g., workshops for community members, families, educators, and school board staff). The experience was my first foray into the field of KMb as I worked closely with diverse education stakeholders to develop KMb products and tools.

Although the project team consistently made concerted efforts to produce evidence, disseminate research, and collaborate with community members, little is known about the impact of the UEY Malton project activities. External research consultants conducted surveys and focus groups to learn about community, service provider, and educator experiences with the project. However, it remains unclear what was done with the results of those findings to apply the lessons learned. This is largely because once the project funding ended, the support of the project sponsor was minimal and the ability for the community to carry forward recommendations from the research was too great to take on with limited resources. Apart from funding and resources, stronger capacity-building efforts were needed to use the research findings to carry out the recommendations of the project. From the UEY Malton project, I learned about the importance of building trust, relationships, and capacity among community members to facilitate evidence-informed policy and programming.

In my work as Senior Knowledge Mobilization Coordinator and Project Lead at the Ontario Ministry of Education, I collaborated with provincial partners in a multi-year endeavor to improve KMb efforts across Ontario. The Knowledge Network for Applied Education Research (KNAER) exemplified efforts to build KMb partnerships between and among different kinds of education organizations such as school boards, universities, and nonprofit organizations. Although different in composition, these projects used a range of community-based strategies to engage different partners (e.g., service providers, universities, school boards) in mobilizing target audiences to use research findings. From the KNAER project, I learned that while educators are engaging in KMb efforts, these efforts are largely uncoordinated with varying understandings and misconceptions about KMb, and limited understandings about what actually works in a long-term, sustainable way.

As program manager of the Research Supporting Practice in Education (RSPE) KMb program during my doctoral studies at OISE, I managed projects with active efforts to bridge the frequently acknowledged cultural gap between the academic and practice worlds. As part of my work on the Elementary Teachers' Federation of Ontario (ETFO) Research for Teachers project, I coordinated plain-language summaries and podcasts with renowned scholars on a range of current educational issues. All in all, the aforementioned experiences gave me first-hand insight into considerable research-informed efforts across the province as well as the gap between the "rhetoric of evidence-based policy and what happens on the ground" (Nutley et al., 2007, 8).

My interest in research use has evolved from my early career as a teacher in the PDSB, and through all my subsequent roles in the education sector. In my current role as Chief Research Officer at the PDSB, I work with a team of researchers and collaborate with school district leaders, administrators, community members, and educators to facilitate the use of "big data" to improve the use of research to inform school success planning with the ultimate goal of reducing achievement gaps and improving well-being, equity, and outcomes for all students. My field experience coupled with evidence from my research conducted in education organizations provide me with insights into KMb lessons discussed in this chapter.

## A FRAMEWORK FOR KNOWLEDGE MOBILIZATION IN EDUCATION ORGANIZATIONS

The conceptual framework from my research on education organizations (Malik, 2020) in figure 8.1 builds on the knowledge transfer strategy of Lavis et al. (2003). Five questions guide the conceptual framework for understanding KMb in Ontario education organizations: 1) Why are the organizations engaging in KMb? (purpose); 2) What knowledge are they producing? (evidence production); 3) Who are the organizations seeking to engage through their KMb efforts? (target audiences); 4) How are organizations engaging in KMb? (products, events, networks, and capacity building [PEN-C], and mediation strategies); 5) What are the implications of these efforts? (impact and challenges). The KMb approaches to these dimensions vary according to contextual factors such as the organizational mission, organizational context, organizational capacity, and social and political context (Malik, 2020). Appendix 1 includes definitions of the key terms found in the conceptual framework.

From the literature, numerous concerns are evident about the research–policy–practice divides in the public sector with unclear solutions about how to mitigate this gap. For example, although widely acknowledged as an essential function of KMb, mediation functions continue to be an underexplored area within KMb (Cooper, 2012; Sin, 2008; Tseng, 2012).

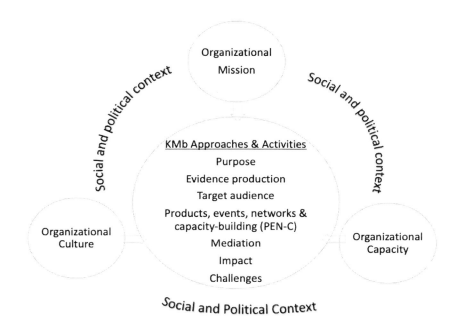

Figure 8.1. Conceptual framework of education organizations engaging in knowledge mobilization (KMb) in Ontario.

## WHAT ARE THE BARRIERS?

As a secondary school French as a Second Language and English teacher in Ontario and abroad, I worked with diverse learners in a variety of school communities. For me, the demands of teaching were all-consuming, and any interest in research was trumped by my daily pressures of lesson planning, assessments, administrative duties, and classroom management. Peer-to-peer sharing was the most common way for the teaching staff to develop strategies and use resources.

However, educators are facing increasing pressure to use data to inform their practices and improve the organization, particularly in times of diminishing resources (Brown et al., 2017; Farrell, 2015). Capacity-building efforts in school districts focus on supporting school administrators in understanding and using data for decision making mainly at the local school level and less so on educators directly.

Commonly cited barriers to research use by practitioners include teachers' own lack of expertise and capacity to acquire, interpret, and apply research; time constraints; and the volume of research evidence available (Nelson & Kohlmoos, 2009). Teachers have expressed a need for brief reports written in nontechnical language, suggesting they were more likely to use research evidence if it was introduced to them or approved by trusted, "unbiased" intermediaries, such as professional organizations, partners, coalitions, networks, peers, and constituents.

Several other studies (Caplan, 1979; Galway, 2011; Honig & Coburn, 2008; Nutley et al., 2007; Serenko et al., 2007; Tseng, 2012) cite numerous barriers that may inhibit KMb processes. Some of the more commonly cited challenges include the divide between researchers and practitioners, limited fiscal resources, KMb not being considered an organizational priority, and a lack of consensus about the meaning of KMb. Understanding these challenges can lead to the development of better strategies to improve KMb efforts in organizations.

Moreover, the issue of trust is a recurring challenge. Coburn et al. (2013) argued that developing and maintaining trust challenges research-to-practice partnerships, such as in relationships between and among research organizations and schools or school districts. In other cases, school district leaders criticized researchers for promising to share research findings and failing to follow up with those findings. The concerns from other studies also indicate perceptions among practitioners that research evidence may be manipulated to suit certain social and political agendas (Nutley et al., 2007; Tseng, 2012; Weiss et al., 2005).

## HOW DO YOU SUCCESSFULLY MOVE RESEARCH INTO PRACTICE?

While reflecting on the multi-pronged approaches to KMb in education organizations, I share the following key recommendations about how systems and structures can support the movement of research into practice:

- Cultivate organizational culture and leadership infrastructure that support research use.
- Build relationships among knowledge brokers, intermediaries, partners, and networks.

- Develop, define, and measure impact.

I discuss each of these recommendations below with consideration from evidence and practice.

### Cultivate organizational culture and leadership infrastructure that support research use.

The social and political context influences the organizational processes in their entirety. These factors may include technological developments, the legal system, changes in government, and public beliefs about KMb practice (Levin, 2012). Although dedicated leadership is essential to supporting KMb at the top levels of organizations, simultaneously cultivating distributed leadership is essential. According to Northouse (2016), "distributed leadership involves the sharing of influence by team members" (390). Distributed leadership can facilitate engagement throughout the system by building capacity to share, understand, and use research at different levels. In this way, engagement at all levels of the system can occur, as Campbell (2014, para 7), asserts:

It is important to cultivate distributed leadership to engage people throughout the education system, government, provincial partners, and research and stakeholder communities in the development, valuing, understanding and use of research and other evidence for educational improvement.

Distributed leadership has been found to have more consensus, trust, and cohesion than teams without shared leadership (Bergman et al., 2012). I suggest that both dedicated and distributed leadership ought to be seen as complementary rather than mutually exclusive in order to promote a wider reach and buy-in among stakeholders.

Furthermore, valuing research services and departments in an organization can influence the culture of research evidence.

A central structural feature, first, is about whether a research department or even a department with a dedicated KMb function exists. Second, the reporting structure influences the value placed on KMb in the organization. An informant from the largest school board in Canada (Malik, 2016) expounded on the virtues of research in the organization:

I think that what I would say is that you have to put Research and Information Services as the prime, a key area to priority and stature in the organization. It has to be arms-length and separate from other departments so that they can be seen as a critical friend, a guide with constructive direction and that to the CEO that piece there in terms of the department must be seen as something that the CEO can access readily and challenge assumptions readily. You have to invest in it. You have to give it a platform.

These observations from the Malik (2016) study of education organizations highlight the investment required not only in the structural processes but also in the open dialogue and information flow encouraged within the school board.

### Build relationships among knowledge brokers, intermediaries, partners, and networks.

Many scholars suggest that knowledge brokers and intermediary organizations play an important role in influencing research uptake (Cooper, 2012; Davies & Nutley, 2008; Levin, 2012; Nutley et al., 2007; Tseng et al., 2007). Sin (2008) provides an insightful theory for understanding intermediaries, in particular the role of cross-pollinators, with connections to many sectors that can often leverage opportunities to share useful information within and across sectors. By understanding the different kinds of mediation functions, it becomes possible to identify intermediary functions, strengths, weaknesses, and areas for improvement.

In general, schools and school districts have a particularly weak capacity to find, share, and apply research to practice (Coburn & Talbert, 2006; Sheppard et al., 2013). Findings from studies on school district uses of research suggest that practices need to strongly align with the district purpose and vision for using the data to improve student outcomes (Honig & Coburn, 2008; Wohlstetter et al., 2008). School boards predominantly engage in research related to school-based data and student achievement. Capacity-building efforts tend to center on building capacity for school administrators to understand and use data for decision making at the local school level. Attempts to implement evidence-based reforms are often highly vulnerable to traditional hierarchical and highly political practices (Datnow, 2000).

Altogether, efforts to engage teachers in research use continue to pose ongoing challenges even when KMb is a priority endeavor for the board. The daily challenges of administrative and curricular tasks can overtake dedicated time and resources needed toward the deep collaboration required for effective and collaborative evidence use for decision making.

## Develop, define, and measure impact.

Because KMb happens in instrumental, conceptual, and symbolic ways, there are also multiple ways of measuring impact. Conceptual use, according to Nutley et al. (2007), relates to the complex, indirect ways that research changes ways of thinking, alerting policy makers to an issue, or general "consciousness-raising" (36). Instrumental use refers to specific pieces of research use and the "direct impact of research on policy and practice decisions" (Nutley et al., 2007, 36). Symbolic use refers to ways of using research to validate preexisting notions or suppositions (Nutley et al., 2007). Understanding research use in its various forms can inform how impact is measured.

Many scholars acknowledge the shortcomings of impact measurement and the highly complex and intangible nature of tracing research use (Malik, 2020). Keeping impact and successful strategies at the forefront is key, as an informant (see Malik, 2016) at the Ontario College of Teachers suggested:

> What are we doing? What research is out there? What is informing practice and keep that on the agenda and connecting those various communities? We have individuals who are researchers. We have individuals whose research would have a real impact. I think continuing to connect those groups is key in looking for the natural networks where that can happen is a strong element.

However, the aspects of what research to mobilize, to whom, and for what impact are riddled with tensions in the KMb field. These tensions are augmented by a general lack of understanding about impact measurement.

Research impact is the overall goal of KMb efforts and it occurs when research evidence is used in practice (Davies & Nutley, 2008; Knott & Wildavsky, 1980). The UK's Teaching and Learning Research Program defines impact in the following way: "We conceive of impact not as a simple linear flow but as a much more collaborative process: interactive, iterative, constructive, distributive and transformative" (Pollard, 2010, 30). This definition reflects the complexity of measuring impact and the importance of collaborative processes. Davies and Nutley

(2008) define impact as "how and where research-based knowledge gets used by policymakers and practitioners and the consequences (i.e., impacts) of that use" (3). In particular, Davies and Nutley (2008) call for a greater focus on the conceptual and enlightenment (see Weiss, 1979) functions of research use when examining organizations. Scholars widely acknowledge the challenges of measuring impact and recognize the limitations of seeing the immediate impact of research use.

## CONCLUSION

During the past decade, there has been a growing interest worldwide in the ways in which organizations incorporate research evidence into policy and practice (Burns & Schuller, 2007; Cooper et al., 2009; Nutley et al., 2007; Qi & Levin, 2013). The strong interest in the betterment of our education systems drives concerns for a greater reliance on research for decision making and practice. There is increasing pressure on educators, policy makers, and government officials to manage and allocate their resources in a way that maximizes the effectiveness of research knowledge.

When considering research-informed teaching, district leaders hold the responsibility for creating the conditions for success for what is practical and possible to implement. First, consultative processes with teachers, parents, and students can guide effective, collaborative decision-making processes. This often requires open dialogue about research evidence, regardless of what the findings suggest, with the common aim of reducing gaps and improving student achievement, well-being, and equity outcomes. Second, engaging and accessible ways of communicating and disseminating research evidence with the public can contribute to the sharing, uptake, and use of research. Finally, knowledge brokering processes across disciplines, communities, and partners require greater active efforts with user audiences in mind.

Altogether, research-informed practice realizes greater success when incorporating collaborative processes and understandings of research use in user communities (Davies & Nutley, 2008). Although the proposed areas sound practical, the actual prioritization and implementation require intentional efforts, values, and resources.

## TOP TIPS FOR DISTRICT LEADERS: RESEARCH-INFORMED PRACTICE

- Support experienced teachers to participate in data literacy learning and opportunities;
- Implement dedicated and distributed leadership cultivating teacher professional learning and exemplary practices; and
- Facilitate knowledge exchange for relationship building across schools, districts, and partnerships.

## TOP TIPS FOR TEACHERS: RESEARCH-INFORMED PRACTICE

- Understand processes and systems to develop agency in finding and applying research evidence;
- Be active in understanding your role as a change agent using evidence to inform classroom practice; and
- Seek opportunities for cross-pollination to engage more broadly with other educators, system leaders, and education partners.

## REFERENCES

Bergman, J. Z., Rentsch, J. R., Small, E. E., Davenport, S. W., & Bergman, S. M. (2012). The shared leadership process in decision-making teams. *The Journal of Social Psychology, 152*(1), 17–42.

Brown, C., Schildkamp, K., & Hubers, M. D. (2017). Combining the best of two worlds: A conceptual proposal for evidence-informed school improvement. *Educational Research, 59*(2), 154–172.

Campbell, C. (2014, October 8). Navigating the road ahead: (Re)visioning Alberta's approach to evidence-informed educational improvement. *Alberta Teachers' Association Magazine, 95.*

Caplan, N. (1979). The two-communities theory of knowledge utilization. *American Behavioural Scientist, 22*(3), 459–470.

Coburn, C. E., Penuel, W. R., & Geil, K. E. (2013). *Research-practice partnerships: A strategy for leveraging research for educational improvement in school districts.* W.T. Grant Foundation.

Coburn, C., & Talbert, J. (2006). Conceptions of evidence use in school districts: Mapping the terrain. *American Journal of Education, 112,* 469-495.

Cooper, A. (2012). *Knowledge mobilization intermediaries in education: A cross-case analysis of 44 Canadian organizations* [Doctoral dissertation, University of Toronto]. https://hdl.handle.net/1807/32688

Cooper, A., Levin, B., & Campbell, C. (2009). The growing (but still limited) importance of evidence in education policy and practice. *Journal of Educational Change, 10*(2-3), 159-171.

Davies, H., & Nutley, S. (2008). *Learning more about how research-based knowledge gets used: Guidance in the development of new empirical research.* William T. Grant Foundation.

Datnow, A. (2000). Power and politics in the adoption of school reforms. *Educational Evaluation and Policy Analysis, 22*(4), 357-374.

Favaro, P., & Malik, S. (2010). *Malton on the move: Report to the community.* Peel Board Printing Services.

Farrell, C. C. (2015). Designing school systems to encourage data use and instructional improvement: A comparison of school districts and charter management organizations. *Educational Administration Quarterly, 51*(3), 438-471.

Galway, G. (2011). From the bureaucracy to the academy: Reflections on two communities. *The Morning Watch – Educational and Social Analysis, 38*(3-4).

Honig, M. I., & Coburn, C. (2008). Evidence-based decision making in school district central offices: Toward a policy and research agenda. *Educational Policy, 22*(4), 578-608.

Knott, J., & Wildavsky, A. (1980). If dissemination is the solution, what is the problem? *Science Communication, 1*, 537–578.

Lavis, J. N., Robertson, D., Woodside, J. M., McLeod, C. B., & Abelson, J. (2003). How can research organizations more effectively transfer research knowledge to decision makers? *Milbank Quarterly, 81*(2), 221-248.

Levin, B. (2012). To know is not enough. *Review of Education, 1*(1), 2-13.

Malik, S. (2009). *Knowledge mobilization report: Understanding the Early Years Malton.* Peel Board Printing Services.

Malik, S. (2016). *Knowledge mobilization in Ontario: A multi-case study of education organizations* [Unpublished doctoral thesis]. University of Toronto.

Malik, S. (2020). Knowledge mobilization for impact: A multi-case study of education organizations. *International Journal of Education Policy & Leadership, 16*(6). https://journals.sfu.ca/ijepl/index.php/ijepl/article/view/945

Northouse, P. G. (2016). *Leadership: Theory and practice* (7th ed.). Thousand Oaks, CA: Sage.

Nutley, S., Walter, I., & Davies, H. (2007). *Using evidence: How research can inform public services.* Policy Press.

Owens, R. G., & Valesky, T. C. (2011). *Organizational behavior in education: Leadership and school reform* (10th ed.). Pearson.

Pollard, A. (2010). Directing the teaching and learning research programme or 'Trying to fly a glider made of jelly.' *British Journal of Educational Studies, 58*(1), 27–46.

Qi, J., & Levin, B. (2013). Assessing organizational efforts to mobilize research knowledge in education. *Education Policy Analysis Archives, 21*(2). https://doi.org/10.14507/epaa.v21n2.2013

Sá, C., Li, S., & Faubert, B. (2011). Faculties of education and institutional strategies for knowledge mobilization: An exploratory study. *Higher Education, 61*(5), 501-512.

Serenko, A., Bontis, N., & Hardie, T. (2007). Organizational size and knowledge flow: A proposed theoretical link. *Journal of Intellectual Capital, 8*(4), 610–627.

Shaxson, L., Bielak, A., Ahmed, I., Brien, D., Conant, B., Fisher, C., ... Pant, L. (2012). *Expanding our understanding of K\* (KT, KE, KTT, KMb, KB, KM, etc.). A concept paper emerging from the K\* conference held in Hamilton, Ontario, Canada, April 2012.* Hamilton, Canada: UNU-INWEH.

Sheppard, B., Galway, G., Wiens, J., & Brown, J. (2013). School boards matter: Report from the pan-Canadian study of school board governance. Canadian School Boards Association.

Sin, C. H. (2008). The role of intermediaries in getting evidence into policy and practice: Some useful lessons from examining consultancy–client relationships. *Evidence & Policy, 4*(1), 85–103.

Tseng, V. (2012, Summer). Sharing child and youth development: The uses of research in policy and practice. *Social Policy Report, 26*(2), 1–24.

Tseng, V., Granger, R., Seidman, E., Maynard, R., Weisner, T., & Wilcox, B. (2007). *Studying the use of research evidence in policy and practice.* The William T. Grant Foundation.

Weiss, C. H. (1979). The many meanings of research utilization. *Public Administration Review, 39*(5), 426–431.

Weiss, C. H., Murphy-Graham, E., & Birkeland, S. (2005). An alternate route to policy influence: How evaluations affect D.A.R.E. *American Journal of Evaluation, 26*(1), 12–30.

Wohlstetter, P., Datnow, A., & Park, V. (2008). Creating a system for data-driven decision making: Applying the principal-agent framework. *School Effectiveness and School Improvement, 19*(3), 239–259.

## APPENDIX 1

Table 8.1. Definition of terms in conceptual framework

| TERM | DEFINITION |
|---|---|
| Organizational mission | The mission is the long-term objective and overall reason for the organization's existence. |
| Organizational capacity | Capacity is about the roles, structures, routines, resources, and internal processes of an organization. |
| Organizational culture | Culture refers to the norms, assumptions, and beliefs of an organization (Owens & Valesky, 2011). |
| Social and political context | Social and political context is about the external societal and political pressures that influence the way organizations operate. |
| Knowledge mobilization (KMb) purpose | The KMb purpose is about why the organization is engaging in KMb efforts. The purpose may be to share knowledge among individuals, co-produce knowledge, draw knowledge into an organization, and disseminate knowledge (Shaxson et al., 2012). |
| Evidence production | Evidence production is what knowledge the organization aims to mobilize. Evidence is the empirical data collected by organizations. |
| Target audience | Target audiences are the end users whom organizations seek to engage through their KMb approaches and activities. |
| PEN-C | Products, events, networks, and capacity building are the main aspects of organizational KMb strategies (Cooper, 2012; Sá et al., 2012). |
| Mediation | Mediation activities occur through multiple means, such as through the creation, translation, sharing, and understanding of research-based evidence (Sin, 2008). |
| Impact | Impact is about measuring whether and to what extent intentional KMb efforts are reaching target audiences to influence policy and/or practice. |
| Challenges | Challenges are defined as any barriers to KMb processes. |

# BECOMING A SECOND LANGUAGE ACQUISITION RESEARCH-INFORMED TEACHER

## BILL LANGLEY

**Bill is a middle school and high school Spanish teacher. He has a bachelor's and a master's in world language education and is currently pursuing his PhD in Educational Leadership from Miami University (Oxford, Ohio) while also in the classroom full time, leading professional development at state, regional, and national language teacher conferences. He is also in the Chair track for the Comprehension-Based Communicative Language Teaching Special Interest Group of the American Council for the Teaching of Foreign Language (ACTFL).**

If our goal for our language learners is to develop communicative ability in a new language, it is important that we as language teachers enact best practices in our classroom based on second language acquisition (SLA) research. There is so much that the research can tell us not only about how humans learn language, but also tips that can make our day-to-day teaching lives more manageable by helping us let go of preconceived notions

In the research that I have read, I have learned that teaching a language is not the same as teaching any other class. History, science, literature classes, and so forth, are concerned with teaching subject matter and skills; in other words, transferring knowledge from the teacher to the learner. In history class, for example, learners focus on content and analytical skills because they already know the language in which the instruction is provided. They are there to learn about history and to learn from it. However, in a language class, ability with the language is the object, not knowing about language. As language teachers, we aren't trying to teach facts about language that learners can later recite; we are trying to develop our learners' communicative ability, giving them opportunities to process and acquire language so they may communicate across a wide array of topics, subjects, and time frames. In a language class, we focus on language first so that learners can acquire new information through language. We teach intercultural skills, we make connections to other content areas, and we learn about the world around us. Building language to learn about those topics is at the core of our classes.

Becoming an SLA research-informed language teacher implies a number of different things. It means that we have a foundation of how languages are learned as well as general pedagogy. It means that we have developmentally reasonable expectations when assessing learner performance, and we know that when we create language learning activities, we are enacting best practices that encourage language acquisition. Thus, becoming a research-informed language teacher starts with understanding what language is and how it is learned, and that knowledge then trickles into instructional strategies and assessment techniques.

## RESEARCH-INFORMED INSTRUCTIONAL PRACTICES

Many scholars agree that comprehensible input (language that contains messages spoken or written in a way such that learners understand those messages) is a key ingredient in developing learners' communicative ability (Krashen, 1981; Lichtman, 2018; Mason & Krashen, 2004). Whether or not comprehensible input is the only necessary ingredient to language learning is a question that many teachers have, and it deserves attention. I implore the reader of this chapter to investigate methods and approaches that focus on input yet still align with their beliefs of what a language class looks like. Ellis and colleagues (2002) discuss that focus on form (i.e., focusing on form as it relates to meaning in context, rather than explicit practice of grammatical forms) might be necessary to improve accuracy of language even though communicative ability can only be acquired by engaging in communicative experiences. Waltz's (2015) solution to this possible need of attention to form is to use "pop-up" grammar, very brief grammatical explanations that support the meaning of the input. An example of pop-up grammar would be if I use the word "caminó" in class I would very quickly draw attention to the accented *o* and tell learners that the "-ó" tells us the action is in the past. We can also draw attention to form by using input enhancement (Sharwood Smith, 1993) using word-processor editing or different prosody when speaking. However, Lichtman's analysis of research shows that learners in classrooms that employ input-based strategies, such as Teaching Proficiency through Reading and Storytelling (TPRS), performed just as well or better than learners in grammar-centered classrooms on grammatical accuracy, vocabulary acquisition, and reading and writing skills. Printer (2021) has done action research on the motivational pull of TPRS with learners, which could aid teachers in their decision to include TPRS-style strategies in their repertoire of instructional strategies. Printer used a lens of self-determination theory (SDT) to gauge the motivational pull of comprehension-based methods, finding that they can meet the different tenets of SDT, which help learners feel motivated to develop their autonomy, relatedness, and competence. Taking this research into consideration can help teachers select methods and approaches to language teaching that fits their personality and upholds research-based practices.

In considering comprehensible input as a key ingredient in language learning, we can develop activities and strategies that engage learners in the language learning mechanisms responsible for acquisition (Waltz, 2015). There is a plethora of online resources such as demonstration videos and step-by-step instructions on activities that center input while focusing on learner interests and personalization. (Shameless plug, I discuss a lot of different activities on my blog, hhttp://languageley. wordpress.com, and link to other creative, research-interested teachers.)

Another topic discussed in the field of SLA is that of interaction. Input and interaction are often paired in the research, and the two can be used as a lens to examine our lesson plans. Interaction helps us make input comprehensible by drawing learners' attention to specific parts of the input. Interaction can be anything that allows learners to do something with language that they have comprehended. Learners interact when teachers ask questions to clarify the content of what is being said or read, when they search a text for specific information, or when they attempt to produce language (Swain, 1985). All of these ways of interacting with language give teachers an opportunity to expand on learners' language or to engage in formative assessment to observe what input is being comprehended and what input is incomprehensible.

Although learner interaction with language users is important, the teacher's interaction with a learner's language is also important. A practice supported by research that may help teachers reclaim their personal time and provide a better work–life balance is putting down the red pen when grading compositions. A lot of language teachers tend to correct every mistake a learner makes in their writing, which can take countless hours to do when you have, like I do, 150 learners. Truscott (1996) makes a case against grammar correction as a means of pushing learners to higher levels of accuracy, which should bring a sigh of relief to all those who have felt they bring too much grading home. Although Truscott makes the case that grammar correction is not effective, that is not to say that no feedback should be given on learner work. In a small study, Semke (1984) suggested that learners got better at writing and were encouraged to write more when the teacher gave content comments only rather than marking errors. In doing this kind of content feedback, teachers can focus on communication to see if the learner is expressing meaning in an appropriate way or when that meaning is not clear, and the teacher can use this as an opportunity to learn more about their learners and make important connections with a learner on a more personal level.

## RESEARCH-INFORMED ASSESSMENT
An SLA research-informed language teacher will have reasonable expectations of what learners can do. Lightbown (1985) argues that making reasonable expectations for learner performance is exactly what language teachers should take from the research. In her piece titled *Great Expectations*, Lightbown lays out 10 generalizations about SLA research and the role that research plays in language teaching. Among her generalizations are three points derived from a much larger pool of research that can give us a better understanding of what we can expect from learners and thus assess learning in a more research-aligned way.

One of the generalizations that aids us in how we assess learners involves sequences of acquisition. That is, some language features have a clear and predictable order in which they develop. For example, VanPatten (2010) lays out a predictable four-stage sequence of the development of Spanish copular verbs *ser* and *estar*. If you have taken a Spanish class, you may remember how difficult it was to differentiate between the two *to be* verbs. VanPatten states that learners will progress through the four stages during their acquisition and that instruction will do little, if anything, to change that. Lightbown (1985) also claims that practice does not make perfect, in that practice and explicit knowledge of grammatical features do not mean that learners can use the practiced feature or access their explicit knowledge in the moment of interacting with another language user or when producing language for other reasons. In terms of assessing, knowing that there are stages of development and that declarative knowledge of grammar rules does not mean that accuracy will be guaranteed in learner output or become part of the learners' implicit system of language, we can assess learners' output based on how well meaning is conveyed.

## BECOMING AN SLA RESEARCH-INFORMED TEACHER

First, I want to acknowledge my privilege in that being part of an academic institution, it is very easy for me to access information about anything I want to study. I also acknowledge that not everyone has the same access to resources that I do. So, in this section, I want to be clear that these tips on becoming a more research-informed teacher are accessible to anyone with an internet connection.

In the 21st century, it is easier than ever to engage in discussions about research and best practices online. Specific to World Language teachers, there are numerous podcasts that deal with discussing SLA research. Podcasts such as *Talkin' L2 with BVP, Tea with BVP, We Teach Languages*, and *The Motivated Classroom* give teachers easy access to relevant research in the field of SLA and offer discussion on the topics in a teacher-friendly way, often citing their references in their episode descriptions. These podcasts provide easy listening with enjoyable hosts that make becoming an SLA research-informed teacher an straightforward and pleasurable experience.

Social media also gives teachers access to relevant, research-based discussions. On platforms such as Facebook, it is relatively easy to use the search bar to find discussion groups that discuss SLA research. On Twitter, there is a host of language teaching–related chats. Twitter chats have been of particular interest to me because they can be in-depth but also can be fast moving which, at least for me, can be a nice change of pace. Getting started with interacting on a Twitter chat can seem overwhelming. There is usually a host who will tweet to a hashtag (an easy way to access similar discussions). Participants then reply to the hashtag, where they can see all of the other responses. A great tool to use for better interaction with Twitter chats is TweetDeck. For language teachers, I suggest looking at #LangChat, #MFLTwitterati, and #SLAChat.

## CONCLUSION

To me, being an SLA research-informed teacher has made my life so much easier. Because I understand that a large part of language learning is access to and interaction with comprehensible input, my lesson and assessment planning has become much less cumbersome. I've been able to reclaim some of my personal time by not stressing over correcting every single "error" a student makes because I know that the research suggests that intensive error correction does not affect acquisitional processes. In my journey to become an SLA research-informed teacher, I also have found a lot of joy in listening to podcasts and interacting with people all across the world through social media. Social media has pushed me to become more research informed but has also given me a reliable support system when I do have questions about my practice. I hope on your journey to becoming a more research-informed teacher, you get to have the same experiences that I have had that have revitalized not only my teaching life but my personal life.

## BILL LANGLEY'S TIPS FOR TEACHERS INTERESTED IN SLA-INFORMED PRACTICES

1. Allow research to inform your practice so that you can let some weight off of your shoulders. Teaching is hard enough, and there is research that supports practices that make our lives as teachers easier—and generally more fun.

2. Find podcasts. There are so many options for language teachers, and the podcast hosts do an admirable job of aggregating information in a way that is accessible to all.

3. Utilize social media to find Personal Learning Networks, check out #LangChat and #SLAChat on Twitter, or look on other social media networks to connect with other teachers who are looking to enhance their practice with research-informed methods.

## REFERENCES

Ellis, R., Basturkmen, H., & Loewen, S. (2002). Doing focus-on-form. *System, 30*(4). 419–432.

Krashen, S. (1981). *Second language acquisition and second language learning.* Pergamon Press.

Lightbown, P. (1985). Great expectations: Second-language acquisition research and classroom teaching. *Applied Linguistics, 6*(2). 173–189. https://doi.org/10.1093/applin/6.2.173

Lichtman, K. (2018). *Teaching proficiency through reading and storytelling: An input based approach to second language acquisition.* Routledge.

Mason, B., & Krashen, S. (2004). Is form-focused vocabulary instruction worthwhile? *Regional Language Centre Journal, 35*(2), 179–185.

Printer, L. (2021). Student perceptions on the motivational pull of Teaching Proficiency through Reading and Storytelling (TPRS): A self-determination theory perspective. *Language Learning Journal, 49*(3), 288–301. https://doi.org/10.1080/09571736.2019.1566397

Semke, H. D. (1984), Effects of the red pen. *Foreign Language Annals, 17,* 195–202. https://doi.org/10.1111/j.1944-9720.1984.tb01727.x

Sharwood Smith, M. (1993). Input enhancement in instructed SLA. *Studies in Second Language Acquisition, 15,* 165–179. https://doi.org/10.1017/S0272263100011943

Swain, M. (1985). Communicative competence: Some roles of comprehensible input and comprehensible output in its development. In S. Gass & C. Madden (Eds.), *Input in second language acquisition* (pp. 235–256). Newbury House.

Truscott, J. (1996). The case against grammar correction in L2 writing classes. *Language Learning, 46*(2), 327–369.

VanPatten, B. (2010). Some verbs are more perfect than others: Why learners have difficulty with *ser* and *estar* and what it means for instruction. *Hispania, 93*(1), 29–38.

Waltz, T. (2015). *TPRS with Chinese characteristics.* Squid for Brains Educational Publishing.

# THE LEARNING (AND UNLEARNING) OF OAKLAND'S EARLY LITERACY COHORT

MARGARET GOLDBERG AND LANI MEDNICK

## Margaret Goldberg

For Margarets's first few years in the classroom, teaching fourth grade in a high-performing school where her students came to her already reading, she had no idea how ill prepared she was to teach reading. When she was hired as a literacy coach and interventionist at a low-performing school where less than 3% of students were proficient readers, she faced a sobering reality. In her site-based role, she was tasked with supporting Oakland Unified's Balanced Literacy initiative, including the rollout of newly purchased curricula. While she was initially eager to bring to this work the Reader's Workshop practices she knew and loved, she quickly learned that the instructional support she had to offer students and teachers was not enough. Over the next five years, she scrambled to learn all she could about how to teach rather than to simply expect children to read.

## Lani Mednick

Like Margaret, Lani began teaching with an open mind but without an understanding of how to teach a child to read. As a Teach for America (TFA) corps member, she learned about crafting lessons, engagement strategies, and backward planning but not about core content or about how children learn. She began teaching in sixth grade and then switched to third, and in each placement she discovered students who had not yet mastered basic reading skills.

Lani moved to kindergarten, hoping to set a solid foundation for her students. However, without an instructional coach or proper training, she leaned on the more experienced teachers around her and on peer-to-peer resources like Teachers Pay Teachers. Taking cues from her colleagues, she taught guided reading with leveled books.

When 70% of her students were deemed to be "meeting expectations" and her efforts were labeled "exceptional" by the administration and district, she could not ignore the inequities reflected in these shockingly low expectations. Lani knew she had more to learn. It wasn't until she left the classroom to become a literacy coach, and met Margaret, that she had the opportunity to learn about the cognitive processes underlying skilled reading, explore the implications for instruction, and understand what it takes for teachers to become truly effective reading teachers.

Margaret and Lani followed radically different paths into teaching. One graduated from a two-year combined credential-master's program, whereas the other completed TFA boot camp. What their teacher prep experiences had in common was that neither of them learned how reading skill develops or how to ensure that all children learn to read. Their paths converged when they found themselves in literacy coaching roles in the same district. What follows is the story of how they discovered the world of reading research and how they led a grant-funded project to implement evidence-based reading instruction in primary grade classrooms.

## OUR REALIZATION

We were hired to support our respective schools in implementing the district's vision of Balanced Literacy. Working in hybrid roles—part literacy coach and part reading interventionist—we quickly began to see holes in the logic of Balanced Literacy. Our curricula and training centered around the belief that children learn to read by reading, but in the low-performing schools where we worked, students who could not yet read were not benefiting from the long stretches of independent reading time typical of Balanced Literacy classrooms.

While students "read" independently, we were expected to teach guided reading. Our lessons included phonemic awareness and phonics, but we lacked a scope and sequence for that instruction, and in the leveled books we used, students rarely had opportunities to apply what we taught. Our foundational skills instruction seemed irrelevant to our students; they could use the predictable sentence structure and pictures to recite leveled books from memory rather than apply phonics to decode words.

The more we prompted our guided reading groups—"Does that look right?" "Does that sound right?" Does that make sense?"—the more we realized that we had turned reading into a game of guess-and-check. Our kids were losing that game. Despite our good intentions and hard work, we were not actually teaching children to read. Our students exhibited reading behaviors—turning pages, even pointing to the words—without actually reading. More than once we heard first-graders say, "I can read this book with my eyes shut!" We were delivering intervention to primary-grade readers and providing coaching to their teachers, but we were not actually helping our struggling students or improving the schools that were failing them.

We were cautioned (by our curricula and in the training provided by our district, commercial publishers, and Teachers College) away from "teaching students to focus too much on the words and too little on the meaning of what they are reading." But we wondered, if we, as reading teachers of first-graders, didn't teach our students how to read unfamiliar words, who would?

And so, we began to ask questions like, "How do children learn to read words?" and "What instruction will ensure our students go to the next grade *really* reading?" As we searched for answers, we stumbled upon a vast body of research that explained how the theories of reading underlying Balanced Literacy had been thoroughly discredited. This spurred us to learn how the brains of skilled readers process text and what instruction provides the most reliable path to skilled reading for all children. We began to make a series of shifts in our thinking, instruction, and materials.

## OUR UNDERSTANDING OF SKILLED READING

from: There are many ways to recognize a word.

to: **Reading requires decoding.**

| FROM: MSV THREE CUEING | TO: SCARBOROUGH'S READING ROPE |
|---|---|

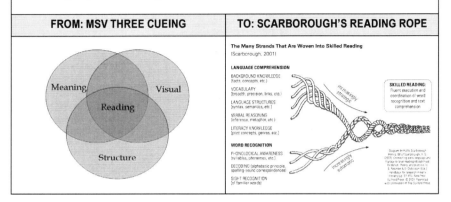

## OUR INSTRUCTIONAL FRAMEWORK

from: A literacy block filled with activities

to: **A literacy block with targeted lessons and evidence-based practices**

| FROM: ACTIVITIES | TO: TARGETED INSTRUCTION |
|---|---|

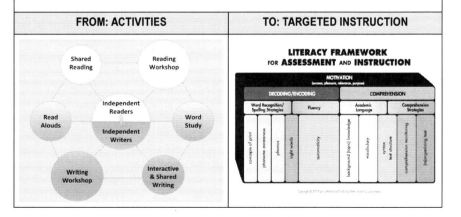

## PRACTICE FOR BEGINNING READERS

from: Books written to teach students to predict words

**to: Books written to teach students to decode words**

| FROM: PREDICTABLE TEXTS | TO: DECODABLE TEXTS |
|---|---|

### Homes

Here is a tree. This tree is a home for an owl.
Here is a log. This log is a home for a fox.
Look at this shell. The shell is a home for a crab.
Look at this cave. The cave is a home for bats.
This is a hive. The hive is a home for bees.
Here is a web. The web is a home for this spider.
Look at this hole. The hole is a home for a mouse.
This house is a home for a dog!

### We Have Homes

A hen will have eggs. A nest is a home for the eggs.
Here is a home for a cub. It is a den.
A web is a home. A web will have a bug in it.
Ducks can swim well. They have a wet home.
A dam is a wet home. A dam will have logs and mud.
A pen is a home for a pig. You can have a pig for a pet!

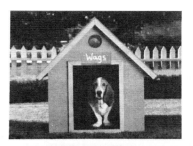

This house is a home for a dog!

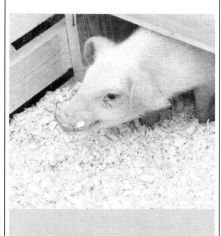

A pen is a home for a pig.
You can have a pig for a pet!

## COMPREHENSION FOR BEGINNING READERS

from: Mini-lessons based in read alouds

to: Intentionally building vocabulary and knowledge through books read aloud

### RICH READ ALOUDS:

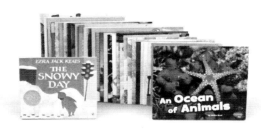

## OUR PROFESSIONAL READING

from: Authors of Balanced Literacy curricula

to: Authors of research

| FROM: FAMILIAR VOICES & CURRICULUA | TO: NEW IDEAS GROUNDED IN RESEARCH |
|---|---|
| | |

The learning and unlearning process was both exciting and stressful, but we were inspired by the potential we discovered in *Teaching Reading Is Rocket Science* by Dr. Louisa Moats:

> Researchers now estimate that 95 percent of all children can be taught to read by the end of first grade, with future achievement constrained only by students' reasoning and listening comprehension abilities. (2020, p.5)

## WHAT WE DID

We made it our mission to share this learning from research as widely as possible, going on to become the leaders of a grant-funded project called the Early Literacy Cohort. Our work included building a community of learners, providing training in how reading works, supporting systems for implementation, and establishing collaboration structures in order to make evidence-based structured literacy instruction an integrated part of the school system. Figure 10.1 and the following tables show the cohort's organizational structure, define the roles within it, and summarize the professional development (PD) program we put in place.

Figure 10.1
**Early Literacy Cohort Organizational Chart**

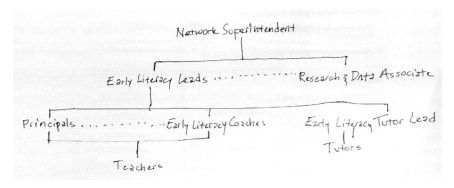

Table 10.1. Early literacy cohort roles and responsibilities

| ROLES | RESPONSIBILITIES |
|---|---|
| Network Superintendent (1) | • Direct and lead the grant-funded project.<br>• Ensure grant fund recipients' fidelity to job agreements.<br>• Direct and support participating school principals.<br>• Hold triannual project planning sessions. |
| Early Literacy Leads (2) | • Plan and lead cohort PD.<br>• Facilitate monthly site visits.<br>• Assist coaches in supporting teachers and tutors.<br>• Manage early literacy assessment calendars.<br>• Coordinate with partner organizations.<br>• Support principals in collaborating with early literacy coaches.<br>• Manage early literacy tutor coach. |
| Research and Data Associate (1) | • Support and manage data collection.<br>• Develop and maintain dashboards and reports for data analysis.<br>• Assist coaches, principals, and teachers in using data collection and analysis tools.<br>• Complete an evaluation of the grant-funded project.<br>• Report progress to grant funder and district leaders. |
| Early Literacy Tutor Coach (1) | • Plan and lead PD for early literacy tutors.<br>• Regularly observe each tutor.<br>• Collect implementation data (fidelity to program, instructional pacing, etc.). |
| Early Literacy Tutors (allocated based on school size, 1–5 per site) | • Work three (3) hours per day.<br>  ○ Prep for and deliver instruction to a minimum of four (4) small groups per day.<br>  ○ Implement the SIPPS (Systematic Instruction in Phonological Awareness, Phonics, and Sight Words) program as designed.<br>  ○ Enter attendance and progress monitoring data.<br>• With guidance from coach and classroom teachers, flexibly group students based on data.<br>• Participate in bimonthly coaching cycles (planning, observation, debrief) with coach and/or early literacy tutor coach. |

| Early Literacy Coaches (allocated based on school size, each managing 1–2 sites) | • Use a coaching and feedback cycle grounded in data to support teacher growth and development.<br>• Observe, co-plan, coach, and model effective literacy instruction for primary-grade teachers and tutors.<br>• Manage screening, diagnostic, and progress monitoring data of primary grade students.<br>• Collaborate with principal to articulate expectations for teachers and tutors re: schedules, instructional content and delivery, planning, and data collection/analysis. |
|---|---|
| Principals (15) | • Develop a schoolwide theory of action to establish instructional best practices in transitional kindergarten to second-grade classrooms.<br>• Communicate student performance goals and progress monitoring expectations.<br>• Create the conditions for early literacy coach's coaching and PD of primary-grade teachers.<br>• Meet biweekly with the coach.<br>• Collaborate with the coach to articulate expectations for teachers and tutors re: schedules, instructional content and delivery, planning, and data collection/analysis. |
| Primary Grade Teachers (all teachers of transitional kindergarten to second grade at cohort sites) | • Coordinate with the early literacy coach and tutors to ensure all students receive targeted, differentiated instruction in foundational skills.<br>• Deliver SIPPS instruction to at least two groups of students per day.<br>• Participate in bimonthly coaching cycles (planning, observation, debrief) with a site-based coach. |

## PROFESSIONAL DEVELOPMENT

|  | Community of Practice | Early Literacy Coach PLC | Cross-site PD | Early Literacy Tutor PLC |
|---|---|---|---|---|
| WHO | Principals and site-based coaches of the 15 elementary schools | Site-based coaches of the 15 elementary schools | Primary-grade teachers from multiple school sites, often grouped by grade level | Community members hired by each school site to deliver differentiated reading instruction |
|  | Led by two early literacy leads and the supervisor of principals | Led by two early literacy leads | Led by pairs of early literacy coaches | Led by early literacy tutor coach |
| WHAT | Guide instructional leaders in the components of evidence-based early literacy instruction and in data analysis. | Develop proficiency in data collection/ analysis, instructional coaching, and practice/planning for cross-site PD. | Build understanding of evidence-based early literacy instruction and how to use curriculum and student data to deliver effective instruction. | Develop the ability to follow the foundational skills curriculum with fidelity and understand why doing so benefits students. |
| WHEN | Three hours, once a month | Three hours, roughly twice a month | Two hours, once a month | Three hours, once a month |
| FOLLOW-UP | Monthly site visits with classroom observations led by early literacy leads and/or the principal's supervisor | Data brought to community of practice and PD delivered at cross-site PD | Observations by coaches and principal and early literacy leads during monthly site visits | Observations by early literacy tutor coach, site-based early literacy coach, and early literacy leads |
|  |  |  | Observation/ debrief of PD with early literacy leads | Observation/ debrief of PD with early literacy leads |

Note: PD = professional development; PLC = professional learning community.

## WHAT MADE IT HARD

Helping schools shift to evidence-based instruction within a Balanced Literacy district was logistically, politically, and emotionally difficult. We faced leaders and teachers who were confused and sometimes frustrated by the differences in messaging, terminology, and expectations between our grant-funded project and the district as a whole.

According to the district, success for kindergarten teachers meant having their students use pictures and repeating sentence structure to recite a predictable book. To meet this goal, teachers followed lessons from the district-adopted curriculum. They taught students to use "picture power" to guess words by looking at the pictures in the books they read. In "guess the covered words" lessons, teachers would cover words with sticky notes so young readers could practice using context to guess unfamiliar words. These lessons were fun, engaging, and easy to prepare. They were also, as we learned in our Early Literacy Cohort, impediments to students' reading progress.

In our Early Literacy Cohort, success meant ensuring that kindergarteners knew their letter-sounds and that they could blend sounds to read words and read decodable texts accurately. Instruction aligned with these goals included phonemic awareness drills, explicit phonics instruction following a scope and sequence, and reading practice that required students to attend to every letter in every word of their books.

Faced with incompatible objectives, school leaders found themselves in the precarious position of telling teachers either to ignore district benchmarks or to attempt both kinds of instruction, thereby confusing students about what it means to "read."

The members of the Early Literacy Cohort pressed district administration to change its primary grade assessments and to allow waivers so that teachers would be free from the expectations of Balanced Literacy. Tensions began to rise as it became clear that although our project was framed as a "pilot," the district had not intended or expected our work to have a district-wide impact. The members of our cohort were actively unlearning Balanced Literacy beliefs and practices, while the district was simultaneously providing Balanced Literacy trainings and promoting Balanced Literacy practices to those outside our project.

Navigating the political landscape was challenging, but seeing the students in our cohort schools benefit from instructional changes gave our work purpose. Kindergarten teachers explained that they had never seen students with reading and writing skills so high, first-grade teachers expressed relief over finally having a plan to help students who had previously seemed unreachable, and second-grade teachers were thrilled every time they received students who could truly read.

## WHAT MADE IT WORK

From the earliest days of our quest to understand how children learn to read, it was clear to us that the findings of reading research had implications for classroom instruction. As we learned more, we came to recognize that widely accepted instructional practices, by ignoring those implications, were harming our schools' most vulnerable students—and doing a disservice to all our students. We knew instruction needed to change, and we felt tremendous urgency to make change.

Our experience leading the cohort taught us that the leadership moves that enable shifts in instruction are no less important than the shifts themselves. We raised expectations for the amount of time principals were to spend in classrooms, the time and attention devoted to analyzing instruction, and the amount and quality of feedback focused on improving teacher practice and student data. We helped principals and coaches understand the importance of valid, predictive, reliable assessments and to analyze the resulting data to determine teacher efficacy. No longer was a well-managed class considered evidence of "good teaching" if student data weren't strong. Perhaps most important, we built cohort-wide awareness of how big a role the kindergarten and first-grade data played in determining school-wide reading success (and failure). Principals who had, at one time, placed lower-skilled teachers in the primary grades in order to stack effective instruction at the grades required to take state tests began to see the repercussions of those decisions.

In our work with principals and coaches, we adopted a process:

- Learn it (develop new understandings about reading and instruction)
- Expect it (clearly articulate the classroom practices that will be required)
- Support it (provide ongoing coaching and feedback to align classroom instruction with best practices)

- Monitor it (collect information about classroom and school implementation, and the resulting student data, in order to determine areas for growth and PD needs)

As principals applied the Learn → Expect → Support → Monitor cycle, instructional shifts began to take hold in cohort schools. The work in our cohort was siloed from the rest of the district, which ultimately made our leadership untenable, but we were able to spur some important changes in the district before the grant-funded project came to an end.

Our project prompted the district to identify early literacy as a district-wide instructional focus, to adopt new assessments, and to quietly end the Balanced Literacy initiative. The school board signed, unanimously, onto a parent-led petition to improve reading instruction by embracing evidence-based practices; a committee has been formed to review new curricula; and stakeholders have been asked to provide input on a new district-wide framework for literacy instruction.

## TIPS FOR REPLICATION

- Establish a coalition of the *willing*. Some people may not be interested in learning or changing their practice, but if you find those willing to do the work, the results speak for themselves and more people will opt in to change.
- Look at your data. Do you have valid, predictable, reliable assessments to find out exactly what instructional needs your students have? Data drives instruction, so you need to get the right kind of data to identify skills gaps to target.
- Look at your curriculum. What is the theory of reading that drives your curriculum? If it is based on the belief that learning to read is a magical process or one of discovery learning, you can expect to have large numbers of students (and teachers) who will struggle. If your materials systematically build a solid foundation, you'll have the tools to minimize an achievement gap.
- Keep learning. Science doesn't stand still, and neither should we. There is still a vast body of research that has yet to be translated to instructional practices. We owe it to our students to continue to learn, grow, and refine our practice as new evidence-based strategies come to light.

## WHY IT MATTERS

Every teacher enters the profession with the intention of doing right by their students, but so many of us are taught to believe that good teaching involves very little direct instruction. We are conditioned to be wary of practices that "drill and kill" or programs that expect us to spend too long on "low-level skills." Shifting instruction to provide phonemic awareness drills, explicitly teaching students spelling patterns that our profession had not expected us to consciously understand, and realizing that reading comprehension is a condition that we create by strengthening decoding and language comprehension skills (not simply a series of strategies we teach)—these are not simply instructional shifts; these require rethinking the teacher's role in the classroom.

When we come to understand that written English is a code that can be unlocked for students with methodical instruction and sufficient practice, our perceptions of our language and of our job descriptions begin to change. Making this shift requires extensive PD, ongoing coaching, and support from school and district leadership. Changing the way we do things is a lot of work. Changing children's lives is worth every bit of effort.

## REFERENCES

Adams, M. J. (1994). *Beginning to read: Thinking and learning about print* (Reprint ed.). Bradford Books.

In F. Lehr & J. Osborn (Eds.), *Literacy for all: Issues in teaching and learning* (pp.77-99). Guilford Press.

Dehaene, S. (2010). *Reading in the brain: The new science of how we read.* Penguin Books.

Foorman, B. R. (1995). Research on "the Great Debate": Code-oriented versus whole language approaches to reading instruction. *School Psychology Review, 24,* 376–392.

Hempenstall, K. (2002). The three-cueing system: Help or hindrance. *Direct Instruction News, 2*(2), 42–51. http://www.nifdi.org/research/esp-archive/volume-2-series-2

Kilpatrick, D. A. (2015). *Essentials of assessing, preventing, and overcoming reading difficulties.* John Wiley & Sons.

Moats, L. C. (2000). *Speech to print: Language essentials for teachers.* Paul H. Brookes.

Moats, L. C. (2007). *Whole-language high jinks: How to tell when "scientifically-based reading instruction" isn't.* Thomas B. Fordham Institute. https://files.eric.ed.gov/fulltext/ED498005.pdf

Moats, L. C. (2020). *Teaching reading is rocket science (2020): What expert teachers of reading should know and be able to do.* American Federation of Teachers.

National Reading Panel (U.S.) & National Institute of Child Health and Human Development (U.S.). (2000). *Report of the National Reading Panel: Teaching children to read: An evidence-based assessment of the scientific research literature on reading and its implications for reading instruction.* U.S. Dept. of Health and Human Services, Public Health Service, National Institutes of Health, National Institute of Child Health and Human Development.

National Early Literacy Panel (U.S.) & National Center for Family Literacy (U.S.). (2008). *Executive summary: Developing early literacy: Report of the National Early Literacy Panel.* National Institute for Literacy.

Scarborough, H. S. (2001). Connecting early language and literacy to later reading (dis)abilities: Evidence, theory, and practice. In S. Neuman & D. Dickinson (Eds.), *Handbook for research in early literacy* (pp. 97–110). Guilford Press.

Seidenberg, M. (2017). *Language at the speed of sight: How we read, why so many can't, and what can be done about it.* Basic Books.

Wolf, M., & Stoodley, C. J. (2007). *Proust and the squid: The story and science of the reading brain.* HarperCollins.

# BUILDING AND LEVERAGING

## HOW TO USE NETWORKS TO SUPPORT EVIDENCE USE

**ELIZABETH FARLEY-RIPPLE**

**Elizabeth Farley-Ripple is a faculty member in the School of Education at the University of Delaware. She studies, teaches, and supports the use of research evidence in educational decision making, and she is an advocate for change in the relationship between researchers and educators. Currently, she co-directs the Center for Research Use in Education, which is rethinking research for schools.**

One of the misconceptions about using research to inform practice is that it is about individuals reading research and implementing research findings as part of their day-to-day activity. This largely instrumental view of research use is misleading, suggesting that this is an individual practice rather than a social one. In fact, research use is profoundly social and relies deeply on relationships within and outside of one's school.

One way of thinking about the social dimensions of research use is in terms of networks. Networks are a means by which information and ideas, as well as other kinds of resources, flow. When we think about research use in schools, two kinds of networks matter: networks that create pathways for new research-based ideas to flow *into* schools, and networks that create pathways for ideas to move *around* and *within* schools.

Many studies have demonstrated the importance of networks for the implementation of reform, professional learning, and instructional improvement (e.g., Brown & Poortman, 2018; Coburn & Russell, 2008;

Daly & Finnegan, 2011; Moolenaar, 2012; Penuel et al., 2009; Spillane et al., 2009; Yoon & Baker-Doyle, 2018). Furthermore, school networks are also powerful tools *for educators and leaders*, particularly when managing change (Farley-Ripple & Buttram, 2013). Educators can leverage teacher networks to promote and support the adoption of new programs or practices, and leaders who understand the power of teacher networks are better positioned to be successful in their improvement efforts.

The power of networks is just as salient in improving research use as it is in broader school improvement. In the rest of this chapter, I talk about the role of both external and internal networks in strengthening research use in schools and what you can do to promote evidence-informed networks in your school. In doing so, I draw on national survey and case study data from the Center for Research Use in Education[2] as examples that help make some common issues and processes less abstract.

## USING NETWORKS TO ACCESS RESEARCH

The first reason networks matter for improving research use is because they provide a potential avenue for access to research. In the US, as well as elsewhere, there exists a gap in the larger education system that connects education researchers to education practitioners; there are often no formal mechanisms for helping researchers connect with practitioners about their work or for practitioners to share needs with researchers. Therefore, educators' individual networks are often the primary means by which new information, ideas, and innovations—and research—flow into schools.

Much of what we know about educator networks from prior studies, and from our own experience, suggests that educators tend to go to specific

---

2.   The Center for Research Use in Education (CRUE) is a knowledge utilization center funded by the US Institute for Education Sciences, charged with the measurement and description of research use in schools. At the core of the Center's work is the development and administration of the *Survey of Evidence in Education*, a pair of instruments—one designed for school-based practitioners and one for researchers—seeking to capture decision-making and research production processes, respectively; perspectives on key gaps between research and practice; networks for connecting with research or practice, respectively; and perceptions of capacity to engage with research or practice, respectively. We are also examining what we call the "third space" between research and practice, in which individuals and organizations serve as brokers between the two communities. We draw on this work in outreach and engagement activities designed to build awareness of the need for and about strategies for building stronger ties between research and practice. For more information, please visit www.research4schools.org.

types of resources for new ideas, including those related to research. These include, first and foremost, other educators. Mostly, we turn to those within our school or district, but also to other places that feature educator expertise, such as teachers' unions, professional associations, and teacher-curated websites. In fact, in our national survey of more than 4,800 school-based educators, the most frequent organizations to which educators turn for research-based information are professional associations, including content-specific organizations (e.g., National Council for Teachers of Mathematics), labor organizations (e.g., National Education Association and local affiliates), and broader professional membership communities (e.g., the Association for Supervision and Curriculum Development). Among the most popular media-based sources are Teachers Pay Teachers and Pinterest.

Other sources of information include organizations and websites with special or trusted content, such as curriculum publishers, program providers, and professional development organizations. For example, educators reported valuing resources from programs implemented in their schools, such as Fountas and Pinnell or Lucy Calkins for literacy, and Positive Behavioral Intervention Supports (PBIS) or Leader in Me for school culture and classroom management, as examples.

At the same time, most educators have few direct ties to the research community, whether accessing peer-reviewed publications or tapping relationships with researchers or research centers—less than 5% of the individuals to which educators turn are researchers (or even professors), and only 15% of the organizations to which they turn are research centers. This means that most of the external networks that educators rely on for new ideas have, at best, indirect connections to research. We'll call this *intermediated* or *mediated* access. In other words, educators rely on sources of research that have already searched for, interpreted, synthesized, and maybe translated into something that is useful for educators.

Information shared through these sources is accessible in multiple ways. That information is either free or available as part of a membership to an organization (which many educators have). It is also likely in a usable format—tools, models of a practice or strategy, or summaries of main points to shape educators' thinking. These features overcome longstanding challenges about how research is produced and communicated. Technical jargon, articles behind paywalls, complex or conflicting findings, and lack of practical implications for educators have long made direct use of research time consuming and challenging for educators.

These are, of course, critical considerations. The fact that access to research is mediated by a broad range of people, organizations, and media sources is, however, something that we need to consider when thinking about research use in schools. Whether or not particular information is research based may be a secondary consideration to whether it is usable and comes recommended by someone you trust. Further, we often don't know a lot about the processes those sources engage in to help make research accessible. Sometimes, we don't know if the information is research based at all.

So, how can you help ensure that research is centered in the external networks on which your school relies?

- *Figure out how to identify research-based resources.* A good first step is to identify criteria for evaluating the evidence base behind resources that you use. Our data show that most educators are not particularly confident in their ability to critically evaluate and consume research, so setting up some criteria for evaluating the evidence base might therefore present its own set of challenges. A starting point might be advice from Willingham's (2012) book, which offers four steps:

  1. **Strip it.** Consider what exactly the claim is suggesting you should do and what outcome is promised.
  2. **Trace it.** Consider who created this idea and what others have said about it.
  3. **Analyze it.** Consider why you should believe the claim is true, including the evidence and, of course, your own experience.
  4. **Should I do it?** It might not make sense to adopt every scientifically backed practice.

- *Evaluate your network (or your school's) for finding research.* Where do you go for ideas? What are their criteria for sharing high-quality information? For example, it is quite easy to examine a professional association's website to assess their explicit commitments to promoting evidence-informed practice or to find evidence of how they use research to inform their guidance (e.g., Are there reference lists? Do conferences include any researchers?). Assess the balance of your network and determine opportunities to be more inclusive of resources that explicitly or directly promote research for practice.

- *Make new connections.* This doesn't mean that you suddenly read the top 10 academic journals or ignore useful professional guidance from colleagues. There are many intermediary organizations and even research or practice organizations that make research available to and useful for educators. Some examples in our work and in other studies (e.g., Malin et al., 2018) are the Collaborative for Academic, Social, and Emotional Learning (CASEL), the Education Resources Information Center (ERIC), Digital Promise, Harvard's Usable Knowledge, and the Marshall Memo. We also note that local research institutions—often but not always institutions of higher education—can be a great resource, whether simply reaching out to a former professor or building a partnership (see Penuel & Gallagher, 2017, for a helpful resource). A shift to include even a few direct connections to research can provide you with a wealth of information that can inform how you think about your practice.

## USING NETWORKS TO BUILD SCHOOL CAPACITY

Whereas external networks offer a means to access research-based information, internal school networks are important for different reasons. They form the social structure of schools, and they are central to the flow of ideas and resources across the organization, which are important to creating change and improving practice (Daly et al., 2010; Farley-Ripple & Buttram, 2015; Hopkins et al., 2018; Penuel et al., 2018).

Because we know educators turn to a wide range of external resources to support their practice, school networks can be an important resource for supporting and sustaining research use in schools. In fact, as noted above, the most common resource educators rely on is other educators. Central actors in those networks—those to whom members of the school turn for advice or resources—can therefore be highly influential in shaping the work of schools. When central actors have external networks that include research-based resources, their influence in schools can help spread research-based information. These individuals are often called research brokers. Some studies find that the principal is an important source of research-based ideas (e.g., Finnigan et al., 2013), whereas others have found that the role of broker is played by teachers, coaches, and others as well (Farley-Ripple & Grajeda, 2019).

No matter who is a research or knowledge broker in your school, they are positioned to help bridge the gap between research and practice and may do so in a couple of ways. In addition to sharing research-based ideas, research brokers can also share strategies for finding and using research. In our survey data, half of educators who share research also share strategies for accessing, reading and understanding, and implementing research. Sharing these skills helps build research-use capacity school-wide and may, as Brown (2018) notes, make a difference in whether and how education research shapes decision making in their context. Second, educators that share research are likely to have more positive attitudes about research in general and to believe its use improves student learning and positively influences their work as an educator. Therefore, school networks that include educators that broker research-based information may also be contributing to their colleagues' capacity and to a school culture of evidence use.

However, not all educator networks—even *within* a school—will include someone with ties to research, and as a result, few if any research-based ideas will flow through that network. Our data suggest a third or less of teachers share research with others in their schools. Yet, these networks may still contribute to the organization in many ways, including building important dimensions of social capital, such as trust, that support professional learning, innovation, and the flow of other important resources—and might represent an opportunity to strengthen the role of research through intervention.

So, how can you leverage your school's network to strengthen research use?

1. *Map current school networks.* In order to take advantage of networks, an important first step is to map the networks that currently exist in their schools, Researchers have tools for mapping networks, but most educators understand who is the "go to" for particular resources or can find out in a few conversations. Some key questions to keep

in mind are: Which members of the school community rely on research-based resources? Which ones are frequently turned to for advice? Which members have strong connections? Which members are relatively isolated? With knowledge of the school structure, you can identify who are influential research brokers, which teachers might not have a broker in their immediate network, and where untapped capacity might lie.

2. *Strategically intervene.* There are many ways to leverage your new knowledge of networks to support research use. For example, create professional learning opportunities around research use for those educators who are influential in their networks but might not be strong users of research. Their peers will likely benefit from their new knowledge, either as recipients of research-based information or by shifts in beliefs about the role of research in education. Alternatively, creating opportunities for sustained interaction and collaboration between groups with and without strong ties to research may help promote stronger networks across the school and create new pathways for research-based resources to flow.

3. *Add research brokers to your staffing plan.* One way to bolster internal networks for research use is to explicitly seek out educators with the background or disposition to serve in such a broker capacity. Our prior work (Farley-Ripple & Grajeda, 2019) suggests that some of the differentiating characteristics of knowledge brokers are observable—they have been part of a research project or been in a program that emphasized research, or they have engaged with research in professional learning communities (PLCs), professional development, or a research conference. They may also demonstrate different beliefs about the value and role of research. Although few schools have the resources to hire staff specifically for research use support roles, these prior experiences can be "look-fors" when hiring for *any* position.

4. *Use your position.* If you are reading this book, odds are that you are a formal or informal school leader, and if you have built stronger ties to research, as suggested previously, you are likely also to be a research broker. Therefore, you are in an influential position in your school. Think about your school network and how you can

support research use more broadly. Whom do you share resources with? Whom do you seek resources from? Seek out opportunities to infuse your interactions with not only research-based information but also your new strategies for accessing and using research, as well as your perspectives on how research can help improve practice and, more important, learning. Further, build out your personal network to include those who might not have ties to research. *Not a leader or broker?* Within your school community, it is likely that there is a research broker (our data show that many are out there!) with whom you can build a relationship or whose ideas you can help promote in faculty meetings and decision opportunities. This helps build a culture of evidence use and sets norms for using research as part of decision making.

## BUILDING AND LEVERAGING CONNECTIONS

This chapter is organized around the idea that networks are powerful tools for supporting the use of research in schools. External networks provide access to research-based resources, whereas internal networks create opportunities for sharing resources and promoting an evidence-use culture. However, networks won't naturally improve research use. They need to be built and leveraged, which, as described in the prior sections, amounts to a few key actions:

- Assess the ways that external and internal networks support research use.
- Take action to address gaps in those networks by making new connections inside or outside of your school
- Build and sustain capacity for research use by becoming an advocate, leader, and broker in your school.

Whether you are looking to grow your own network or facilitate a stronger network within your school community, or advocating for a more evidence-centered set of external resources to inform your school's practice, I have offered a few key steps to take that will build your research-use capacity, and subsequently build others' capacity as well. Building and leveraging evidence-informed networks are important steps in making the research-use revolution a reality.

# REFERENCES

Brown, C. (2018). Research learning networks: A case study in using networks to increase knowledge mobilization at scale. In C. Brown & C. L. Poortman (Eds.), *Networks for learning: Effective collaboration for teacher, school and system improvement* (pp. 38–55). Routledge.

Brown, C., & Poortman, C. L. (Eds.). (2018). *Networks for learning: Effective collaboration for teacher, school and system improvement*. Routledge.

Coburn, C. E., & Russell, J. L. (2008). District policy and teachers' social networks. *Education Evaluation and Policy Analysis, 30*(3), 203–235.

Daly, A. J., & Finnegan, K. (2011). The ebb and flow of social network ties between district leaders under high stakes accountability. *American Education Research Journal, 48*(1), 39–79.

Daly, A. J., Moolenaar, N., Bolivar, J., & Burke, P. (2010). Relationships in reform: The role of teachers' social networks. *Journal of Educational Administration, 48*(3), 20–49.

Farley-Ripple, E. N., & Buttram, J. L. (2013). Harnessing the power of teacher networks. *Phi Delta Kappan, 95*(3), 12–15.

Farley-Ripple, E. N., & Buttram, J. (2015). The development of capacity for data use: *The role of teacher networks in an elementary school. Teachers College Record, 117*(4), 1–34.

Farley-Ripple, E. N., & Grajeda, S. (2019). Avenues of influence: An exploration of school-based practitioners as knowledge brokers and mobilizers. In J. Malin & C. Brown (Eds.), *The role of knowledge brokers in education: Connecting the dots between research and practice* (pp. 65–89). Routledge.

Finnigan, K. S., Daly, A. J., & Che, J. (2013). Systemwide reform in districts under pressure: The role of social networks in defining, acquiring, using, and diffusing research evidence. *Journal of Educational Administration, 51*(4), 476–497.

Hopkins, M., Spillane, J. P., & Shirrell, M. (2018). Designing educational infrastructures for improvement: Instructional coaching and professional learning communities. In S. A. Yoon & K. J. Baker-Doyle (Eds.), *Networked by design:* Interventions for teachers to develop social capital (pp. 192–213). Routledge.

Malin, J. R., Brown, C., & Trubceac, A. S. (2018). Going for broke: A multiple-case study of brokerage in education. *AERA Open, 4*(2), 2332858418769297.

Moolenaar, N. M. (2012). A social network perspective on teacher collaboration in schools: Theory, methodology, and applications. *American Journal of Education, 11*, 7–39.

Penuel, W. R. de los Santos, E., Lin, Q., Marshall, S., Anderson, C. W., & Frank, K. A. (2018). Building networks to support effective use of science curriculum materials in the carbon TIME project. In S. A. Yoon & K. J. Baker-Doyle (Eds.), *Networked by design: Interventions for teachers to develop social capital* (pp. 192–213). Routledge.

Penuel, W. R., & Gallagher, D. J. (2017). *Creating research practice partnerships in education*. Harvard Education Press.

Penuel, W. R., Riel, M. R., Krause, A., & Frank, K. A. (2009). Analyzing teachers' professional interactions in a school as social capital: A social network approach. *Teachers College Record, 111*(1), 124–163.

Spillane, J. P., Hunt, B., & Healey, K. (2009). Managing and leading elementary schools: Attending to the formal and informal organization. *International Studies in Educational Administration, 37*(1), 5–28.

Willingham, D. T. (2012). *When can you trust the experts? How to tell good science from bad in education*. John Wiley & Sons.

Yoon, S. A., & Baker-Doyle, K. J. (Eds.). (2018). *Networked by design: Interventions for teachers to develop social capital*. Routledge.

# RESEARCH-INFORMED TEACHING AT SCALE
## THE PROMISE OF CROSS-DISTRICT COLLABORATION

**JOEL KNUDSON**

Joel Knudson is a principal researcher at the American Institutes for Research. Joel's work has focused on facilitating and documenting the work of cross-district partnerships. He is currently the Deputy Director of the California Collaborative on District Reform.

School districts can play an instrumental role in bringing research-based practice into classrooms on a broad scale. In service of high-quality instruction, cross-district collaboration can help provide access to expertise and accelerate the learning process across school systems.

## CROSS-DISTRICT COLLABORATION AS A VEHICLE FOR EQUITY AND SCALE

Instructional improvement requires effective practice from highly skilled classroom teachers. Any exploration of research-informed practice therefore rightly focuses on the role of individual teachers. However, if every student is to experience a world-class education, an exclusive focus on teachers is insufficient. Variation in teacher knowledge and skills, as well as comfort with accessing and making use of research, contribute to a wide range of instructional quality. Moreover, because teacher assignment policies typically match the most experienced teachers with our most advantaged students, those teachers who are best equipped to apply evidence from research to their teaching may be the furthest removed from students who need the most support (e.g., Goldhaber et al., 2015; Sass et al., 2012, Mayer et al., 2000).

Enter school districts, which can play a vital role in promoting and supporting the broad implementation of effective teaching practice. Local school systems have evolved from their primarily administrative origins to embrace increasing levels of responsibility for the quality of the instructional core. Indeed, research consistently attests to district-level contributors to school improvement, and even to the incorporation of evidence-based practices (e.g., Honig et al., 2010, 2017; Sykes et al., 2009). With respect to instruction, districts shape what students learn and how they learn it through decisions about curriculum adoption, course offerings, and instructional frameworks. They also influence the composition of the teaching force through recruitment, hiring, compensation, and retention. Instructional quality further relies on district approaches to building teacher capacity through professional development, feedback, coaching, and time and structures for educator collaboration.

For all the potential that exists in school districts, barriers inside and outside of school systems frequently stand in the way of progress. In the face of these challenges, cross-district collaboration offers an opportunity to accelerate the learning process. By turning to their peers for examples, district leaders can capitalize on promising evidence-based practices without having to reinvent the wheel in addressing their problems. By understanding the missteps that slowed progress in other contexts, district leaders can forge more efficient pathways to implementing proven strategies in their own school systems. By engaging a broader community of learners to navigate shared problems, district leaders can realize that—as one California superintendent frequently claimed—none of us alone is as good as all of us together.

## THE CALIFORNIA COLLABORATIVE ON DISTRICT REFORM AS ONE MODEL OF COLLECTIVE LEARNING

One example of productive cross-district learning comes from the state of California. Launched in 2006, the California Collaborative on District Reform joins district leaders, researchers, policy makers, support providers, advocates, and funders in ongoing, evidence-based dialogue to improve outcomes for all students in California's school systems, with particular attention to equity and access for historically underserved students in the state. The group typically convenes three times per year for two-day meetings nested in the context of a host district. The meetings are an opportunity for education leaders from a variety of professional backgrounds to learn about the promising practices underway in the district. They also create the space for the host district to gather feedback and advice about some of their most persistent problems. In the process, the meetings elevate lessons that apply to all Collaborative members, regardless of their context.

A meeting focused on mathematics instruction illustrates the ways in which exchanges of ideas through the California Collaborative help to foster research-informed teaching. Sanger Unified School District had achieved dramatic district-wide improvement through a series of cultural and behavioral shifts, including an approach to student learning grounded in Explicit Direct Instruction (David & Talbert, 2013). As the district transitioned to a new set of academic standards in mathematics, however, district leaders recognized that their emphasis on mastery of basic skills would be insufficient to achieve the deeper learning, student-centered instruction, and more active student engagement called for in the new standards (Talbert & David, 2019).

A California Collaborative meeting enabled Sanger leaders to incorporate knowledge from research by bringing in one of the authors of the new standards, Phil Daro. Daro offered an overview of teaching practices in Japan that had informed the development of the new standards, and he also helped to translate how features of Sanger's existing use of Explicit Direct Instruction could be incorporated as a vital components of the district's instructional shifts. By engaging in dialogue with subject matter experts, district leaders benefited from a more thorough exploration of an evidence base and its translation to district practice than what is possible from consuming the static words of a peer-reviewed study. As a cross-organizational group, the collective influence of multiple districts and the communities they represent helped provide access to influential and respected voices that a single district might not have been able to arrange alone.

Moreover, dialogue among leaders from multiple districts and among respected voices from policy, research, and technical assistance helped to unpack key implementation challenges. Leaders in Sanger faced the challenge not only of understanding and promoting high-quality mathematics instruction but also of fostering changes in practice among a teaching force that felt overwhelmed by a wave of new expectations and that had high levels of investment in their existing instructional approach. By engaging peers across systems and roles, Sanger leaders and other participants explored not only *what* quality instruction could look like but *how* it might be achieved.

More recently, meetings during the COVID-19 pandemic helped position district leaders to apply evidence-based practices in response to unanticipated challenges. One such challenge was the inequities in traditional grading; the pandemic provided opportunities for better aligning grading policies to content mastery. A growing body of research demonstrates the flaws of traditional approaches to grading, including the disproportionately negative impact on historically underserved students of policies that reward behaviors like homework compliance over content mastery (Feldman, 2019). In fall 2020, these disparities came into sharp relief as disruptions to in-person schooling forced transitions to remote learning. Many districts across the country saw an increase in the number of students receiving low grades during remote learning. For example, the percentage of students earning a D or F at the 10-week mark in Los Angeles Unified School District grew by 16 points in grades 6–8 and 13 points in grades 9–12 relative to performance in the previous year. More troubling was the increase in academic struggles among the district's most vulnerable students: The rates grew by 25 and 22 points for homeless students, by 22 and 18 points for foster youth, and by 20 points for English learners in both grade spans.

A California Collaborative meeting provided a forum for members to engage in dialogue about how to respond to students' immediate needs and to take advantage of the pandemic to spark conversation and action around long-term changes. Some districts had already taken action in the past to redesign policies around grading, whereas others were engaging in serious discussions with their teachers for the first time. Through this cross-organization collaborative discussion, district leaders were able to exchange ideas and lessons learned from their respective efforts to revisit grading practices. They also had an opportunity to examine the implications of research on grading—most of which had been conducted in the context of typical schooling conditions—and apply it to the novel context of widespread remote learning.

For Los Angeles Unified School District, the conversation affirmed the recognition that students' prospects for postsecondary preparation were being seriously threatened and that the dilemma required urgent action. Building in part on the insights from this conversation, the district announced shortly after the meeting that it would temporarily convert students' "no pass" or "fail" grades to an "in progress" rating, granting them additional time to increase proficiency for their permanent grade. Although the district is careful not to post a causal relationship, approximately 10,000 students subsequently improved their marks from "in progress" to a passing grade in fall 2020, and an additional 2,000 improved their grade from a D to a higher grade with an additional opportunity to complete work.

## FEATURES OF EFFECTIVE COLLABORATION

In the work of the California Collaborative and other cross-district learning communities, some key features have helped to foster the examination and incorporation of evidence-based practices.

First, grounding conversations in concrete problems of practice can help bring research to life. Any intervention designed to improve student learning emerges from a specific learning context. The student population, capacity of the teaching force, community and organizational history, political dynamics among system and community leaders, and myriad other factors shape the approaches that educators take and the degree to which they can achieve success. Driven perhaps by a desire to present an evidence base as impartial, however, much of the research base on instructional improvement is—at least on its face—agnostic about these critical contextual factors. By using the lens of specific challenges district leaders are navigating, educators and their partners can develop a deeper understanding of how knowledge from research can respond to and integrate with the many other dynamics that shape student learning.

Second, cross-role groups introduce expertise from multiple perspectives. District leaders offer an evidence-based perspective from their own experience that can inform the work of their peers—whether or not that experience is supported through rigorous peer-reviewed studies. Teachers and teacher leaders can help keep the conversation grounded in the realities of classroom instruction and teacher capacity. Researchers themselves bring insights about what works in school systems, including the application of a broader body of knowledge to the particular circumstances in which any one district operates. Policy makers can learn about and work to create the kinds of supportive conditions that enable evidence-based practices to grow, expand, and thrive. Advocates can call attention to the needs of historically underserved students, and the adaptations to strategies that may be necessary to meet them. By pulling many voices together, learning communities like the California Collaborative can help their members identify opportunities, recognize blind spots, and deepen their own understanding of the challenges schools face and the potential solutions for addressing them.

Third, trust among partners in a learning community fosters the honest exchange of ideas. Too often, conference presentations or other convenings of professional associations feature "dog-and-pony shows" of the brilliant approaches underway in a school or district. In an effort to draw attention to work about which they are justifiably proud, educators sometimes gloss over or even ignore the inevitable imperfections, unanticipated challenges, and persistent flaws of their approaches. There is value in learning from promising practices, to be sure, but more powerful learning experiences occur when colleagues across organizational lines can dig deeply into the most pressing obstacles to success. When group organizers bring together participants with a learning stance, conversations can focus on challenges and opportunities for growth. When education leaders can share their experiences in a safe space, authentic learning can occur. When a room of peers recognizes that effective leadership is defined not by achieving immediate success, but by asking difficult questions and refining strategies when success is elusive, the power of collaboration is strongest. Careful attention to building relationships and establishing trust to the point that people feel comfortable with vulnerability has been an important foundation for learning to take place.

## TOP TIPS

1. Organize discussions around concrete problems of practice to explore the application of evidence-based practices in the concrete realities of schools and districts.

2. Strategically assemble learning communities to provide access to expertise—both through group membership and opportunities to interact with respected guests.

3. Take time to select participants, establish relationships, and build the trust that can foster an honest exchange of ideas about bright spots and areas of struggle.

## REFERENCES

David, J., & Talbert, J. (2013). *Turning around a high poverty district: Learning from Sanger.* S.H. Cowell Foundation.

Feldman, J. (2019). *Grading for equity.* Corwin.

Goldhaber, D., Lavery, L., & Theobald, R. (2015). Uneven playing field? Assessing the teacher quality gap between advantaged and disadvantaged students. *Educational Researcher, 44*(5), 293–307.

Honig, M. I., Copland, M. A., Rainey, L., Lortin, J. A., & Newton, M. (2010). *Central office transformation for district-wide teaching and learning improvement.* Center for the Study of Teaching and Policy, University of Washington.

Honig, M. I., Venkateswaran, N., & McNeil, P. (2017). Research use as learning: The case of fundamental change in school district central offices. *American Educational Research Journal, 54*(5), 938–971.

Mayer, D. P., Mullens, J. E., Moore, M. T., & Ralph, J. (2000). *Monitoring school quality: An indicators report.* US Department of Education, National Center for Education Statistics.

Sass, T. R., Hannaway, J., Xu, Z., Figlio, D. N., & Feng, L. (2012). Value added of teachers in high-poverty schools and lower poverty schools. *Journal of Urban Economics, 72*(2–3), 104–122.

Sykes,G., O'Day, J., & Ford, T.G. (2009). The district role in instructional improvement. In G. Sykes, B. Schneider, D. Plank, & T.G. Ford (Eds.), *Handbook of Education Policy Research* (pp., 767-784). Routledge.

Talbert, J., & David, J. (2019). *Sanger Unified School District: Positive outliers case study.* Learning Policy Institute.

# MOVING RESEARCH INTO PRACTICE
## IT'S A COLLABORATIVE EFFORT

**MICHAEL FAIRBROTHER AND JACQUELINE SPECHT**

Dr. Michael Fairbrother is an adjunct professor in the Faculty of Education at the University of Ottawa, in Ottawa, Ontario, Canada. He teaches in the Faculty of Education's bachelor and graduate programs and is a former elementary classroom and special education teacher. His research focuses on inclusive literacy practices, professional learning, and the processes of teacher change. He is a research associate for the Canadian Research Centre on Inclusive Education collaborating to expand, develop, and mobilize knowledge of research-informed inclusive practices.

Dr. Jacqueline Specht is a professor in the Faculty of Education at Western University in London, Ontario. She teaches in initial teacher education and the graduate programs in Applied Psychology. She is the Director of the Canadian Research Centre on Inclusive Education and was the South Ontario lead of the Réseau de Savoir sur l'Équité/ Equity Knowledge Network (RSEKN). Her research focuses on the development of inclusive practice for both beginning teachers and school leaders. She brings to her work an emphasis on the ways in which we can mobilize knowledge in education to support research-informed practice.

The notion of research-informed practice in education is one that has been well debated in the research literature over the years (Abukari & Kuyini, 2018), and the fact that researchers are not practitioners may be a barrier to moving that research into practice (Dagenais et al., 2012; Datnow & Hubbard, 2016). Our definition of research-informed borrows from Campbell (2017) "to indicate the use and adaptation of empirical evidence from research, evaluation, and data, plus ... professional knowledge, expertise, and judgement" (8).

As a teacher, one might ask why it is important to be research informed. Is it not enough to gather my own information and decide what to do based on that? Although we agree that experience is important and teacher knowledge can inform research, it is not enough. We often have our own biases that can interfere with our ability to be objective (e.g., Dagenais et al., 2012). If we think that something might work, we only look for the outcomes that support that thinking; we tend to ignore those outcomes that go against our thinking or do not appear relevant to the particularities of our classrooms (Vanderlinde & van Braak, 2010). This bias may be especially problematic when we are working with students who struggle with their learning in our classrooms. We want to make sure that any of the teaching and learning tools we utilize have research evidence to support their use; at least then we have a chance of success. When there is no research to support these practices, it can take time away from effective instruction and may lead to further disappointment for learners and teachers when success is not evident. One such example is the ubiquitous notion of learning styles. There are a number of concerns with this concept: (a) there are reportedly 70 different constructs that use this term, meaning that many people can be thinking of different definitions (Papadatou-Pastou et al., 2021); (b) there is no scientific research upon which these constructs are based (Papadatou-Pastou et al., 2021); and (c) the energy teachers spend creating many different lessons based on the notion that certain students can only learn in certain ways is exhausting (Rohrer & Pashler, 2012).

As researchers and educators, we are of the belief that research-informed practice is indeed necessary and possible in enhancing the teaching and learning in elementary and secondary schools. What is important to stress is that for practice to be research informed, it must be usable by the practitioners, promoted by the policy makers, and supported by the findings of the researchers. Current thinking is that research-informed practice is not merely practitioners doing what researchers say, but rather it is a collaboration of stakeholders in education and therefore a systemic responsibility (Brown & Zhang, 2016; Nelson & Campbell, 2017; Pollock et al., 2019). This collaboration includes an extensive learning network to connect pre- and inservice teachers, schools, school boards, and educational partners through mobilizing research, data, and instructional practices across the education system.

## CREATING AN ETHOS OF RESEARCH-INFORMED PRACTICE

### Initial Teacher Education

For teachers to be effective, there must be harmony between their beliefs and values, their knowledge and skills, and their practice. Sharma (2018) posits that pre-service teacher education is key in beginning to develop this harmony. We believe that there is a need for a deliberate focus on research-informed practice in all coursework. As teacher educators, it is important that we model the use of research in teaching. One of the barriers that we see is the different approaches to knowledge—what counts as research and whose knowledge is valued. At times, it may be confusing for teacher candidates when they hear two very different approaches to teaching the same subject. For example, the teaching of reading is an area of concern. Findings from research with classroom teachers exemplifies important gaps in initial teacher education reading coursework and its limited influence on teacher reading instruction (Fairbrother, 2019, 2020; Joshi et al., 2009; Stark et al., 2016; Washburn et al., 2011). In initial teacher education, there is not time to get into all the nuances of research and so teacher candidates end up being confused, often only being introduced to distinct bodies of knowledge (e.g., whole reading or code-based instruction) that themselves are shallow overviews about literacy and learning to read. Interestingly, this results in many teachers entering the profession perceiving that they know more than they do (Stark et al., 2016). Fairbrother (2020) and Stark et al. (2016) acknowledge that pre-service reading instruction often prioritizes how to set up the reading environment and lacks code-based learning experiences for teaching beginning and struggling readers. This research indicates how ineffective practices prevail across time, unfortunately instilling a sense of teacher efficacy that is not research informed and that clearly emphasizes the crucial role of teacher education for beginning teachers in helping them avoid the research-to-practice gap.

Our goal in initial teacher education ought to be to graduate people who understand that teaching is not a list of prescriptions to be followed but a vast array of knowledge that we can use to support our practice. Cain (2019) discusses the need for teacher candidates to determine their own needs in improving practice. They are encouraged to read research and reflect on their own practice. Western University's Faculty of Education has recently implemented a pass/fail system for teacher education using this rationale. We want teacher candidates to build their competencies over the 16-month program. Using the expectations of the profession, coursework engages them in content-specific and general pedagogical processes where they can engage in building competencies of the future. In many ways, this process is what we would expect of practicing teachers, and creating these opportunities at the initial teacher education phase is ideal.

## Practicing Teachers

Our experiences as researcher, teacher educator, and professional teacher indicates that teachers must have opportunities to engage with research in professionally meaningful ways and learn how to consume and translate research findings (see also Datnow & Hubbard, 2016). Graduate school provides opportunities for discussion of the broader aspects of the research experience and what it means to be consumers, practitioners, and contributors. For example, a Master of Special Education beginning in the third year of teaching would provide a necessary catalyst for merging levels of professional knowledge and awareness of the context of school and community with a newfound understanding of research to balance teaching practices with a research-informed stance (Nelson & Campbell, 2017). Adding to the Canadian context is Canadian census data indicating that nearly three quarters of full-time teachers in Canada do not have a graduate degree and therefore face barriers to accessing current literature and research-informed practices to help them meet their students' needs (Wall et al., 2018). It appears, then, that although graduate studies could support educators in becoming research literate, graduate school is not a reality for many Canadian teachers. Therefore, we also need to count on professional learning to address teachers' needs for developing practices informed from empirical research and guided in local data.

Campbell (2017) indicates that, in Canada, professional learning for teachers appears to be evidence informed although not necessarily data driven. This distinction suggests that although many elementary and secondary teachers know what research indicates, they do not necessarily use the data specific to their own context (whether that be a student, the class, or the school) to guide their practice (Nelson & Campbell, 2017). There is a culture in Canadian professional learning where evidence is used to support teacher learning but it is not necessarily used enough to meet the particular needs of one's teaching context—and specifically in relation to supporting the learning needs of those students who traditionally struggle in our school system.

Although there appears to be no shortage of research summaries (e.g., What Works Clearinghouse, Ministry reports, websites, best practice pamphlets), the divide continues between what gets practiced and what research suggests (Brown & Zhang, 2016; Datnow & Hubbard, 2016). Until this divide is bridged, too many classroom practices will remain separate from researchers' findings. Research indicates the paramount importance for teachers is to be a part of professional learning that relates to their state and stage of experiences and to the context of their students, and to be supported by the learning systems in which they work (Fairbrother, 2020; Hargreaves, 2005). For example, shifts in a school board's professional learning priorities, the ability to access the funds and time to undertake professional learning, and the availability of contextually relevant professional learning (particularly urban and rural) are factors that influence how well teachers perceive that their professional learning helps them to meet their students' needs (Fairbrother, 2020). This list scratches the surface but demonstrates the complex concerns influencing teachers' learning opportunities and experiences. A professional learning approach that fuses opportunities for teachers to incorporate research evidence with local data are ingredients toward ensuring research-informed practices.

## CREATING RESEARCH COLLABORATIONS

Creating change within education requires a collaboration from teachers in classroom to policy makers in the ministry. If practitioners are engaged in research and understand how the results relate to their contexts, they are more likely to implement them in the future. (Pollock & Campbell, 2021). An example of this type of work was evident in the Réseau de Savoir sur l'Équité/Equity Knowledge Network (RSEKN) (see https://rsekn.ca). We were funded by the Ontario Ministry of Education to mobilize the knowledge on equity related to ability, gender, language, immigration, income, race, and sexuality. The excitement of those involved with the different projects was contagious. Events such as associate teacher day brought in teacher candidates and their associate teachers for a day to learn about equity and its effect on the learning of students. The day provided time for the teacher candidate and their associate teachers to discuss research and the importance of bringing it back to their classroom practice. Community member involvement was also highlighted in one of the groups. We know that when communities collaborate with the school, there is success. By focusing on what works and how to best implement it in the schools, all voices are heard and teachers and families work for the best of the students. School board personnel were involved in the creation of videos related to equity. These short five-minute videos were written using real-life experiences and were created with school board members to share with their colleagues. An accompanying discussion guide is a springboard for action. As this one example illustrates, there are many ways to immerse those in practice with research other than having to read about it in written articles. Involvement with research and understanding its relation to practice is key to its use.

## CONCLUSION

It is paramount for teachers and students to work as effectively as possible in the time in which they are in school. It is important that as educators we have sound reasons to act as we do. Relying on research evidence and our professional judgment informed by data provides the solid foundation on which to act. This chapter has outlined why it is important to move research to practice and ways in which we hinder and help that movement. To end, we provide three important ideas to ensure that we are on the road to moving research into practice:

- Be familiar with the research that guides your practice, both broadly and specifically related to your particular context.
- Use the research to promote your competencies.
- Discover the opportunities to work with researchers and learning networks to add to the knowledge of informed practice.

# REFERENCES

Abukari, A., & Kuyini, A. B. (2018). Using research to inform practice: The teacher as a practitioner researcher. *Journal for Researching Education Practice and Theory, 1*(2), 1–5.

Brown, C., & Zhang, D. (2016). Is engaging in evidence-informed practice in education rational? What accounts for discrepancies in teachers' attitudes towards evidence use and actual instances of evidence use in schools? *British Educational Research Journal, 42*(5), 780–801. https://doi.org/10.1002/berj.3239

Cain, T. (2019). Research-informed initial teacher education. In D. Godfrey & C. Brown (Eds.), *An ecosystem for research-engaged schools: Reforming education through research* (pp. 123–137). Routledge.

Campbell, C. (2017). Developing teachers' professional learning: Canadian evidence and experiences in a world of educational improvement. *Canadian Journal of Education, 40*(2), 1–33.

Dagenais, C., Lysenko, L., Abrami, P., Bernard, R., Ramde, J., & Janosz, M. (2012). Use of research-based information by school practitioners and determinants of use: A review of empirical research. *Evidence & Policy, 8*(3), 285–309. https://doi.org/10.1332/174426412X654031

Datnow, A., & Hubbard, L. (2016). Teacher capacity for and beliefs about data-driven decision making: A literature review of international research. *Journal of Educational Change, 17*(1), 7–28. https://doi.org/10.1007/s10833-015-9264-2

Fairbrother, M. (2019, June). Complexity theory and implications for teacher learning research [Paper presentation]. *Canadian Society for the Study of Education*, Vancouver, Canada.

Fairbrother, M. (2020). *Exploring teachers' perceptions of the complex contextual factors influencing decisions to participate in professional learning on early reading and their uptake of classroom strategies.* [Doctoral dissertation]. University of Ottawa.

Hargreaves, A. (2005). Educational change takes ages: Life, career and generational factors in teachers' emotional responses to educational change. *Teaching and Teacher Education, 21*(8), 967–983. https://doi.org/10.1016/j.tate.2005.06.007

Joshi, R. M., Binks, E., Hougen, M., Dahlgren, M., Ocker-Dean, E., Smith, D., Joshi, R., & Cunningham, A. (2009). Why elementary teachers might be inadequately prepared to teach reading. *Journal of Learning Disabilities, 42*(5), 392–402. https://doi.org/10.1177/0022219409338736

Nelson., J., & Campbell, C. (2017). Evidence-informed practice in education: Meanings and applications. *Educational Research, 59*(2), 127–135. http://doi. org/10.1080/00131881.2017.1314115

Papadatou-Pastou, M., Touloumakos, A. K., Koutouveli, C., & Barrable, A. (2021). The learning styles neuromyth: When the same term means different things to different teachers. *European Journal of Psychology of Education, 36*, 511–531. https://doi.org/10.1007/s10212-020-00485-2

Pollock, K., & Campbell, C. (2021). Guest editorial. *Journal of Professional Capital and Community, 6*(1), 1–6. https://doi.org/10.1108/JPCC-01-2021-083

Pollock, K., Campbell, C., McWhorter, D., Bairos, K., & van Roosmalen, E. (2019). Developing a system for knowledge mobilisation: The case of the Knowledge Network for Applied Education Research (KNAER) as a middle tier. In D. Godfrey & C. Brown (Eds.), *An ecosystem for research-engaged schools: Reforming education through research* (pp. 22–40). Routledge.

Rohrer, D., & Pashler, H. (2012). Learning styles: Where's the evidence? *Medical Education, 46*, 34–35.

Sharma, U. (2018, May 24). Preparing to teach in inclusive classrooms. *Oxford Research Encyclopedia of Education*, 1–20. https://doi.org/10.1093/ acrefore/9780190264093.013.113

Stark, H., Snow, P., Eadie, P., & Goldfeld, S. (2016). Language and reading instruction in early years' classrooms: The knowledge and self-rated ability of Australian teachers. *Annals of Dyslexia, 66*(1), 28–54. https://doi.org/10.1007/ s11881-015-0112-0

Vanderlinde, R., & van Braak, J. (2010). The gap between educational research and practice: Views of teachers, school leaders, intermediaries and researchers. *British Educational Research Journal, 36*(2), 299–316. https://doi. org/10.1080/01411920902919257

Wall, K., Zhao, J., Ferguson, S. J., & Rodriguez, C. (2018). *Results from the 2016 Census: Is field of study a factor in the payoff of a graduate degree?* https://www150.statcan.gc.ca/n1/pub/75-006-x/2018001/article/54978-eng. pdf. Statistics Canada Catalogue no. 75-006-X.

Washburn, E., Joshi, R., & Binks Cantrell, E. (2011). Are preservice teachers prepared to teach struggling readers? *Annals of Dyslexia, 61*(1), 21–43. https:// doi.org/10.1007/s11881-010-0040-y

# UNLEASHING GREATNESS
## BUILDING A RESEARCH CULTURE IN YOUR SCHOOL

**JEREMY HANNAY**

Jeremy is a Canadian who has lived and worked in the United Kingdom for the last 11 years. He started his career in Ottawa, Canada, in the province of Ontario, where teacher agency, professional research, and collaboration are embedded parts of the edu-culture. He completed his doctoral research at the University of Exeter, investigating lesson study (a Japanese form of action- and practice-based teacher development) and its associations with school climate, teacher self-efficacy to use inclusive practices, teacher learning, and pupil outcomes. He is the head teacher of Three Bridges Primary School in Southall, an award-winning, diverse community school serving a remarkable community known for its counter-culture approaches to school improvement, teacher development, and whole-school well-being.

## ALIGNMENT: NAVIGATING COMPLEXITY

When I started working at my current school, none of the staff had ever been involved in action or practice-based research. Many of the staff were in their first five years of teaching and/or new to the school, and the standard practice was that some*one* would decide on what was best. Often, this person was a team or subject leader, had been on some training at the local authority, and was tasked with informing everyone of what they had learned.

Learning and teaching are complex; developing a culture to examine and enhance them is even harder. In the ever-changing nature of staff makeup and teaching teams, this is often the easiest approach to making sure that everyone is on the same page. Be told and then tell. When your staff is constantly in its infancy, it is difficult to deal with complexity. This means that diving straight into more formal approaches to research is likely to cause more anxiety than answers, more fear than fruit.

In establishing a culture of research, it is important for the school to start where it is rather than where it wants to be. This means immersing staff in the kinds of activities that lead to constructive collaboration, meaningful discourse, and the freedom to try new things without fear. More deeply, this involves looking at how research, professional agency and decisional capital align with your structures, systems, and policies in place at the school already. Creating a culture means aligning everything. Enacting action and practice-based research can change the culture of a school—but in harmony not in isolation. "Inquire today, inspected tomorrow" is not the mantra of any successful school. The values that underpin research and inquiry are about internal responsibility, reflection, individual and collective agency, depth of thinking, and the generation and application of knowledge and understanding. Performative management practices are driven by external accountability, convenience, explanation, absorption, and basic knowledge and data.

## CREATING THE CULTURE

To create a sustainable and healthy research culture, it must align with the systems and structures in place at the school. At Three Bridges, we have used a model of professional capital (Hargreaves & Fullan, 2012) to align our practices with the values and culture of research.

| Professional Capital Theory PC = f(HC, SC, DC) | Human Capital | Social Capital | Decisional Capital |
|---|---|---|---|
| The development of Professional Capital is the function of three distinct types of capital in a school or school system: human capital, social capital and decisional capital. | > attracting excellent teachers<br>> develop capacity of groups, teams, communities of teachers<br>> development over time<br>> make teaching desirable | > teachers working in teams with a specific focus on learners and learning<br>> organized and intentional<br>> shared responsibility for learners and learning | > informed agency to make instructional decisions impacting upon learners and learning<br>> competence, insight, judgement<br>> collective decision making |

Table 14.1. Professional capital theory

Source: Hargreaves & Fullan, 2012.

From 2012, we examined the structures and systems in place at the school in order to align seemingly unrelated policies and practices to the values that underpin a research culture. This is the difference between adoption and engagement—altering the course of other practices that misalign. If you see research in isolation, it will happen that way; if you see research in harmony, you must make it that way. This means looking at traditional approaches to school development and improvement, pedagogy and practice, and policies that may have outlived their usefulness.

At Three Bridges, developing a research culture started with the removal of practices like written marking and mandated proforma-based planning. Written marking is an age-old practice that involves the teacher telling and the student absorbing (if, in primary school, they can read and understand the comments at all!). It makes assumptions about meaning and understanding. It relays basic information about a student's work based on a snapshot. However, we didn't say, "no more marking." We investigated alternative approaches to feedback collaboratively and collectively decided on approaches that were stronger (Hannay, 2016a, 2018).Proforma-based planning is another practice that found its way from the England's Newly Qualified Teacher program into the folders of experienced teachers. It is often a template that was designed by someone in the school. It has specific boxes that must be completed with the teacher's plans. Sometimes, they are collected in advance of the lessons and scrutinized by someone else, requiring amendments and resubmission.

In truth, what both of these practices say, loud and clear to your professional staff, is that we value external accountability over internal responsibility, simple explanation or information over more nuanced discussion, the absorption of someone else's knowledge over individual and collective inquiry, distance over depth, and simplicity over complexity (Hannay, 2019). Although it sounds odd to be discussing making and planning practices when looking at developing a research culture, they are absolutely connected when addressing the systems and structures for a professional research culture.

## MOVING RESEARCH INTO PRACTICE

Determining how you will both disseminate the findings from research and commit to enacting those findings in classroom practice is essential to building buy-in from staff and getting the best value from the investment of time and resources. In the initial stages of informal research at the school, the approach we took was "go away and have a play" (Hannay, 2017), which involved staff reading and collectively reflecting on articles that focused on best practice in a subject area before going away and having a play with it in their own classrooms. They would then reconvene as a group and discuss the impact of these strategies with their learners before ultimately committing it to collective practice. As the research opportunities at the school became more formalized through lesson study and performance growth and development (in place of performance management), staff had times scheduled to disseminate their findings with the rest of the school and then an opportunity to publish their findings on the school's website. This allowed a focus in one group to be spread across the school to other groups. However, simply telling others about your findings does not necessarily move it into practice in your own classroom or that of others.

Providing the staff with the flexibility to investigate both school aims and their own professional aims (which may or may not be aligned with those of the school's development plan) is important here. Staff are more likely to change their practice as a result of interrogating a combination of things that matter to them and items that matter to the school at large. When investigating a school aim, it is important that if research uncovers that something the school is doing could be changed or made better (even if it wasn't what was expected by the Senior Leadership Team!), the teachers must have the freedom to make those changes—even if it falls on its face and needs to be changed back. When asking questions that matter to them as professionals (e.g., a Key Stage 1 [ages 5–7] teacher interested in fine arts projects with children in Key Stage 7–11), every effort must be made to allow for flexible working patterns to make this happen; perhaps having the teacher swap classes with another on certain afternoons to pursue their question. Being creative and flexible as school leaders is at the heart of moving research into practice.

## SEEING SUCCESS

When we first engaged in research and collaborative enquiry at the school in 2012, it was almost immediately clear that this was not seen as a robust and rigorous enough approach to school or professional development and improvement. I was told that the only way to improve results and get the coveted badge from Ofsted (England's national accountability and inspection body) was to move research and inquiry to the back burner and focus on relentlessly monitoring the staff.

Nothing could be more wrong.

Prior to initiating a research culture, staff discussed planning, lesson sequences, and resources; they were compliant, not courageous (Hannay, 2016b). New ideas were scarce and there was a distinct strategy in use by most staff: "wait to be told." In addition, the school rested in the image of the most senior staff—what they thought, what they believed, what they expected.

After initiating both informal and formal approaches to research over time, I immediately heard more focused conversations about learners and learning; those conversations were not limited to meeting times. They began to permeate all aspects of school life: the corridors, the PPA (planning, preparation, and assessment) room, the staff room, and formal meetings. Although staff still talked about their lessons, their conversations focused on what approaches worked and for whom; they discussed the impact of their teaching and how it was changing to meet the needs of the learners. When a lesson went poorly, they no longer discussed the children and their deficits, but the teaching and how it could be made better. Excitingly, new ideas from staff at all stages of their careers began flooding into meetings and office chats. Teachers began feeling like their voices had volume. The truth is, the school I hoped we would be in five years' time paled in comparison to the school we were able to uncover with the teachers leading their own learning. Nearly 10 years on (5 of more formal research and enquiry), we have a fancy Ofsted badge, our pupils' results are strong, staff retention is excellent, and everyone is generally happy. Our staff is now mature and thrives on complexity. You can mandate mediocrity. You can only unleash greatness.

## TOP TIPS

**A – Alignment:** Creating a culture of research means aligning everything to its values: internal responsibility, reflection, individual and collective agency, depth of thinking, and the generation and application of knowledge and understanding. Otherwise, it is a bolt-on and won't fit nicely or sustainably.

**B – Get Out of the Way:** Creating a research culture means giving some of the responsibility for vision, pedagogy, practice, and values over to your staff. Do not be so stuck to one way of doing something that it stifles the excitement of asking and answering bold questions.

**C – Start Small:** Don't jump into full-blown, formal research practices if your team isn't ready. Small, incremental steps are the sure way to sustainability. It sounds simple, but wherever *they* are, start *there*.

## REFERENCES

Campbell, C., Lieberman, A., Yashkina, A., Alexander, S., & Rodway, J. (2018). *Executive summary: Teaching learning and leadership program.* https://www. otffeo.on.ca/en/learning/teacher-learning-and-leadership-program/

Fullan, M., Rincon-Gallardo, S., & Hargreaves, A. (2015). Professional capital as accountability. *Education Policy Analysis Archives, 23*(15), 1–22.

Gillen, S. (2018). Plan on a Post-it note? *Education Leader & Manager.* https:// www.threebridgesprimary.co.uk/docs/Other%20Docs/ELMJAN16117.pdf

Hannay, J. (2016a). How to stop marking taking over your life. *Teach Primary.* https://www.teachwire.net/news/how-to-stop-marking-taking-over-your-life

Hannay, J. (2016b). We cannot have courageous and confident teachers if they are simply passive and compliant. *Teach Primary.* https://www.teachwire. net/news/we-cannot-have-courageous-and-confident-teachers-if-they-are-simply-passive

Hannay, J. (2017). Creating a successful school is not as simple as ticking the right boxes. *Teach Primary.* https://www.teachwire.net/news/creating-a-successful-school-is-not-as-simple-as-ticking-the-right-boxes

Hannay, J. (2018). Are you looking at your wellbeing the right way? https:// www.twinkl.co.uk/blog/jeremy-hannay-guest-post-are-you-looking-at-your-wellbeing-the-right-way

Hannay, J. (2019). Lose the learning walks. *The Headteacher.* https://www. theheadteacher.com/attainment-and-assessment/lose-the-learning-walks

Hannay, J. (2020). Inspiring learning. *NAHT Leadership Focus, 53.* https://www. threebridgesprimary.co.uk/docs/Published_Works/NAHT_article.pdf

Hargreaves, A., & Fullan, M. (2012). *Professional capital: Transforming teaching in every school.* Ontario Principals' Council.

Howard, K. (2020). *Stop talking about wellbeing.* John Catt.

Lieberman, A., Campbell, C., & Yashkina, A. (2015). Teachers at the centre: Learning and leading. *New Educator, 11*(2), 121–129.

Lieberman, A., Campbell, C., & Yashkina, A. (2016). *Teacher learning and leadership: Of, by, and for teachers.* Taylor & Francis.

Lightfoot, L. (2016). Tips on reducing teacher stress from the "happiest school on earth." *Guardian.* https://www.theguardian.com/education/2016/mar/22/teaching-crisis-school-what-keep-them

Rincon-Gallardo, S., & Fullan, M. (2016). Essential features of effective networks in education. *Journal of Professional Capital and Community, 1*(1), 5–22.

Watson, M. (2018, March/April). If you're happy and your know it... *The Teacher,* 12–13. https://www.threebridgesprimary.co.uk/docs/Other%20Docs/The_Teacher_March_3AApril_2018_for_web.pdf

# COURAGE TO CHANGE
## BRINGING READING SCIENCE TO THE CLASSROOM

**LINDSAY KEMENY**

**Lindsay Kemeny has been teaching for 10 years and is an IDA certified Structured Literacy Classroom Teacher. She has a master's degree in Curriculum and Instruction, and currently teaches second grade. She lives in northern Utah with her husband and four children.**

### THE PROBLEM

I will never forget the day my nine-year-old son looked me in the eyes and said, "I wish I was one of those babies that got left in a hot car." It took my breath away...I couldn't fathom the depths of his pain. However, my beautiful little boy wanted to *die* because of the humiliation he felt with his inability to read. I knew from the time he was very young that he struggled to learn. When he entered kindergarten, I felt a sense of desperation when I realized that I, a teacher, had no idea how to help him. I had tried everything I was taught in college and my early years of teaching. I read to him constantly from the time he was a baby. I did picture walks, surrounded him with books, asked what would make sense, and practiced with flash cards. Nothing seemed to help. Eventually, he was diagnosed with severe dyslexia. His diagnosis sparked a flame inside me to find out all I could about dyslexia and effective reading instruction. I needed to help him, and I needed to prevent others from experiencing the shame and embarrassment that he did. So, I learned all I could about what is now referred to as the science of reading.

It was a pivotal moment in my teaching career when I realized that the ways I had been taught to teach reading were not in line with research. I was outraged, embarrassed, and haunted by the thought that I had failed previous students. Why wasn't I taught the science of reading? As I have gradually changed and improved my instruction, a passion for sharing what I have learned with others has been ignited. I decided to write a blog post where I revealed what I consider "deadly errors" of teaching reading. The post sparked praise but also controversy in many teacher groups on social media. One teacher scoffed and remarked that she highly doubted that learning to read created a life-or-death situation for students. I disagree.

The ability to read is so tightly connected to how people feel about themselves. It is also closely connected to how our society views intelligence. The pressure is often too much. Students with learning disabilities such as dyslexia have a three times higher risk of suicide (Daniel et al., 2006), and 89% of suicide notes have dyslexic-like spellings (McBride & Siegel, 1997). In addition, a study of a Texas prison showed that 80% of the inmates were functionally illiterate. There seems to be a direct school-to-prison pipeline for those with reading problems. I visited a classroom in my district where a little third-grader kept his head down on his desk and refused to do anything. When he was approached by an adult, he would lift his head and remark, "I'm illiterate. I'm illiterate." Then he would put his head back down. He had completely shut down. This is what is happening to these students—they are shutting down. Every day they are forced to be in an environment that constantly reminds them they are failing. The pressure is often too much. The gap gets wider and wider, causing their self-esteem to plummet lower and lower. They feel lost and forgotten. They trudge through the school system, haunted by feelings of inadequacy and worthlessness. So, yes, I do think reading is a life-or-death situation.

We greatly underestimate the impact reading can have. Don Meichenbaum, a psychotherapist and expert on trauma, noted that one of the characteristics of resilient children is academic competence, especially in reading and math (Meichenbaum, 2018). Expanding on this, the most powerful thing we can do for traumatized children, as teachers, is to teach them to read (Dykstra, 2018). We have the ability to unlock this power in our students.

## GROWING SUSPICIONS

The year my son was diagnosed was also the first year I taught kindergarten. I had previously taught second grade and was excited for this new challenge. However, I soon became frustrated as I started teaching these kindergarten students to read. Despite spending so much time on letter-sound instruction, the books that I was given from our big-box curriculum did not reinforce what I had been teaching my students. These stories were not decodable but relied on repetitive patterns and picture cues to figure out the words. I had been so excited to show my students that knowing letters and sounds would help them learn to read. Instead, these books forced me to tell students to stop sounding out the words.

I felt as though I had to ask them to throw everything they had been learning out the window. "Oh, this word you can't sound out." "Uh, look at the picture. Does it give you a clue?" I was so frustrated that the words in these books could not be read without me providing their repetitive sentence patterns or instructing them to look at the pictures for cues. I hated that students weren't putting their letter-sound knowledge to use. I hated that they were basically going through the motions of "reading," but really they were just guessing.

I had used balanced literacy approaches and these same cueing prompts when I taught second grade earlier in my career. My students would read their books by using context clues, pictures, and thinking about what would make sense, as I instructed them to do. The damage these cueing habits caused was never apparent to me until I was teaching kindergarten. This wasn't reading! I wanted my kindergarten students to practice their letter sounds. I wanted to show them how they could put those individual sounds together to make words. I wanted them to apply all the phonemic awareness and phonic knowledge they had gained. I wanted them to decode. Instead, I was giving them a false idea of what reading was.

That same year, I had a student who struggled severely. By the end of the year, she had learned only a few letters. I was unsure how to help her. I remember placing a book in front of her as I administered our state-mandated end-of-year kindergarten test. She vaguely looked at the words on the page and then studied the picture. She looked back down at the words and found the word "I." Then she looked at the picture again and said, "I like the dog." She turned the page and continued in the same fashion. She "read" the whole book perfectly, even though she only knew a few letters and sounds. I knew she could not really read, but she certainly gave the appearance of reading. I began to grow uneasy about the reading methods I had been taught.

## THE REALIZATION

Between my son's diagnoses and these experiences with my kindergarten students, I began to question everything. Dyslexia? What exactly is it? As I began to investigate dyslexia and ponder my teaching methods, things began to click. I not only learned about the science of reading, but I discovered a wealth of research that I had never been exposed to before. I became obsessed with getting my hands on every book imaginable: Kilpatrick, Moats, Seidenberg, Henry, Shaywitz, Birsch, Eide, and Wexler. I could not stop reading! I felt like a starved animal. I couldn't get enough. All my workouts at the gym turned into mini professional development (PD) sessions: I watched videos of The Reading League's Live Events, lectures on phonics and explicit instruction on YouTube, Orton-Gillingham demonstrations, and more.

The more I learned, the angrier I became. Why was I never taught about dyslexia? It is the most commonly diagnosed learning disability, yet it's barely mentioned in teacher preparation programs or in schools' PD offerings. I was a certified teacher and yet I knew nothing about it. Why was I never taught about the National Reading Panel? Why was I never taught about structured literacy? Why was I never taught about explicit, systematic phonics and phonemic awareness? Why wasn't I told there was an approach that could reach *all* learners and not just the top 40%? Why aren't teachers given this vital information? I felt betrayed. I felt misled. Who are the proponents of balanced literacy and why are they promoting it? Why is the science of reading being largely ignored?

## APPLICATION

Armed with this knowledge, I began my second year of teaching kindergarten in a much different way. I was bound and determined to teach more explicitly and systematically. I wrote a grant for high-quality decodable books, removing predictable texts from my classroom. I asked my principal to purchase a phonemic awareness curriculum and she graciously agreed. There was no more guessing from pictures, no more guessing from context clues, no more coding running record errors with an *M*, *S*, or *V*. I continued to increase my knowledge by taking a five-day training in structured literacy.

I began applying all the things I was learning with the students in my classroom, and my students responded. Even the students with the most difficulty in my class began learning to read well. I recall one student literally shouted, "Mrs. Kemeny! I am actually reading the words!" His joy and excitement were overflowing. My students felt so much confidence and success, and our reading scores began to climb.

I also began working intensely with my son. Shocked to find that his special education teachers were not trained in dyslexia or the science of reading, I began to take over the responsibility of teaching him to read. I worked with him each day. We started at the end of his third-grade year and continue even now as he is in fifth grade. As his reading steadily improves, so does his self-esteem. He is not only coming to terms with his disabilities, but he is fully embracing them. The fractures in his heart are healing and his confidence is growing.

## CHALLENGES

Now that I have this information, I am passionate about sharing it with others. However, I have found that bringing this knowledge to teachers is so much harder than I thought. There are so many layers involved and walking into a room of teachers and telling them that there is no evidence to support the three-cueing system or that learning styles is a myth is akin to walking into a church and saying there is no God. People get deeply offended. It is so hard for us to separate the person or teacher we are from the practices that we use. However, it is vital for us to make the distinction and have the bravery we need to change our instruction if it is not aligned with research.

An important point for teachers to realize is that when we learn new research findings, it is not always a matter of adding things into our teaching repertoire. Sometimes, applying research means abandoning techniques we've come to rely on for years. This is often the hardest part of bringing research to practice: untangling the web of misinformation from our practice.

## INFORMING PRACTICE

With that in mind, I'd like to share some of the key points I have learned about reading over the past couple of years. There's a wrong way to teach reading and, unfortunately, it is the most popular way. I am frustrated that so many teacher preparation courses and PD classes are teaching reading methods not supported by science. As teachers learn the errors of their ways, it is easy to feel surprised, guilty, and even defensive. I plead with teachers to take a moment to step back, take a deep breath, and use this information as a springboard to start their journey into learning more about the science and research of reading. It helps to focus on the steps ahead rather than dwell on the mistakes in the past. Instead of feeling denial, guilt, or anger, I encourage teachers to simply learn more and do better.

I call these mistakes the seven deadly errors of teaching reading, because I truly believe they can be life changing for students.

## DEADLY ERROR 1: THREE-CUEING STRATEGIES

Many teachers know these as the "Beanie Baby strategies." They scour dozens of thrift stores to find Beanie Baby toys to represent these different reading "strategies." These include tactics like "Skippy the Frog," where you simply skip over a word if you don't know it, read the rest of the sentence, and then guess what word would make sense. Or "Eagle Eye," where you examine the pictures for clues to help you figure out the words. "Lips the Fish" reminds us to get our mouth ready, say the first sound of the word, and guess the rest. There is no research to support these Beanie Baby strategies. They are based on the three-cueing system, which has been completely debunked by science (Adams, 1998; Hempenstall, 2006; Primary National Strategy, 2006). In fact, what the research *does* tell us is that these are strategies that *poor* readers use, *not* good readers. So, when we teach our students these strategies, we are actually teaching them to read like a struggling reader.

## DEADLY ERROR 2: USING PREDICTABLE TEXTS

I'm not talking about beautiful, authentic books like *The Napping House*. I'm talking about those contrived early readers with repetitive patterns such as, "We cleaned the garage. We cleaned the house. We cleaned the school," and so forth. The only way for brand new readers to get through these texts is by memorizing the patterns and using the three-cueing strategies I warned about previously. This is not reading! This is guessing and memorizing. It creates damaging habits that are extremely tough to break.

## DEADLY ERROR 3: HEAVY EMPHASIS ON SIGHT WORDS

I visited another kindergarten classroom the very first week of school. The teacher was attempting to teach the sight word *from*. After quite a bit of labored instruction and activities, she excitedly exclaimed, "So what's our sight word of the day?" The bewildered students simply stared at her, until one excitedly shouted, "F!" Young students are still learning the difference between a letter and word, and yet, many insist on teaching them a certain number of "high-frequency words." I am disheartened when I see the pressures some districts place on their kindergarten students (and teachers!), demanding that they memorize 50, 75, even more than 100 sight words. Instead of focusing our efforts on getting these students to memorize words, we need to intensify our focus on phonemes and the graphemes that represent them. There is a limit to how many sight words a child can memorize. However, if they are able to orthographically map these words, the number is endless. "If a child memorizes ten words, the child can only read ten words, but if the child learns the sounds of ten letters, the child will be able to read 350 three sound words, 4,320 four sound words, 21,650 five sound words" (Kozloff, 2002, para. 19).

## DEADLY ERROR 4: NOT TEACHING PHONEMIC AWARENESS TO MASTERY

Many educators think of phonemic awareness as a "kindergarten skill," but it goes much beyond that. David Kilpatrick (2016) states that phonemic awareness should be explicitly taught to *all* students until at least the *second grade*, and then beyond for those who haven't mastered it yet. Older, struggling readers almost always have weaknesses in this area that were never addressed. Because the most common source of reading difficulties is phonemic awareness, every teacher needs to make this a priority. We should teach it to the whole class through second grade and in small groups for those who need it in all other grades. A student is never too old to learn this skill, and studies show that as phonemic awareness improves, reading ability improves as well.

## DEADLY ERROR 5: INCIDENTAL PHONICS

The National Reading Panel (2000) advocates not only for phonics but also for *systematic* phonics. Some reading approaches encourage the teacher to teach phonics incidentally, only when an opportunity presents itself. For example, a child stumbles upon a word he/she doesn't know in a text, and *then* the teacher decides to teach that particular grapheme. In contrast, systematic phonics is much more explicit. The teacher follows a planned sequence of phonics skills. This ensures that students will have a strong foundation, without holes or the need to rely on guessing strategies.

## DEADLY ERROR 6: PHONICS IN ISOLATION

Teaching systematic and explicit phonics is very effective as long as it is not taught in isolation. Most of the instruction time should be spent applying the phonics skill you are teaching in authentic reading and writing experiences.

## DEADLY ERROR 7: NEGLECTING VOCABULARY AND BACKGROUND KNOWLEDGE

Sometimes, we work so hard teaching our students basic decoding skills, it can be easy to neglect vocabulary and background knowledge. However, it is important not to forget the other side of Scarborough's (2001) Reading Rope. Many curriculum programs neglect these areas by focusing too much on "skills" and not enough on actual content. Natalie Wexler (2020) talks about this in her book, *The Knowledge Gap*. Teaching comprehension skills such as "finding the main idea" and "text features" does not necessarily lead to improved comprehension. Teaching a student to find the main idea in one text will not lead to being able to find the main idea in other text. Cognitive scientists have known for years that the most important factor in good reading comprehension is how much vocabulary and content knowledge you have of the subject. Instead of focusing so much of our attention on these comprehension "skills," we need to make sure we build their vocabulary and background knowledge.

## CONCLUSION

Using research and science to provide students with the most effective reading instruction is the greatest gift we can give them. There is a right and wrong way to teach reading, and the sooner we can come to grips with that fact, the sooner our nation's reading proficiency rates will improve. We, as educators, have a moral obligation to teach our students to read. The ability to read will open up countless opportunities for them. I feel strongly that teachers do the very best with the knowledge they have. It is unfortunate that most of us have not had access to this knowledge. Even worse, we have been taught ways that are not in line with what cognitive scientists have learned about reading and the brain.

It takes a lot of courage to take a hard look at your teaching and determine if the way you are teaching is effective for all students. Yet, I see teachers doing this all over the world, and I am bolstered by their examples. They are turning their backs on the ineffective reading strategies that have been taught to them. Sometimes, it's hard when you feel like an island. It can be scary to speak up. Just know that there is an invisible army behind you, cheering you on and supporting your efforts. I know that we can help these discouraged learners, and I have gradually recognized that my reach can extend beyond the four walls of my classroom. So, yes, I will share, I'll write, I'll speak, and I'll present. And, oh my, will I teach! Our students deserve it.

## KEY TAKEAWAYS:

- Have courage! Focus on the steps ahead instead of dwelling on past mistakes. Know better, do better.

- Bringing research to the classroom can sometimes mean abandoning practices we've come to depend on.

- Teaching students to read is the most powerful thing we can do for them.

## REFERENCES

Adams, M. J. (1998). The three-cueing system. In F. Lehr & J. Osborn (Eds.), *Literacy for all issues in teaching and learning* (pp. 73–99). Guilford Press.

Daniel, S. S., Walsh, A. K., Goldston, D. B., Arnold, E. M., Reboussin, B. A., & Wood, F. B. (2006). Suicidality, school dropout, and reading problems among adolescents. *Journal of Learning Disabilities, 39*(6), 507–514. https://doi.org/1 0.1177/00222194060390060301

Dykstra, S. (2019, February 3). *A developmental model of trauma, growth, and resilience: The place for language and reading* [Video]. https://www.youtube.com/watch?v=kovadVljoPA

Hempenstall, K. (2006). The three-cueing model: Down for the count? *Education News.* www.ednews.org/articles/4084/1/The-three-cueing-model--Down-for-the-count/Page1.html

Kilpatrick, D. (2016). *Equipped for reading success: A comprehensive, step-by-step program for developing phonemic awareness and fluent word recognition.* Casey & Kirsch.

Kozloff, M. (2002). *A whole language catalogue of the grotesque.* UNCW. http://people.uncw.edu/kozloffm/wlquotes.html

McBride, H. E., & Siegel, L. S. (1997). Learning disabilities and adolescent suicide. *Journal of Learning Disabilities, 30*(6), 652–659. https://doi.org/10.1177/002221949703000609

Meichenbaum, D. (2018, May). *The nature of the challenge: Incidence and impact of trauma and implications for interventions* [Paper presentation]. Melissa Institute 22nd Annual Conference, Miami, FL.

National Reading Panel. (2000). *Teaching children to read: An evidence-based assessment of the scientific research on reading and its implications for reading instruction.* National Institute of Child Health and Human Development.

Primary National Strategy. (2006). *Primary framework for literacy and mathematics.* Department of Education and Skills. http://www.standards.dfes.gov.uk/primaryframeworks/

Scarborough, H. (2001). Connecting early language and literacy to later reading disabilities: Evidence, theory and practice. In S. B. Neuman & D. K. Dickinson (Eds.), *Handbook of early literacy research* (Vol. 1, pp. 97–110). Guilford Press.

Wexler, N. (2020). *The knowledge gap: The hidden cause of America's broken education system—and how to fix it.* Avery.

# WHEN LEARNING MOVES ONLINE, WHAT CAN BE IMPROVED?

ANDREW LYMAN-BUTLER

Andrew taught biology and chemistry at every level from middle school through Advanced Placement/International Baccalaureate for 11 years, at a variety of American schools: urban and suburban, low and high socioeconomic status, public, private, and charter. In 2019, he left teaching to pursue a second career as a physician. There is a vast chasm between the learning strategies used by most secondary teachers and the techniques used by medical students, for whom the stakes could not be higher.

Equity in education is one of the most compelling moral issues of our time, but the gulf between our approach to equity and the strategies that actually promote equity appears to be growing. Indeed, the greatest affront to equity is that we continue to promote the use of ineffective feel-good instructional and assessment strategies (Kirschner et al., 2006) in the schools serving our most disadvantaged student populations.

I taught chemistry at a high school where the poverty rate is nearly 90%. I surveyed my students at the beginning of every school year to get to know them as individuals but also to construct a profile of the student body as a whole. The statistics are striking: They report working an average 7.5 hours per week for pay, and 11 hours on unpaid duties like caring for siblings, both of which are significant risk factors for school failure (Hammond et al., 2007). Many of my students had out-of-school responsibilities totaling 40 or more hours every week. Despite these and other formidable obstacles, 85% planned to pursue higher education after graduation. If we are to keep that door open for students, it is essential that we hold them to high academic standards while also improving the graduation rate; one must not come at the expense of the other. How, then, can we best support meaningful academic success for our most at-risk students?

## WHAT IS BLENDED ASSESSMENT?

Blended learning—a mode of instruction in which some elements are delivered face-to-face and some online—yields superior student outcomes relative to either traditional classroom-based instruction alone or online learning alone (Means et al., 2009), but it remains unclear specifically which component is responsible for these gains. This question has become particularly urgent with the shift toward online instruction with COVID-19. Students have limited access to expert in-person teaching—this has always been the case, but it is especially true now—but virtually unlimited access to technology. I contend that supplementing effective in-person instruction with a robust online assessment platform is the combination most likely to produce measurable growth without compromising academic standards. I call this approach *blended assessment*.

With so many existing online learning models, why introduce yet another? I am concerned that the current blended learning paradigm effectively serves as a smokescreen for practices that undermine equity: increased class sizes, reduced student access to expert instructors, and funneling of public education funds to for-profit software and curriculum companies (McRae, 2015).

I do not believe that blended learning models with heavy emphasis on online instruction are effective. Despite a paucity of evidence, this approach is a common feature of alternative high school and "credit recovery" schemes. I was once asked to supervise a credit recovery program, and the curriculum and assessment were atrocious. It was a canned commercial offering with forgettable videos and quizzes that were trivially easy to cheat at, with unlimited retake options with the same questions every time. If the instruction delivered by computers is not the piece most responsible for student growth from blended learning, then it suggests that high-quality online assessments may be doing the heavy lifting. This view is consistent with an abundance of literature from the past 20 years on the science of learning. Despite the frequent lofty claims for blended learning (e.g., personalization for everyone, 21st-century skills), something much less sexy—but much more powerful—is at work under the hood in a blended assessment classroom: retrieval practice.

## CHARACTERISTICS OF THE ONLINE ASSESSMENT PLATFORM AND WHY THEY WORK

My quizzes and tests are on a Moodle server and include the following features, which are absent from many commercial software packages often used for online learning:

*They end the distinction between formative and summative assessment, and between assessment and practice.* Traditional education theory demarcates formative assessment, which is intended to give student and instructor a snapshot of current performance and to guide instructional decisions, from summative assessment, which is done to evaluate a student's learning and assign a grade. This distinction has outlived its usefulness in the digital age. Students who take online quizzes can re-attempt them many times over without any extra time commitment on the part of the teacher, and they can receive immediate feedback rather than waiting for papers to be graded. Scores on these quizzes can and should be used to calculate a student's grade, with the explicit understanding that the grade is fluid and may always be improved if the student invests additional effort and demonstrates growth. This makes every quiz attempt low stakes for the student in that quiz failure does not have adverse grade consequences. This model can properly be described as *retrieval practice.* The US Department of Education's Institute of Education Sciences recommends "quizzing with active retrieval of information at all phases of the learning process to exploit the ability of retrieval directly to facilitate long-lasting memory traces" (Pashler et al., 2007, p.2), noting that quiz-based retrieval practice is one of the few learning strategies for which there is "strong" evidence of efficacy. Agarwal et al (2017), in a review of three studies ranging from middle school to medical school, noted a significant benefit to long-term retention, with effect sizes greater than $d = .80$. Although the quiz/test format is not the only way to promote retrieval practice, it has the advantage of encouraging maximum effort from students (who naturally want to perform well on anything that's considered an assessment) and providing data that can inform grading and response to intervention.

*Multiple assessment attempts on the same course material.* More and more schools are implementing the practice known as *standards-based grading* (or *proficiency-based grading* or *assessment for learning*), which awards no grade points for homework and behavior but also requires that students be given multiple attempts to demonstrate proficiency. Clymer and Wiliam (2007) contrast this modality with traditional grading systems:

> Grades based on the accumulation of points over time are counter-productive for several reasons. First, this approach encourages shallow learning. In most classrooms, if students forget something that they have previously been assessed on, they get to keep the grade. When students understand that it's what they know by the end of the marking period that counts, they are forced to engage with the material at a much deeper level. Second, not altering grades in light of new evidence of learning sends the message that the assessment is really a measure of aptitude rather than achievement. Students who think they will do well will engage in the assessments to prove how smart they are, whereas students who think that they are likely to fail will disengage. When assessment is dynamic, however, all students can improve. They come to see ability as incremental instead of fixed; they learn that smart is not something you are—it's something you become. (p.2-3)

In addition, the data afforded by multiple reassessments provide for analysis of interventions or changes in instruction. The biggest problem with allowing multiple attempts, of course, is the enormous time commitment for generating new versions of tests and marking papers. This is the greatest potential advantage of computer assessment.

*Considerable variation in assessment items between students and between attempts.* Numeric questions make use of Moodle's "calculated" question type, in which random numbers within set limits are generated for each question, and student responses are evaluated using a teacher-supplied formula and a margin of error. Further variation is incorporated by using an item bank with multiple variants of each question type, which are sampled at random every time a new assessment attempt is generated. Two students sitting next to each other will have completely different quizzes, and a student re-attempting a quiz will have it regenerated from scratch. This makes copying or cheating effectively impossible. For example, one question reads "In the compound $C_5H_{11}O_3$, what percent by mass is carbon?" The subscripts (5, 11, and 3) are replaced with random numbers (within reasonable limits) every time the question is attempted. Additional variation is generated by asking for the percent mass of hydrogen or oxygen instead of carbon.

Another example illustrates some of the unlimited variation built into a different question type:

Use this balanced equation to solve the following problem:

$$2\,HCl_{(aq)} + Mg_{(s)} \rightarrow MgCl_{2\,(aq)} + H_{2\,(g)}$$

How many liters (at STP) of hydrogen gas would be produced by the reaction of 0.18 grams of magnesium?
Do not include units in your answer.

Answer:

Use this balanced equation to solve the following problem:

$$2\,HCl_{(aq)} + CaCO_{3\,(s)} \rightarrow CaCl_{2\,(aq)} + H_2O_{(l)} + CO_{2\,(g)}$$

How many moles of hydrochloric acid (HCl) would be needed to completely react with 0.34 grams of $CaCO_3$?
Do not include units in your answer.

Answer:

I have seen students attempt this problem a dozen (or more!) times throughout a school year without ever encountering the same question or even the same format. Unlike multiple-choice assessments with invariant question stems, the only way for a student to earn the point is to understand how to solve the problem.

*Throwback questions.* Every quiz and exam are cumulative, with a typical assessment consisting of around 20% items from past units. This results in assessments that are both interleaved (involving a diverse set of problems from across the curriculum) and spaced through the year on an expanding schedule (i.e., with more elapsed time between subsequent reviews of a given concept, because the chances of any particular question type appearing diminish as more content is included). This combination of spaced rehearsal and interleaved practice is supported by robust findings in cognitive science (Cepeda et al., 2006; Mozer et al., 2009; Rohrer et al., 2014).

*Teacher feedback involving worked examples.* Students are encouraged to ask for help following an unsuccessful quiz attempt. When they do, I provide them with a detailed solution to each problem they solved incorrectly. Students know that re-attempted quizzes will contain entirely new problems, so memorizing the answer will be no use—they must understand how the solution is arrived at.

*Lab work.* Blended assessment can be applied to practical exercises as well. I have written quiz questions that actually serve to check students' pre-lab calculations and results. In this example, I prepared potassium chloride solutions with a range of concentrations and used a conductivity tester to generate a standard curve; then, I programmed Moodle to use the curve to check students' empirical values. This allows every student to work on their own unique lab problem and to receive instant feedback on their results—and most importantly, to re-attempt the procedure an unlimited number of times (with a different random assigned concentration each time) until they are satisfied with the results.

Go to the lab and prepare a 0.056 M solution of **potassium chloride**.

Some things you will need to know:

- the volume of the flask you are using; don't forget to convert to liters
- the correct formula and molar mass of your compound
- the formula for molarity (look at your homework packet for example problems)

You should show all you work on a piece of notebook paper so Mr. LB can help you if you get stuck.

After you've made your solution, follow the directions on your lour lab handout to test its conductivity. Type in your conductivity number here. Do not include units.

Answer:

Students then receive feedback depending on the accuracy of their results, ranging from this:

You did not set up your calculations correctly, or you had major errors in your lab technique. Please show your calculations to Mr. LB for help.

When you were preparing your solution, did you:

- Weigh your solute correctly, including remembering to zero the balance?
- Use deionized water as your solvent?
- Swirl the flask to completely dissolve the solute?
- Add water up to the line on the flask?
- Invert the flask several times to mix the solution thoroughly?

To this:

> Outstanding! You really nailed it. Your answer was within 1% of the expected value, which is the limit of the accuracy of the conductivity tester. In other words, you got the best possible result.

Another implementation of this strategy provides students with immediate feedback on each step of their lab calculations and checks their final results for accuracy:

Enter your lab data and calculation resulta for the Hydrate Lab. You don't need to include units with your answers when you type them in here.

| | |
|---:|:---|
| empty_crucible: | 10 |
| crucible_and_hydrate: | 12.5 |
| crucible_after_heating: | 11.5 |
| mass_of_anhydrous_CuSO4: | 1.5 |
| mass_or_water_evaporated: | 1 |
| moles_of_anhydrous_CuSO4: | 2 |
| moles_of_water: | .01 |
| coefficient_for_H2O: | 5 |

Mass of empty crucible looks good

Good, you used enough copper (II) sulfate

Good, you didn't use too much copper (II) sulfate

Good job, you heated your crucible long enough to drive off all the water

You might have overheated your crucible or spilled something, or made a weighing mistake

You calculated the mass of anhydrous copper (II) sulfate correctly

You calculated the mass of evaporated water correctly

You made a mistake calculating the moles of anhydrous copper (II) sulfate

You made a mistake calculating the moles of water evaporated

You made a mistake calculating your coefficient

*Accessible anywhere.* This was important before, but it is essential with COVID-19. Students can log on to the class website from any device; it works well with smartphones. They have the option to work on assessments at home, at the library, on the bus, while waiting in line, and so forth. In the past, fears of the "digital divide" exacerbating equity issues may have prevented serious consideration of blended learning, but in 2018, 92.5% of my students reported owning their own smartphone, and 95% were able to access the internet at home. Before the pandemic, many lower-income students were saddled with responsibilities or inconveniences (e.g., public transit) that prevented them from meeting with teachers outside the school day to re-attempt assessments; now, everyone must figure out how to accommodate testing at a distance. The blended assessment strategy bridges this gap.

## HOW IT ADVANCES EQUITY

Blended assessment should be considered a viable equity strategy in secondary education for a number of reasons. Most important, additional learning time and multiple assessment opportunities can be provided to a much greater extent than is possible with traditional pencil-and-paper assessment. This disproportionately benefits disadvantaged categories of learners, including English language learners, immigrants, refugees, students with individualized education programs, and students who are below grade level in their math skills. (My own anecdotal classroom experience is that immigrant students often score below proficient on first attempts, but enthusiastically seek help and retake quizzes, sometimes accumulating 10 or more attempts on a single learning objective.) Using retrieval practice as both a learning strategy and a low-stakes assessment strategy also promotes a growth mindset, which has a protective effect against poverty (Claro et al., 2016). Students with lower working memory capacity also benefit disproportionately from retrieval practice (Agarwal et al, 2017), and so do students with test anxiety (including, potentially, stereotype-threat-induced anxiety) (Agarwal et al., 2014; Smith et al., 2016.

The benefits of computer-mediated retrieval practice and proficiency-based grading are clear, and the dual emergencies of systemic inequity and COVID-19 demand that we start leveraging this high-yield strategy immediately. I offer three action items to this end:

1. Incorporate retrieval practice into daily lessons beyond the online assessment platform. For example, I interrupt lectures regularly with pop-up quiz questions, or have students practice drawing molecules, chemical formulas, and so on, on a class set of whiteboards.

2. Start using, sharing, and promoting open assessment resources. I've posted my chemistry item bank at lymanbuttler.com/moodle.

3. Persuade your school to stop purchasing expensive proprietary learning content management software. Moodle provides much more powerful assessment functionality than the commercial platforms and is infinitely extensible and customizable. Schools can self-host and hire information technology staff with Moodle expertise (or the willingness to learn it) for a fraction of the cost of a typical software contract.

## REFERENCES

Agarwal, P. K. (2018). *Retrieval practice improves learning more than reviewing classroom content.* https://www.retrievalpractice.org/research/

Agarwal, P. K., D'Antonio, L., Roediger, H. L., McDermott, K. B., & McDaniel, M. A. (2014). Classroom-based programs of retrieval practice reduce middle school and high school students' test anxiety. *Journal of Applied Research in Memory and Cognition, 3*(3), 131–139.

Agarwal, P. K., Finley, J. R., Rose, N. S., & Roediger, H. L., III (2017). Benefits from retrieval practice are greater for students with lower working memory capacity. *Memory, 25*(6), 764–771.

Cepeda, N. J., Pashler, H., Vul, E., Wixted, J. T., & Rohrer, D. (2006). Distributed practice in verbal recall tasks: A review and quantitative synthesis. *Psychological Bulletin, 132*, 354–380.

Claro, S., Paunesku, D., & Dweck, C. S. (2016). Growth mindset tempers the effects of poverty on academic achievement. *Proceedings of the National Academy of Sciences, 113*(31), 8664–8668.

Clymer, J. B., & Wiliam, D. (2007). Improving the way we grade science. *Educational Leadership, 64*, 19.

Hammond, C., Linton, D., Smink, J., & Drew, S. (2007). *Dropout risk factors and exemplary programs: A technical report.* National Dropout Prevention Center/ Network (NDPC/N).

Kirschner, P. A., Sweller, J., & Clark, R. E. (2006). Why minimal guidance during instruction does not work: An analysis of the failure of constructivist, discovery, problem-based, experiential, and inquiry-based teaching. *Educational Psychologist, 41*(2), 75–86.

McRae, P. (2015, June 1). Myth: Blended learning is the next ed-tech revolution. *Alberta Teachers Association Magazine, 95*(4).

Means, B., Toyama, Y., Murphy, R., Bakia, M., & Jones, K. (2009). *Evaluation of evidence-based practices in online learning: A meta-analysis and review of online learning studies.* US Department of Education.

Mozer, M. C., Pashler, H., Cepeda, N., Lindsey, R., & Vul, E. (2009). Predicting the optimal spacing of study: A multiscale context model of memory. In Y. Bengio, D. Schuurmans, J. Lafferty, C. K. I. Williams, & A. Culotta (Eds.), *Advances in neural information processing systems 22* (pp. 1321–1329). NIPS Foundation.

Pashler, H., Bain, P. M., Bottge, B. A., Graesser, A., Koedinger, K., McDaniel, M., & Metcalfe, J. (2007). *Organizing instruction and study to improve student learning. IES Practice Guide. NCER 2007–2004.* National Center for Education Research.

Rohrer, D., Dedrick, R. F., & Burgess, K. (2014). The benefit of interleaved mathematics practice is not limited to superficially similar kinds of problems. *Psychonomic Bulletin & Review, 21,* 1323–1330.

Smith, A. M., Floerke, V. A., & Thomas, A. K. (2016). Retrieval practice protects memory against acute stress. *Science, 354*(6315), 1046–1048.